618.92 85836075 HEG

JET LIBRARY

Accession no.
01051974

49.50.

Please collect
CD/ CD-ROM Computer Disc
from the Library Counter.
Disc No. 14

**PLEASE CHECK DISC IS IN
BOOK WHEN ISSUING &
RETURNING**

D1337044

Evaluation of the Sexually Abused Child

Evaluation of the Sexually Abused Child

SECOND EDITION

A Medical Textbook and Photographic Atlas

ASTRID H. HEGER, M.D.

Associate Professor of Clinical Pediatrics
University of Southern California School of Medicine
Executive Director
LAC/USC Violence Intervention Program
Los Angeles, California

S. JEAN EMANS, M.D.

Associate Professor of Pediatrics
Harvard Medical School
Chief, Division of Adolescent Medicine
Co-Director, Center for Young Women's Health
Children's Hospital
Boston, Massachusetts

DAVID MURAM, M.D.

Professor of Obstetrics and Gynecology
State University of New York Health Sciences Center
Brooklyn, New York

CAROLE JENNY, M.D.

Professor of Pediatrics
Brown University School of Medicine
Director, Safe Child Protection Program
Hasbro Children's Hospital
Providence, RI

CAROLYN J. LEVITT, M.D.

Assistant Professor
Department of Pediatrics
University of Minnesota School of Medicine
St. Paul, MN

CATHERINE KOVEROLA, Ph.D.

Assistant Professor of Psychology and Pediatrics
University of Southern California School
of Medicine
Los Angeles, CA

SUSAN POKORNY, M.D.

Chief Department of Obstetrics and Gynecology
Kelsey Seybold Clinics
Associate Clinical Professor of Pediatrics
Baylor College of Medicine
Houston, TX

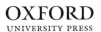

OXFORD
UNIVERSITY PRESS

OXFORD

UNIVERSITY PRESS

Oxford   New York

Athens   Auckland   Bangkok   Bogotá   Buenos Aires   Calcutta
Cape Town   Chennai   Dar es Salaam   Delhi   Florence   Hong Kong   Istanbul
Karachi   Kuala Lumpur   Madrid   Melbourne   Mexico City   Mumbai
Nairobi   Paris   São Paulo   Singapore   Taipei   Tokyo   Toronto   Warsaw
and associated companies in
Berlin   Ibadan

Copyright © 2000 by Oxford University Press, Inc.

Published by Oxford University Press, Inc.
198 Madison Avenue, New York, New York 10016
Oxford is a registered trademark of Oxford University Press

All rights reserved. No part of this publication may be reproduced,
stored in a retrieval system, or transmitted, in any form or by any means,
electronic, mechanical, photocopying, recording, or otherwise,
without the prior permission of Oxford University Press.

Library of Congress Cataloging-in-Publication Data
Evaluation of the sexually abused child :
a medical textbook and photographic atlas/
[edited by] Astrid H. Heger, S. Jean Emans, David Muram ;
Carole Jenny . . . [et al., contributors]. —2nd ed.
p.   cm.   Includes bibliographical references and index.
ISBN 0-19-513126-6
1. Sexually abused children—Evaluation Atlases.
2. Child sexual abuse—Diagnosis Atlases.
I. Heger, Astrid.   II. Emans, S. Jean, Herriot.   III. Muram, David.
[DNLM: 1. Child Abuse, Sexual—Diagnosis.
2. Child Abuse, Sexual Atlases.
3. Interviews—methods.
4. Physical Examination—methods.
WA 320 E915 1999]   RJ507.S49E93   1999   618.92'85836075—dc21
DNLM/DLC   for Library of Congress   99-13480

The science of medicine is a rapidly changing field. As new research and clinical experience broaden our knowledge, changes in treatment and drug therapy do occur. The
author and the publisher of this work have checked with sources believed to be reliable
in their efforts to provide information that is accurate and complete, and in accordance
with the standards accepted at the time of publication. However, in light of the possibility of human error or changes in the practice of medicine, neither the author, nor the
publisher, nor any other party who has been involved in the preparation or publication
of this work warrants that the information contained herein is in every respect accurate
or complete. Readers are encouraged to confirm the information contained herein with
other reliable sources, and are strongly advised to check the product information sheet
provided by the pharmaceutical company for each drug they plan to administer.

9 8 7 6 5 4 3 2 1
Printed in the United States of America
on acid-free paper

Preface

The second edition of *Evaluation of the Sexually Abused Child* brings new challenges to the editors and each of the contributors to this volume. The fundamental challenge, however, remains the same: to evaluate each child and family with an eye to science while maintaining high standards of interviewing, medical evaluation, and diagnosis of child sexual abuse. Since the first edition was published eight years ago, we have learned more about evaluating children for possible sexual abuse. We know the profound implications a diagnosis of sexual abuse can have, and we understand normal genital anatomy and the post-traumatic changes associated with sexual assault in greater detail. Medical professionals, charged with the responsibility of evaluating and protecting children, understand more than ever the importance of peer review and the problems of inexpert diagnosis.

This new edition reflects advances in research and gains in experience. It offers an updated overview of the social system and the psychological impact of sexual abuse, as well as the latest in interviewing techniques, forensics, and the medical diagnosis of sexual abuse and sexually transmitted diseases. In addition, we have more than doubled the color atlas to cover sexual abuse of adolescents, patterns of healing trauma, and further examples of normal anatomical variations and medical conditions. The expanded atlas, with over 250 plates, provides a full range of illustrations to aid medical professionals in the diagnosis of genital variations, disease, and trauma.

On rereading the Foreword to the first edition, we realize that although there has been tremendous progress in the quality of intervention for victims of child sexual abuse, the charge, the warnings, and the challenge remain.

Los Angeles, Calif.   A. H.
Boston, Mass.   S. J. E.
Brooklyn, N.Y.   D. M.
January 1999

Contents

Introduction

RICHARD D. KRUGMAN, S. JEAN EMANS,
AND ASTRID HEGER

The last twenty-five years have been marked by a dramatic increase in recognition of the problem of child abuse—especially sexual abuse. In 1976 there were 35 reported cases of sexual abuse among Colorado children; by 1986, the number of reports had exceeded 3,500. Substantiated cases in 1989 were nearly 2,000. Between 1989 and 1999, reported cases of child sexual abuse in the United States rose to over 500,000 each year. What Kempe called "Another Hidden Problem" in his 1977 C. Anderson Aldrich Award Lecture at the American Academy of Pediatrics Annual Meeting is clearly no longer hidden.

Public and professional response to the problem has been predictable. From denial of its existence through the desire to recognize, rescue, and treat the victim and to find, prosecute, and incarcerate (and occasionally treat) the offender, individuals and communities are grappling with a flood of cases so great that the multidisciplinary child protection system (broadly defined—not just the child protection agency) cannot hope to handle it.

Historically, physicians have been a part of the multidisciplinary approach, and many were somewhat prepared to assist in the diagnosis of "battered children." We had training in recognizing fractures, burns, and bruises, and could ferret out discrepant histories.

Sexual abuse diagnosis was another matter. There were many problems, among them:

1. Many physicians have found it hard to imagine that children in their practice are victims of sexual abuse.
2. Few physicians had received any training in medical school or residency on the subject of sexual abuse.
3. Few physicians had received (or remembered, if they did) training in evaluating the genital and anal anatomy of prepubertal children. The genital exam, especially in girls, has probably been "deferred" more often than the neurological exam in routine pediatrics. Nurse clinicians became actively involved in many practices and centers examining children, with many of the same limitations of training as their physician colleagues, but with the additional handicap of gaining credibility and stature in the medical and legal arenas.
4. When children said they were sexually abused, law-enforcement agencies and prosecutors wanted "physical evidence." A child's word was not enough.
5. Early studies described physical findings in sexually abused children, but in the absence of studies of "control" non-abused children, "certainty" was an elusive concept.
6. Later studies showed that the absence of findings did not mean that a child *was not* abused, and the presence of some findings (e.g., enlarged hymen) did not mean that a child *was* abused.

We have now arrived at the year 2000, and some order has been brought to this chaos. Nationally, we are teaching medical professionals about the diagnosis of sexual abuse. We have created a system of referral centers staffed with multidisciplinary teams, and law-enforcement personnel working on those teams understand that a child's word may very well be enough. In addition, medical research has provided expanded knowledge from which it is possible to interpret physical findings more accurately.

All health care professionals will be better off having this reference volume—provided it is used properly. That means remembering that the diagnosis of sexual abuse is made primarily on the basis of a child's history. Physical findings may lead us to suspect abuse, but they don't often tell us when and if it happened or who did it. These questions are best answered through a coordinated multidisciplinary approach with the physician taking a part.

This book also helps us learn (some of us for the first time) what the variants of normal are to the genitalia and anus of children. It won't answer all of our questions, though, and when questions remain, we need to consult our colleagues and not worry about saying, "I don't know." The stakes are too high for us to guess about sexual abuse—for everyone involved.

Contributors

S. JEAN EMANS, M.D.
Associate Professor of Pediatrics
Harvard Medical School
Chief, Division of Adolescent Medicine
Co-Director, Center for
　Young Women's Health
Children's Hospital
Boston, Massachusetts

KENNETH R. FREEMAN
Judge
Los Angeles Superior Court
Los Angeles, California

WILLIAM FRIEDRICH, PH.D.
Department of Psychology
Mayo Clinic
Rochester, Minnesota

ASTRID H. HEGER, M.D.
Associate Professor of
　Clinical Pediatrics
University of Southern California
　School of Medicine
Executive Director
LAC/USC Violence Intervention
　Program
Los Angeles, California

CAROLE JENNY, M.D.
Professor of Pediatrics
Brown University School
　of Medicine
Director, Safe Child Protection
　Program
Hasbro Children's Hospital
Providence, Rhode Island

CATHERINE KOVEROLA, PH.D.
Assistant Professor of Clinical
　Psychology and Pediatrics
University of Southern California
　School of Medicine
Los Angeles, California

RICHARD KRUGMAN, M.D.
Professor of Pediatrics and Dean
University of Colorado School of
　Medicine
Denver, Colorado

CAROLYN J. LEVITT, M.D.
Assistant Professor of Pediatrics
Department of Pediatrics
University of Minnesota
St. Paul, Minnesota

DAVID MURAM, M.D.
Professor of Obstetrics and Gynecology
State University of New York
Health Sciences Center
Brooklyn, New York

SUSAN F. POKORNY, M.D.
Chief, Department of Obstetrics
　and Gynecology
Kelsey-Seybold Clinic
Associate Clinical Professor of Pediatrics
Baylor College of Medicine
Houston, Texas

DEBORAH C. STEWART, M.D.
Associate Professor of Pediatrics
College of Medicine
University of California, Irvine
Irvine, California

1

MAKING THE DIAGNOSIS OF SEXUAL ABUSE: TEN YEARS LATER

ASTRID HEGER

Over the past ten years many medical professionals have integrated knowledge about the recognition of child sexual abuse into their medical education and practice. This is a 180-degree turn from two decades ago.

Twenty years ago there was little emphasis on the medical evaluation of the sexually abused child. The focus of most child advocacy professionals was on gaining acceptance for the diagnosis of the "battered child." Sexual abuse was ignored by most of the medical community. In 1975, Sgroi called child sexual abuse "the last frontier in child abuse," reminding the medical practitioner that "in order to make the diagnosis of child sexual abuse, one must entertain the possibility that it occurs." During the decade that followed, a number of physicians called for an increased awareness of sexual abuse by medical professionals and appropriate education of all health care professionals. However, training remained primarily focused on the taking of a history from the caretaker and the child, the psychosocial dynamics of sexual abuse, and the responsibility to report and protect.

Although we have made tremendous progress over the past fifteen years, sexual abuse continues to present a unique challenge to the medical professional. Making the diagnosis requires that clinicians first come to terms with their own inner rejection of the fundamental concept that adults use children for sexual gratification. In the early 1980s, with the heightened awareness of child sexual abuse as a common pediatric problem, communities expected the primary medical professional to perform the medical evaluation. However, it soon became clear that most medical professionals were inadequately trained and that the diagnosis required a high level of skill and experience. Recognizing the potential harm to children and families by missing a diagnosis or by over-diagnosing, a system of multidisciplinary centers evolved. In these specialized centers, now often called Child Advocacy Centers (CAC), the medical staff had received enhanced training and kept current by participating in local and national peer review.

The primary medical professional remains an important partner. The community professional is essential to CAC success by recognizing that child sexual abuse is a problem, by referring children to centers of excellence, and by actively integrating prevention programs into community practice. To effectively participate as part of this team, primary medical professionals required an understanding of the dynamics of the child-victim and how to recognize the behavioral and medical symptoms of abuse. For those primary care clinicians who have the original contact with the child or those working in areas geographically distant from a CAC, this book provides guidelines for appropriate medical evaluation and testing.

Children are powerless and vulnerable, and so they are "ideal" victims of sexual abuse. Their vulnerability is compounded by the fact that sexual abuse occurs in private, as part of a dark secret. This secret rapidly becomes guilt: guilt for not telling and guilt for not being able to stop the abuse. If the abuser becomes the child's "only friend," and the child experiences normal pleasurable physiological responses to the sexual stimulation, the associated shame further prevents the child from disclosing the abuse. Often the abuser uses threats to ensure that secrecy will be maintained. Threats may take many forms, including actual violence to the child or loved ones or potential consequences such as the child being blamed or getting in trouble. In incest cases, the additional burden of maintaining the family is placed on the child. This responsibility may not be stated, but it is clearly implied. All of these factors maintain the secret and force the child to accommodate in order to survive.

The child sexual abuse accommodation syndrome described by Summit in 1983 explains the progression through secrecy, helplessness, entrapment and accommodation, disclosure and, finally, retraction. All of these stages result in behavior that makes it even more difficult for adults to accept that abuse occurs. Society expects children to "say no, run, tell." In reality most children do not tell and can't scream, struggle, or run. Dysfunctional or "acting-out" behavior further diminishes willingness by adults to believe any history of abuse. Finally, after living with the abuse for a time, the child may offer an unconvincing, tentative, and incomplete disclosure. Most adults discount such reports, and the child learns not to complain. The adults learn not to listen. And the end result is that society is relieved to learn that sexual abuse does not really occur or, at the very least, not in "nice" neighborhoods.

Other myths surround the secret of child sexual abuse. Generally children are not abused by strangers; most cases involve someone within the family or a person known to the child. Although it is true that most victims are girls, Abel (1987) showed that the majority of fixed pedophiles chose to molest boys. Despite recent attempts to discount children as witnesses, children have been shown to be reliable historians. Non-abused children do not fantasize about sexual contact with adults, or about things that are not part of their experience.

The relationship of the abuser to the victim may vary from a member of the nuclear family to a relative stranger. Individuals who seek sexual gratification from children are described as pedophiles. They may be "regressed pedophiles," individuals with a normal peer sexual orientation who turn to children for sexual satisfaction, especially when they are stressed or disempowered. The "fixed pedophile" is sexually oriented only to children. A third type of abuser has been labeled the "undifferentiated perverse." Such persons appear to be sociopaths, often are substance abusers, and will have forced sexual contact with males and females of all ages. Finally, the juvenile offender who acts out his or her own abuse on younger victims is becoming increasingly familiar to medical and mental health professionals.

An understanding of the victim and the abuser provides the medical professional an objective view of the process of sexual abuse. This is important in correlating a pattern of behavioral and medical complaints with the possibility of sexual abuse. (See Tables 1–1 and 1–2).

Now that medical professionals are aware of the importance of considering the diagnosis of sexual abuse within the context of the

Table 1–1. Role of the Medical Professional: Identifying Behavioral Indicators of Possible Sexual Abuse

ACUTE TRAUMATIC RESPONSE

Newly manifested clinging behavior and irritability in young children

REGRESSION

Loss of bowel and bladder control, thumb sucking, renewed need for a security blanket, withdrawal

SLEEPING DISTURBANCES

Night terrors, sleepwalking, bed-wetting, inability to sleep alone

EATING DISORDERS

Feeding difficulties in infants and pre-schoolers, anorexia nervosa, overeating

SCHOOL PROBLEMS

Change in performance, loss of concentration, easily distracted

SOCIAL PROBLEMS

Anger/acting out among peers, altered levels of activity with shortened attention span and "hyperactivity" or depression and inactivity, poor peer relationships, restricted social life in adolescents, and sexualized behavior inappropriate for developmental level

BEHAVIORAL SEQUELAE

Poor self-esteem, depression; guilt, suicidal gestures; acting out sexually inappropriately for age or excessive preoccupation with masturbation; delinquency; running away; substance abuse; prostitution; and psychosomatic gynecologic and gastrointestinal complaints

Table 1–2. Medical Indicators of Child Sexual Abuse

Male and Female

Bruising, scratches, bites
Sexually transmitted diseases
Blood stains on underwear
Bruising or swelling of genital area not consistent with history
Pain in anal, genital, gastrointestinal and urinary areas
Genital injuries (unexplained, inconsistent)
Injury to inner lips
Grasp marks
Enuresis and encopresis
Anal fissures

Male

Pain on urination
Penile swelling
Penile discharge

Female

Vaginal discharge
Urethral inflammation
Lymph gland inflammation
Pregnancy
Recurrent atypical abdominal pain

primary care practice, they should incorporate prevention information into general well child care. Possibly the most important tool is encouraging parents to communicate with their children. Simple rules surrounding good and bad secrets—"Bad secrets are what another adult tells you not to tell your parents,"— and private zones can help equip even a preschooler to cope with a hostile world. During the general medical examination the examiner can use the opportunity to give correct names to body parts, explain that certain parts should not be touched inappropriately, and include information on "who to tell" if abuse should occur. (See Chapter 4.)

When after behavioral and medical indicators suggest sexual abuse and the medical professional has taken a history from the child, a careful medical examination should be performed by a skilled examiner. This examination must be performed in the best interests of the child (see Chapter 5). The trained examiner should participate as part of a multidisciplinary team and have a thorough understanding of the interpretation of clinical and laboratory evidence. As for any medical diagnosis, it is important to know how to document clinical findings and obtain and preserve laboratory findings. Finally, child sexual abuse is the one diagnosis that the medical professional is asked to make that is going to result in interaction with the legal system. Since most medical professionals have an aversion to any interaction with this system, we need to learn to overcome any personal response and become skilled and powerful witnesses on behalf of children. (See Chapter 6.)

One of the hardest concepts for many professionals to grasp is that most child victims remain free of any significant medical findings. This is because of delayed disclosure and the nature of the abuse. Sexual abuse of the young child rarely involves penetrating trauma. Most often, children are involved in fondling, manipulation, oral, and anal intercourse. When vaginal penetration (across the hymen) does occur, there are usually diagnostic findings consistent with penetrating trauma. Acute injuries (within a few days) to the vagina or anus are easier to document, but children rarely disclose during that phase of the abuse, and such abrasions and lacerations resolve quickly, especially when they involve only the anus. Mucous membranes heal quickly and without significant scarring. Penetrating trauma of the vagina, as well as the anus, of the postpubescent female can heal completely without any changes diagnostic of sexual assault.

Over the past twenty-years, medical knowledge has enhanced physicians' ability to document and interpret normal and abnormal genital anatomy. Although most examiners have understood the need to examine a child-victim of recent assault, there was a natural reluctance to examine the child if there had been delayed disclosure or if the child reported only touching.

Today, most protocols for the evaluation of sexual assault or abuse agree on the need to evaluate patients as an emergency within the first 72 hours. However, few programs have implemented protocols for evaluating children who might be outside the acute phase, but are still in the process of healing. Documentation of both clinical and forensic evidence of a recent assault is important in protecting the child and appropriately prosecuting the offender. More discussion has evolved about the interpretation of possible indicators of abuse in cases with delayed disclosure. In an effort to better understand the medical diagnosis of past or chronic abuse, a wide range of possible indicators has been evaluated. Hymenal openings, measured in millimeters, were perceived by some to be the answer. It has hoped that these findings, described in millimeters, would provide scientific evidence to reassure us that the history from the child was indeed accurate. In time, examiners and researchers came to realize that measurements of this kind are often unreliable and inconsistent and depended on everything from the gender of the evaluator, to the amount of traction placed on the labia, to the position in which the child was placed. Anal relaxation was considered as a possible precise and sensitive indicator of abuse. This too came into question as subsequent researchers looking at a non-abused population, found that it was a common finding in the non-abused child and again depended on a wide range of variables. There were numerous other findings that were considered as the "acute and convalescent" titer for abuse. These included intra-vaginal or peri-hymeneal synechiae, absent hymeneal tissue ventrally, labial fusion, and other measures of hymeneal height or volume.

In 1983 we began the use of the colposcope for the documenta-tion of physical findings in children who had been sexually abused and in comparison non-abused populations. Within months of the initial investigations, photographic documentation became an im-portant component of the clinical and forensic evaluation. Pho-tographs could document trauma associated with sexual assault and provide information regarding normal genital anatomy. Pho-tographs became the basis for much research over the past decade and are now accepted as the standard of care in most referral cen-ters in the world.

Photographic documentation not only became the basis for most research in this field, but was also useful in peer review and in coming to a consensus of what examiners understood to be normal and abnormal. Photographs delineated the extremes of normal and abnormal but also documented a range of nonspecific findings, most of which are congenital and should not be misinterpreted. In parallel with research into the medical findings of abuse grew a very clear understanding of what was normal.

The major research benefits of colposcopy are now obvious, but the most important benefit to the child was the acceptance of the colposcope as a valid diagnostic tool and the photographs as a sub-stitute for repeat examinations. This use of photographs in place of repeat examinations has been validated by the legal system and withstood the scrutiny of the appellate court process (*California* vs. *Mendibles*, 1988).

By 1990, the benefits of colposcopy were accepted by most referral centers and were used to better understand the medical diagnosis of sexual abuse, to provide peer review, to reach consensus, and to protect children. Most recently we have developed a network of centers and professionals who can immediately review cases and find expert photographic consultations through the use of telemedicine.

The true value of the medical examination for possible sexual abuse is for the protection, the treatment, and the reassurance of the child. The capacity to explain the "intactness" of the child is an important part of the positive outcome. Although it is important for medical professionals to continue to emphasize that the history is the most important part of any medical evaluation, we do play an important role in the evaluation, treatment, and healing of the child. Children are injured when abuse involves penetrating trauma or acquiring sexually transmitted diseases. Appropriate treatment such as plastic repairs of serious genital trauma and the prescribing of antibiotics is an essential component of medical interventions. Children and parents still need to know that they will heal, and that they are free from disfigurement and disease. Who better than the medical professional to tell the child and family that the child will be well, will grow up to be normal, and is not responsible for the abuse? Our advocacy and encouragement of parents to keep the abused child in therapy contributes to the ultimate well-being of that child. We have enormous power to provide paths to healing.

Now almost twenty years after Kempe (1978) described child sexual abuse as "another hidden pediatric problem," we are routinely teaching the medical diagnosis of sexual abuse in most pediatric training programs. This training is a dynamic part of most pediatric conferences. Sexual abuse is no longer a hidden problem, we can use what we know to validate the history from the child. We can also use our understanding of the abuse process to explain that most cases of child sexual abuse are free of medical findings.

The medical professional now has enough history and clinical information to act with genuine professional objectivity in the best interests of the child. The history from the family, legal and/or social system, and the child is combined with the medical and laboratory evaluation in coming to a final diagnosis. The medical professional's interaction with the child-victim can be a powerful step in the ultimate healing process. With a calm, reassuring evaluator, such children can learn that they are not marked or different from others. Armed with this stronger, more positive image of themselves, they are ready for psychological treatment, and for a bright, productive future.

BIBLIOGRAPHY

Abel, G, J Becker, M Mittleman, J Cunningham-Rather, J Rouleau, and W Murphy, (1987). Self-reported sex crimes of non-incarcerated paraphiliacs. *Journal of Interpersonal Violence*, 2(1), 3–25.

American Medical Association. Diagnostic and treatment guidelines on child sexual abuse. *Arch. Fam. Med.* 1993; Jan:2 (1):19–27.

Anderson, SC. Psychosocial sequelae in intrafamilial victims of sexual assault and abuse. Abst. *Third International Congress on Child Abuse and Neglect*, Amsterdam, 1981.

Blythe MJ, DP Orr. Childhood sexual abuse; guidelines for evaluation. *Indiana Med.* 1985;78:11–18.

Burgess, AW, AN Groth, LL Homstrom, and SM Sgroi. *Sexual Assault of Children and Adolescents*. Lexington, Mass.: Lexington Books, 1978.

Butler, S. *Conspiracy of Silence: The Trauma of Incest*. New York: Bantam Books, New York, 1979.

Finkelhor, D. *Sexually Victimized Children*. New York: Free Press, 1979.

Goodman, GS and RS Reed. Age differences in eyewitness testimony. *Law and Human Behavior.* 1986;10:317–332.

Goodman, GS, L Rudy, BL Bottoms, and C Aman. Children's concerns and memory: Issues of ecological validity in children's testimony. In Fivush R and J Hudson (eds.). *What Young Children Remember and Know*. New York: Cambridge University Press, (In Press).

Heger, AH. Twenty years of medical evaluation of the sexually abused child; Have we helped or hurt? *Int. Journal of Child Abuse and Neglect.* 1996;10:893–897.

Helfer, RE and RS Kempe. *The Battered Child*. 4th Ed. Chicago: University of Chicago Press, 1987.

Herjanic, B. Sexual abuse of children. *JAMA* 1978;239:331–333.

Hibbard, RA and GL Hartman. Components of child and parent interviews in cases of alleged sexual abuse. *Child Abuse Negl.* 1993; Jul/Aug:17 (4):495–500.

Kempe, CH. Sexual abuse, another hidden pediatric problem. The 1977 C. Aldrich Anderson Lecture, *Pediatrics.* 1978;62:382–389.

Krugman, R. Recognition of sexual abuse in children. *Pediatr Rev.* 1986;8:25–30.

Ladsen, S. Do physicians recognize sexual abuse. *Am. J. Dis. Child.* 141:411–415, 1987.

MacFarlane, K and J Waterman. *Sexual Abuse of Young Children*. New York: Guilford Press, 1986.

May, JG. Sexual Abuse: The undercover problem. *Current Problems in Pediatrics.* 1977 (VII);12:3–39.

Sgroi, S. Sexual molestation of children; The last frontier in child abuse. *Child To-day.* 1975;May-June:18–21.

Summit, R. Sexual child abuse; Helping the physician entertain the diagnosis of child sexual abuse. *Dealing with Sexual Child Abuse.* Chicago, National Committee for the Prevention of Child Abuse, 1978:19–33.

Summit, RC and J Kryso. Sexual abuse of children: A clinical spectrum. *American Journal of Orthopsychiatry.* 1978;48:237–250.

Summit, RC. The child sexual abuse accommodation syndrome. *Child Abuse and Neglect.* 1983;7:177–193.

Teixeira, RG. Hymenal colposcopic examinations in sexual offenses. *Am J Forensic Med Pathol.* 1981;2:209–214.

Woodling, BA and A Heger. The use of the colposcope in the diagnosis of sexual abuse in the pediatric age group. *Child Abuse Negl.* 1986;10:111–114.

2

THE CHILD PROTECTION SYSTEM

RICHARD KRUGMAN AND ASTRID HEGER

Early on, much of the work done in the field of child sexual abuse focused on the recognition, investigation, and evaluation of the physical findings of children presumed to be sexually abused. Over the past decade there has been a dramatic shift in focus to building multidisciplinary teams integrating medicine and mental health with social and legal interventions to create appropriate service plans for children and their families.

Relying only on medical evidence resulted in a screening process by which children were sorted into several cohort populations—the sexually abused, the non-abused, and (if we are honest) the "we don't knows." Often historical information from children and their caretakers was overlooked, and some children were inappropriately labeled non-abused based on "normal" examinations, while others were labeled abused and inappropriately placed in foster homes. Fortunately, there is a growing awareness that medical

examination alone is often an inadequate information base for social service decisions.

Access to a multidisciplinary center of excellence helps social
service workers make appropriate decisions. Professionals associated with these centers provide expert medical examinations and
skilled interviews. Information thus provided can be integrated into
a case management plan fitting the needs of each population of children, and those who are sexually abused can be referred for social
and legal interventions and appropriate mental health services. The
non-abused child, who has been referred for possible abuse (usually
because of an inexpert examination), but gives no history, can be examined by the medical professional, given appropriate medical
treatment and prevention information, and returned home. Those
classified as "we don't know" could be referred to mental health services and followed by the center. Life goes on for the latter two
groups, and the experience of being screened should not have been
harmful, but there is continued concern about what happens to
those children who are victims of sexual abuse. How are sexually
abused children treated by the child protection system? The following is a hypothetical case to better explain the differences between customary practices and those used by a multidisciplinary
team.

J. T. is a first-grade student who was participating in a personal
safety curriculum sponsored by the local law enforcement agency.
During the puppet show she blurted out, "That happened to me!"
at a point where one of the characters said, "If anything like what
happened to Judy (a puppet who was molested by her uncle) has
happened to you, you should tell someone!" The teacher took J. T.
to her office where she asked her some questions. J. T., now frightened, would not respond. The teacher, as required by law, tele-
phoned the county department of social services. The following
events took place over the next 24 hours. *Actions that would be taken
now by a multidisciplinary advocacy center are in boldface type:*

- A social worker and law enforcement officer interviewed J. T.,
  during which time she showed them on anatomic dolls where
  somebody had "touched her." She would not identify "some-
  body" because "he told me not to tell." She also indicated that
  oral–genital sexual activity was involved.
- **J. T. was briefly interviewed by the social worker and taken
  to a multidisciplinary center where a trained professional in-**

terviewed J. T. while medical, law enforcement, and social service workers observed via a one-way mirror or hidden camera. J. T. disclosed that her mother's boyfriend had been putting his penis in her mouth.

- J. T. was taken to a hospital emergency room where she waited two hours to be seen. She was examined by a doctor who "stuck sticks in my bottom—both parts," as well as her mouth, and drew blood from her arm, but never talked to her or explained what was happening.
- **J. T. was examined at the center by a trained pediatric specialist who took a brief medical history, explained the examination, allowed her to choose to have the advocate with her, performed a general examination and genital examination with photodocumentation, and reassured the child that she was fine.**
- She was taken to a crisis center where she spent the night with two other children, both of whom exhibited very angry and violent behavior toward the younger child.
- **She was placed with her maternal aunt, with whom she has a good, long-standing relationship, in an environment where she felt safe, and was allowed to return to her school. She was assigned a case manager who reviewed the case with the advocacy center team.**
- J. T. appeared in court for a temporary hearing where she saw her mother for the first time. After the hearing, she was told she would have to go to a receiving home for a few days. Her mother, crying hysterically, told her that she would get her back, to "be good," and "don't tell them anything."
- **A preliminary detention hearing took place while J. T. waited in the playroom of the children's court with her aunt. The judge spoke with her privately in chambers, at which time J. T. reported what had happened with "Jerry," and said that she wanted to go home to be with her mother, but wanted that "sex stuff" to stop.**

Over the next 24 days, J. T. experienced the following:

- Lived in the receiving home with ten other children
- Attended a new school, because the receiving home and her home were in different school districts
- Began seeing a therapist twice a week to "talk and play," during

which time she identified her mother's boyfriend as the "some-body"

- Was sick and went to another hospital emergency room for care
- Was examined at this hospital by another doctor who "used a machine to take pictures" of her genitalia and rectum and "stuck more sticks" in her bottom and in her mouth (the initial specimens were lost at the first emergency room)
- Met and talked with her intake social worker
- Met and talked with the law enforcement officer twice and again played with the dolls
- Met and talked with her guardian ad litem
- Saw her mother three times in an office with the intake social worker
- Met and talked with the county attorney who would be filing the petition in juvenile court to continue the county's custody of J. T.
- **Was temporarily placed with her maternal aunt**
- **Attended her own school**
- **Started counseling with the advocacy center**
- **Had monitored visitation with her mother**
- **Saw the medical staff of the advocacy center–affiliated health care plan for children in foster care or family preservation**
- **Met with her guardian ad litem**

Over the next 24 weeks, J. T. experienced the following:

- Was ruled "dependent and neglected" by the juvenile court and placed in a foster home that had fewer children than the receiving home
- Was taken to a new doctor close to her foster home for treatment of the flu
- Attended a third school because the foster home and receiving home were in different districts
- Continued to see her therapist twice a week
- Met her ongoing social worker, who would try to reunite J. T. with her family
- Met and talked with the district attorney who would be prosecuting the criminal case against the mother's boyfriend
- Met the victim assistance worker who showed her the courtroom where she would be testifying
- Met the court-appointed special advocate who was gathering in-

formation for the treatment plan to be implemented at the next juvenile court hearing

- Testified in the criminal court at a preliminary hearing
- **Was returned home to her mother, who entered the family preservation program under the supervision of social services**
- **Went to court, where she saw her mother's boyfriend plead no-contest to child endangerment charges**
- **Continued in individual therapy and entered mother–daughter therapy at the center**
- **Saw her school performance improve**
- **Was visited by her social worker every two weeks**
- **Continued to receive medical care at the center-affiliated health care system that monitored her health and safety during the initial phases of family reunification**

Over the next 24 months, J. T. experienced the following:

- Was in the same foster home for six months
- Talked with two more attorneys and a new social worker because the district attorney, ongoing social worker, and guardian ad litem were transferred to another agency or moved
- Testified at the criminal trial of her mother's boyfriend, who was found guilty and sentenced to eight years in prison
- Was returned to her mother after a series of supervised and unsupervised visits
- Continued with her therapist once a week, and then met her mother's therapist and began family therapy once a week

Over the succeeding 24 months, J. T. and her mother actually experienced the following:

- **Completed mother–daughter therapy with the mental health services of the center**
- **Mother disclosed sexual abuse as a child and on-going domestic violence from both J. T.'s father and Jerry**
- **Mother continues in parenting classes and individual and group therapy**
- **J. T. feels safe and supported with her mother and is doing well in school**

- **J. T. is now back with her own pediatrician who is participating in her case management**
- **J. T. was student of the month at school last month**

Under the old regime, J. T. encountered over two dozen professionals, lived in four different centers or houses, attended three different schools, and saw a different medical provider every time she was examined or ill. Yet this case, as presented, is a triumph! She was reunited with her mother and both got treatment services. She was in only one foster home before reunification, not counting the crisis center and receiving home; she didn't have venereal disease; she was protected from further abuse; her assailant went to prison. Not all cases go so well.

Under the new regime, J. T. had access to one of the many *Child Advocacy Centers* in the United States. She spoke with only a few professionals and received only one medical examination, done by a trained professional, with photodocumentation making additional examinations unnecessary. She was protected by a social system that understood the importance of keeping a child in her community with family or friends whenever possible. Her mother had the support of the center and a sympathetic system so that she could provide a protective home and get the help she needed. Because of the excellent forensic work done by the center, the case never got as far as the criminal court, and J. T. never had to testify or see Jerry again.

However, in some parts of the United States and around the world, a case such as this would be treated quite differently. J. T. may never have had access to a program that gave rise to her spontaneous disclosure. Her case might never have been reported or, if it was reported, never opened. If it was opened, it might not have been adjudicated or criminally prosecuted. She and her mother might never have received treatment. She might, in fact, still be in an abusive environment.

Yet from J. T.'s, or any child's, perspective, even when it works, the child protection system in the United States is fragmented, discontinuous, and crisis driven, and its components are understaffed, underfunded, undertrained, and under the gun from public and legislative sectors that may be more attentive to parents who claim mistreatment by the system. To our knowledge, no country or state system publishes, or even collects, data on the outcomes of children in the protection system. That alone continues to be a disgrace.

It is no surprise, then, that in its August 1990 report, the U.S. Advisory Board on Child Abuse and Neglect called the present state of the child protection system in the United States a "national emergency." It should be noted that the term "child protection system" refers to a broad multidisciplinary system including the health, child welfare, law enforcement, mental health, education, judiciary, and legal systems. The board report suggested that it would take a decade of effort to ameliorate the present emergency and build a new, comprehensive, child-centered, neighborhood-based child protection system. Without this effort, the board believed the crisis it saw in 1990 would become chaos and that failure to act in a timely way would lead to loss of any hope of improving the lot of abused children in the United States.

Since 1990, some regional and local social service providers have begun to build comprehensive, child-centered, community-based programs. But changes in the national welfare system indicate a diminished interest in sweeping changes of the child protection system. There is further evidence of loss of interest in that in 1996 Congress abolished the U.S. Advisory Board and the Clinton Administration downgraded the National Center on Child Abuse and Neglect to the Office on Child Abuse and Neglect. So much for responding to an emergency!

When children are protected appropriately, our resources are spent economically. The child protection system works best when engaged in a multidisciplinary program through which participants coordinate their efforts to provide the ultimate protection to the child. These advocacy centers or centers of excellence minimize the trauma to the child and family while protecting society and saving the legal and social systems millions of dollars each year.

There are ranges of multidisciplinary teams that focus on diagnosing and treating abused children. Suspected Child Abuse and Neglect Teams (SCAN) are hospital-based and work particularly well when physical abuse and/or neglect are the presenting problem, but can become strained when the diagnosis is sexual abuse. Physical abuse/neglect cases require social services for the child and family and involvement in the dependency or family court.

Child advocacy centers were established as a prototype for the evaluation, investigation, and treatment of child sexual abuse. In those centers the team members include representatives from medicine, social work, mental health, law enforcement, prosecuting attorneys, and community advocates. These centers work best when they are medically based and are integrated into the SCAN team of the hospital. The development of advocacy center protocols that promote 24 hour, daily access to medical evaluations and team interventions offers the best for the child and the community. The challenge of intrafamilial sexual abuse, involving, as it does, social services and dependency court and interaction with the legal and judicial systems, is best served when evaluation is done at a center of excellence. Because of enhanced outcomes for children and families, communities are establishing these multidisciplinary, child-oriented child advocacy centers and are encouraging expansion of services to include all forms of child abuse and family violence. Cooperation prevents multiple interviews and examinations and keeps children from entering the system inappropriately. When all responsible professionals are required to join in deciding the best course for each child, it is less likely that a case will fall through the cracks.

Regardless of the quality or availability of local resources for protecting the abused child, it is essential and legally required that medical practitioners report suspected abuse promptly. The examiner may feel angry at the lack of appropriate social services for the child and feel that the child is better off out of the system, but this is not a decision the practitioner can make. When resources are inadequate, the medical professional can be a powerful advocate for development of appropriate local multidisciplinary programs. Obviously each center must meet certain goals for protection of the child, but the professionals involved may offer different ideas, depending upon the resources available.

Finally, the locally administered social systems will differ between states and counties. These factors all contribute to "the child protection system," which has thousands of incarnations in the United States and around the world. The lack of uniformity from place to place makes it imperative that practitioners know their own local system, their personal role within it, and the short- and long-term outcomes for the children they wish to protect.

FURTHER READING

Burgess, AW, AN Groth, LL Holmstrom, and SM Sgroi. *Sexual Assault of Children and Adolescents*. Lexington, Mass.: Lexington Books, 1978.

Helfer, ME, RS Kempe, and RD Krugman. *The Battered Child*. 5th ed. Chicago: University of Chicago Press, 1997.

Helfer, RE and CH Kempe. *Child Abuse and Neglect: The Family and the Community*. Cambridge, Mass.: Ballinger, 1976.

Krugman, RD. Future role of the pediatrician in child abuse and neglect. *Pediatr Clin North Am*. 1990;37:1003–1011.

Sgroi, SM. *Handbook of Clinical Intervention in Child Sexual Abuse*. Lexington, Mass.: Lexington Books, 1982.

U.S. Advisory Board on Child Abuse and Neglect. *Critical First Steps in Response to a National Emergency*. Government Printing Office, Washington, D.C., 1990.

3

PSYCHOLOGICAL EFFECTS OF CHILD SEXUAL ABUSE

CATHERINE KOVEROLA AND
WILLIAM N. FRIEDRICH

A description of the psychological effects of sexual abuse is central to understanding its impact. Numerous researchers and clinicians have attempted to establish a classic psychological profile of the sexually abused child, and after two decades of research, what has emerged is not a classic profile, but rather a consensus that there are divergent effects manifested along a continuum. This continuum ranges from children who are seemingly asymptomatic to those who are severely impaired in many areas of their lives. In recent years research in child sexual abuse has focused on numerous contextual variables believed to determine the impact of abuse on a given child. The aim of this chapter is to provide medical professionals with a brief review of empirical research on the impact of sexual abuse upon children, as well as a framework from which to understand the behaviors and psychological functioning of their patients.

DEFINITIONAL ISSUES IN UNDERSTANDING CHILD SEXUAL ABUSE

Most of this volume is devoted to a medical view toward identifying and diagnosing findings defined as being consistent with child sexual abuse. This chapter addresses the psychological and sociological effects of child sexual abuse. Finkelhor (1994) states that the legal and research definition requires two elements: (1) sexual activities involving a child, and (2) "an abusive condition," such as coercion or a large age gap between the participants, indicative of a lack of consensuality. In other words, child sexual abuse is conceived of as the involvement of children and adolescents in sexual activities that they do not fully comprehend, that they are unable to give consent to, and that violate social taboos. Sexual abuse can include a wide range of acts such as fondling of the genitalia, intercourse, oral copulation, sodomy, and obscene or pornographic photographing, filming, or depiction of children. The second component of child sexual abuse, as defined by Finkelhor, is the notion of the power imbalance/coercion between victim and perpetrator. Earlier definitions of child sexual abuse typically accepted a five-year age difference between the victim and the perpetrator. As clinicians have increasingly identified situations of peers/siblings of similar ages engaging in coerced sexual behaviors, the five-year age difference has been reconsidered. Similarly, in situations of date rape there is often not a large age difference between victim and perpetrator. At present there is a lack of consistency among researchers on how child sexual abuse is defined and who is included or excluded in the abuse sample. In some studies sexual abuse between same-aged peers is categorized as child sexual abuse, while in others it is separated out as peer abuse, and in still others it is not categorized as child sexual abuse at all. Furthermore, researchers differ on whether the endpoint of childhood is age 16 or age 18.

PREVALENCE OF CHILD SEXUAL ABUSE

How common is child sexual abuse? Despite almost two decades of research, the answer to this simple question eludes researchers, for a number of reasons. The most salient reason is that child sexual abuse is a secretive, hidden offense, shrouded in fear and, thus, highly under-reported. In the United States there are three official sources of data documenting the reported occurrence of child sexual abuse: (1) the National Incidence Study of Child Abuse and Neglect (NIS), (2) child protection agencies, and (3) law enforcement agencies. These incidence reports, however, reflect only those patients being treated by health and mental health professionals; clearly they do not include unreported cases. Because so much child sexual abuse remains undisclosed, to obtain prevalence data, researchers have relied on retrospective surveys of adults. In a review of 19 survey studies of child sexual abuse prevalence, Finkelhor (1994) reports "considerable evidence exists to show that at least 20 percent of American women and 5–10 percent of American men experienced some form of sexual abuse as children." (p. 31) In an earlier review of prevalence studies, Finkelhor and colleagues had reported ranges of 6–62 percent (1986).

RISK FACTORS FOR CHILD SEXUAL ABUSE

To identify children who may be at risk, it is important first to consider who are the victims of sexual abuse. Sexual abuse is widespread, not a rare childhood experience. Furthermore, sexual abuse occurs in all demographic strata. Sexual abuse is not, however, a random event (Friedrich, 1990). A number of researchers have investigated factors that place a person at risk. Finkelhor (1979) identified a number of predictors of childhood sexual victimization: the presence of a stepfather, living without the mother at some point, not being close to the mother, having a mother who has not finished high school, a sex-punitive mother (sexually repressive), no physical affection from the father, a family income under $10,000, and two or fewer friends in childhood. These risk factors were cumulative, with each additional factor increasing a child's vulnerability between 10 and 20 percent. In view of the fact that many children who have been sexually abused present with psychiatric symptoms, it is interesting to note that there is considerable overlap of risk factors for sexual abuse and risk factors identified for the presence of psychiatric disorders in children. In a Canadian epidemiological study, Offord and colleagues (1989) found nine significant correlates of psychiatric disorders in children: family income under $10,000, urban vs. rural residence (urban children had a higher likelihood of disorder), family dysfunction, a parent treated for psychological disorder, a parent arrested, the age of the child (older children had a higher number of disorders), the sex of the child, the child having failed a grade, and the child having a chronic medical illness.

Neither sexual abuse nor psychiatric disturbance, then, is a random event. Identifiable variables predict a greater likelihood of occurrence. These variables seem to overlap one another. It should be noted that these findings are correlational in nature and thus cannot be interpreted as causative. They are, however, suggestive of the types of issues and situations that the medical professional confronts when dealing with patients who have been sexually abused (Finkelhor, 1979). For example, upon interviewing any number of sexually abused children and their parents, the medical professional often can discern a disturbed mother-child relationship. The mother may exhibit an absence of bonding or lack of empathy for the child. For example, if the perpetrator is a stepfather and the mother a victim of domestic violence, she may have tremendous difficulty providing adequate emotional support to her child. This is further complicated by the mother's own history. Further interviews with the family often reveal that the problems are intergenerational. It is a common scenario for the mother to have been abused by her stepfather and to have had an emotionally absent mother. These problems are not random or coincidental; rather, they are deeply entrenched in a family system that is highly resistant to change and woven into a context of impaired interpersonal relationships and lack of resources. These contextual risk factors are important not only for understanding how the child came to abused, but also for future planning. Intervention for the child without consideration of the contextual predisposing risk factors will likely be met with failure.

INITIAL IMPACT OF CHILD SEXUAL ABUSE

Early research on the initial impact of child sexual abuse was based primarily on anecdotal clinical case reports and chart review methodology. In the past ten years, sounder methodological studies have been completed in which sexually abused children are compared to non-abused children. In a review of 45 such studies, Kendall-Tackett and colleagues (1993) identified the following behaviors/symptoms as the most common effects manifested by sexually abused children: anxiety, fear, post-traumatic stress disorder, nightmares, depression (including despressive symptoms), withdrawal, suicidal behaviors, poor self-esteem, somatic complaints, aggressive antisocial behaviors, cruelty, delinquent behaviors, sexualized behaviors, promiscuity, school and learning problems, hyperactivity, regression or immaturity, illegal acts, self-destructive behaviors, running away, substance abuse, and self-injurious behavior. In many studies, composite symptoms are reported and categorized as follows: internalizing behaviors, such as anxiety and fear, and externalizing behaviors, such as aggressive and antisocial behaviors.

The frequency of these symptoms varied widely according to the Kendall-Tackett review. For example, between 20 and 30 percent of victims presented with a particular symptom at the time of initial assessment. The symptom clusters most commonly identified were those associated with post-traumatic stress disorder (PTSD) 53 percent. However, results of research that examined PTSD was variable, and not all of it utilized DSM criteria. The results also reflect numerous developmental patterns. For example, preschoolers more commonly exhibted symptoms reflective of anxiety, nightmares, PTSD, and sexualized behavior than did older children. School age children were noted to have more fear, neurotic behaviors, aggression, nightmares, school problems, hyperactivity, and regression and immaturity. The data on adolescents was more sparse, but seemed to show the greatest number of problems with depression, withdrawal, suicidal ideation, self injurious behavior, somatic complaints, illegal activities, running away, and substance abuse. The data also found that sexual behavior was specific to sexual abuse. However, recent research has indicated that sexual behavior and PTSD are also associated with other types of child maltreatment and generalized distress in children (Friedrich et al, under review). One a very important finding was that children may be asymptomatic following abuse, as determined by the assessment measures utilized in the study. The rate of asymptomatic victims is typically 30 percent of the total sample.

The absence of observable symptoms can often be explained by the limited range of measures utilized, the developmental non-specificity of the symptom (sexual difficulties may only be noted when the victim is older, for example), as well as the moderating influence of the child's environment.

Comprehensive Model of Trauma Impact

As is evident from the previous review, children who have been sexually abused can present with a broad range of symptoms. Some children present with numerous and severe behavior problems and function poorly; others become overachievers and highly competent. Some children disclose the abuse readily; others deny it. In addition to the broad range of symptomatology that must be assessed, the medical professional is presented with a myriad of potential variables thought to mediate the child's adjustment. How does the medical professional make sense of the multiplicity of interactive variables involved?

In the previous edition of this volume, the Comprehensive Model of Trauma Impact (CMTI) was presented. The model endeavors to delineate these variables and identifies potential interaction pathways (see Figure 3–1). The CMTI has four main components: (1) the nature of the trauma, (2) the individual's areas of functioning, (3) the systemic context, and (4) passage of time/developmental considerations. The CMTI is not based on any particular theoretical viewpoint, but is presented as a framework in which to consider the numerous variables and issues salient to assess and treat victims of child sexual abuse.

Nature of Trauma

Since the first edition of this book, research on the specific details of sexually traumatic events has shifted. Rather than focusing exclusively on the trauma of child sexual abuse, both researchers and clinicians have increasingly recognized that the majority of child

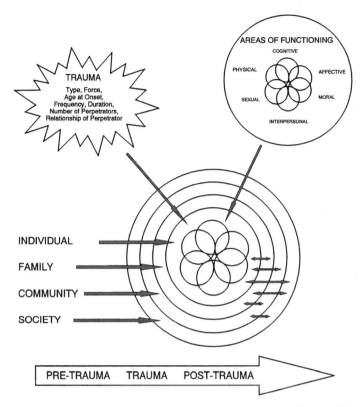

Fig. 3–1. Comprehensive model of trauma impact. (From Koverola, Heger, and Lytle, 1990).

sexual abuse victims have suffered multiple forms of victimization. These forms include the following: physical abuse, neglect, psychological abuse, and exposure to domestic violence and/or community violence. Information on other forms of abuse should be obtained from a victim at the same time as information on the sexual abuse. This includes age at onset, duration, frequency, type of abuse, identity and closeness of perpetrator, and use of force. There are numerous empirical studies documenting wide-spread multiple victimization of children. *Multiple Victimization of Children: Conceptual, Developmental, Research and Treatment Issues* edited by Rossman and Rosenberg (1998) provides an extensive review and analysis of different types of child abuse and the relationships between the type of abuse and the child's adjustment. It is evident from this volume as well as others (eg. Kendall-Tackett et al, 1993; Pearce and Pezzot-Pearce, 1998) that the impact of multiple victimization is not simply additive, but has an exponential impact upon the child's adjustment and behavior.

Sexual abuse encompasses a broad range of experiences. A number of parameters determine the severity of abuse. These parameters include variables such as type of act, frequency, duration, age of onset, use of force, relationship to perpetrator, and number of perpetrators. Clinicians and researchers have speculated as to which variables are linked with the most severe impact. Finkelhor and Browne (1986) found that the empirical data were contradictory for variables related to frequency, duration, and earlier age at onset. They found more consensus on the variables of relationship to perpetrator, type of abuse, and use of force. Children exhibited more symptoms of psychological distress when the father (or father figure) was the abuser, the abuse involved genital contact, and the use of force accompanied the abuse. The relative influence of these variables is generally supported in Kendall-Tackett et al (1993).

Areas of Development

The second component of the CMTI is areas of development in the individual being. The areas of development identified within the CMTI as particularly salient include affective, cognitive, interpersonal, sexual, moral, and physical.

One of the most challenging and simultaneously delightful aspects about children is that they are ever changing. Behaviors that are normal and appropriate at one age can be indicative of significant impairment in functioning at another age. When considering childhood behaviors, the frequency, intensity, and duration of the behaviors must be considered as well as the age at which they occur. For example, frequent temper tantrums and displays of aggression are common among 2-year-olds, yet identical behavior would be considered inappropriate for an 8-year-old. In determining whether a child's behavior is indicative of distress or dysfunction, developmental norms must be considered. The rate of development or change over a specified time is significantly greater for a child than for an adult. This rapid rate of change is what makes the study of the child so challenging.

The child develops across a number of different dimensions, all of which interact with one another. The most notable are the cognitive, affective, interpersonal, moral, sexual, and physical areas of development. The development of the child is determined by the biological constitution interacting with the environment in which the child grows and develops. The child's constitutional components comprise the child's basic temperament and personality style, as well as innate cognitive potential. The child's constitution also includes a set course of development along each of the dimensions noted above. These constitutional factors are continuously interacting with the child's environment, thus determining collectively how the child develops. When the child's environment includes an individual who sexually abuses the child, the normal course of development is halted. The child must process this event on a number of different levels. The developmental level of the child at the time of the abuse, together with the child's basic constitution, determines how the event is processed. The experience then becomes incorporated into the child's sense of self.

Sexual abuse has an explicit impact on each area of development identified in the CMTI. There is considerable evidence to indicate that affective development, the child's ability to experience and express affect in a developmentally appropriate manner, is negatively impacted in children who have been sexually abused. For example, symptoms of depression, anxiety, fear, hostility, and somatization are higher for sexually abused children than for non-abused children (Beitchman et al, 1991; Kendall-Tackett et al, 1993; Gomes-Schwartz et al, 1990; McGrath et al, 1990; Swanston et al, 1997; Wolfe, et al (1989). Sexually abused children are often impaired in their ability to regulate their affect and tend to exhibit intense expressions or present with a blunt affect. The development of behavioral self-regulation is impacted by child sexual abuse. Many sexually abused children are unable to regulate their behavior in developmentally appropriate ways. Delays in behavioral regulation include aggression, hyperactivity, self injurious behavior, running away, and delinquent acts and have been identified in numerous studies. (Beitchman et al, 1992; Kendall-Tackett et al, 1993; McGrath et al, 1990; Pearce and Pezzot-Pearce, 1997, Tong et al, 1987, Tufts New England Medical Center, 1984).

There is evidence to suggest that child sexual abuse interferes with cognitive development. This is manifest, for example, in language developmental delays, academic difficulties (Trickett et al, 1994), and difficulty concentrating, as well as in the cognitive components of post traumatic stress symptoms, such as intrusive thoughts and memory impairments. (Deblinger, et al, 1990; Kendall-Tackett et al, 1993; McLeer et al, 1988; Wolfe et al, 1989).

Typically interpersonal development is severely impacted by child sexual abuse, not surprisingly, in view of the fact that sexual abuse is an intense interpersonal violation. The ability to develop trusting, intimate relationships is often significantly impaired and delayed (Conte and Shuerman, 1988; Tong et al, 1987; Wolfe et al, 1989).

Moral development is an area that has been studied only quite recently in child sexual abuse survivors. There is evidence to suggest that sexual abuse impacts the individual's sense of justice and hopefulness about the future. Janoff-Bullman's (1992) research on shattered world assumptions addresses these concepts. The child's moral development must integrate extremely painful realities at a premature stage of development. Sexual development and subsequent behavior is particularly germane to sexual abuse, and research has pointed to the consistency with which this is a problem for victims throughout their lives (Friedrich, 1998). *The Child Sexual Behavior Inventory* (Friedrich, 1997) was developed with a pediatric normative sample and a clinical sample, and, in cases of alleged abuse, is a useful measure of how typical a child's sexual behavior is.

Finally, sexually abused children's physical development can be impacted in a number of ways, depending on the severity of the abuse. These may include pregnancy, diseases, and physical trauma to genitalia. There is now some research to suggest that sexual abuse can result in early puberty for girls (Trickett and Putnam, 1993) and elevated growth hormore levels for boys. (Jensen et al, 1991). In a study conducted by DeBellis et al (1994) findings showed a urinary catecholamine excretion increase in sexually abused girls, a similar pattern found in individuals with post traumatic stress disorder and depression.

Data relevant to pediatricians indicates more frequent somatic complaints in sexually abused children (Friedrich and Shafer, 1995). A correlate of sexual abuse seems to be the children's reduced ability to describe their feelings accurately. They feel that their bodies are damaged, and express distress via somatic routes.

Children who have been sexually abused may present with delays in development in one or several areas. It is important to bear in mind how these areas and inter-related. For example, cognitive delays or impairment undoubtedly impacts how a child processes issues in the interpersonal realm of her life. The child may begin to experience herself as socially isolated because of impaired social skills, intensifying feelings of sadness and or anxiety. It is instructive to see how the impact on one area of function can have significant deleterious impact on others. Without intervention, the child is clearly on a downward spiral. The child's sense of self, self valuing, and self esteem can be conceptualized as the consolidation of all these areas of development. Not surprisingly, children who have been sexually abused have lower self-esteem than non-abused children (Bagley and Young, 1989). The child's sense of self develops within the context of interpersonal relationships. The child knows herself or himself in relation to others. When a child is sexually abused, that child is forced to incorporate sexuality into a relationship before she or he is developmentally prepared to do so. The experience is further charged with dynamics such as secrecy, powerlessness, fear, confusion, and betrayal. Depending upon the cognitive, affective, interpersonal, moral, sexual, and physical development at that point, the child may be more or less successful in coping with the event. Some children are clearly able to encapsulate the event(s) and do not incorporate it into their sense of self in a destructive manner. Other children are less fortunate. Sexual abuse affects them in a more detrimental manner, and they present with a host of problematic behaviors, ranging from depression, fear, and anxiety to aggression, hostility, and sexual acting out.

It can not be over-emphasized how important it is to consider the impact of child sexual abuse on development in specific areas, as well as overall. It is critical that the health care professional identify potential areas of developmental lag or delay so that intervention can be implemented appropriately. Often it is most efficient to intervene in an area of the child's strength rather than her weakness. Because all of the areas are interrelated, strengthening one area of function typically strengthens development in an area that is lagging behind.

Systemic Context

The third component of the model is the systemic context in which the child develops. This component of the model draws from the work of Belsky (1980, 1993) highlighting the importance of the context in which the child exists. Of most importance to the child is her or his immediate family. Within the family, the child is impacted by the parent's psychological functioning, parent and sibling support or rejection, family communication styles, and generational boundaries.

The community includes friends, school, church, and community groups and law enforcement, child protection, and medical personnel. The relative degree of support or rejection experienced by the child in the community interacts with the child's adjustment. The societal context is the underlying value and belief system that determines how society responds to sexual abuse. The societal context also encompasses cross-cultural differences and beliefs regarding sexuality. The impact of the societal context on the child is more indirect than the others and occurs largely via the community and family.

The family is the child's primary social environment. As such, family variables are a significant factor in determining how sexual abuse impacts on the child. The family can affect the child as a predisposing and negative or as protective and positive factor.

The preceding discussion highlighted the role of the parent-child relationship, particularly the mother-child relationship, in placing the child at risk for abuse. The parent's psychological functioning has been demonstrated to have a powerful impact on the child's adjustment. In addition to the direct impact of the parent on the child, the parent's own psychological adjustment is an important consideration when completing an evaluation.

Psychological assessments of children rely at least in part on parental reports. The assessor must always evaluate the parent's report of a child behavior in light of the parent's own psychological functioning. The question in essence becomes, "Is the child disturbed, or disturbing?" Children are very seldom self-referred to health-care professionals. Children come to the attention of health-care professionals when they are disturbing to adults, usually the parents. One must determine whether the parent is over or underreporting the child's behavior problems. In the case of sexually abused children, both are possibilities. A detached, uninvolved parent may be less attentive, and therefore unaware, of the child's problems, particularly if the child tends to be an internalizer. In contrast, a parent who is rejecting and hostile toward the child, or who is in significant psychological distress, may exaggerate the child's behavior problems and overreport. Numerous researchers have documented that distressed parents report significantly more psychopathology in their children than do nondistressed parents. The reliability and validity of the parent report is critical to assessing a child's level of function. This is a particularly important variable to consider when assessing a child who has been sexually abused because there is a likelihood that a parent is experiencing significant psychological distress. It is particularly helpful to obtain corroborative information from others who know the child well, such as teachers, social workers, and other involved adults.

In addition to the parent-child relationship, there are a number of other salient family variables that may determine the impact of sexual abuse upon the child. For example, the degree to which the family has appropriate boundaries, particularly intergenerational boundaries, serves either to place a child at risk or to protect the child. In cases of father-daughter incest, there is a blurring of intergenerational boundaries, and the child is placed in the role of the father's sexual partner, while the mother has effectively abdicated her sexual role as wife. The functional level of the marital subsystem is a critical variable. In families with high levels of marital discord, parents are emotionally unavailable to the child. This places the child at risk for abuse both within and outside the family. In families in which the intergenerational subsystems are intact, the child can utilize the support of siblings. However, in families who have a disturbance in this dimension, children will not be supportive of one another. This leaves the sexually abused child isolated within the sibling subsystem. It is often not until later in adulthood that many siblings discover, much to their amazement, that they were all abused by the same perpetrator.

Another important family variable is the communication style of the family. This determines whether the abused child has a viable mechanism for sharing the abuse experience with a parent or sibling. In families with a disturbance in communication, there are ambiguous messages about the acceptability of the abuse, and, consequently, the sexually abused child cannot disclose the abuse. In contrast, if a family has open communication, the child can readily tell a family member that abuse has occurred. The type of communication in the family also affects whether the child faces supportive acceptance or hostile denial and rejection. Preliminary findings with 50 sexually abused children indicated that children with supportive mothers were significantly more likely to disclose abuse than those with non-supportive mothers (Koverola et al, 1990).

A child's extended family, much like the nuclear family, serves as both predisposing and protective factors in sexual abuse. For many sexually abused children, the perpetrator is a member of the extended family, and, in such a case, the extended family functions as a significant predisposing factor. Further, the extended family may be protective of the perpetrator, and the child's disclosure of abuse may be met with anger and rejection. However, there may also be important supportive individuals in the extended family who provide both psychological and physical protection for the child. As has already been noted, a child's disclosure of abuse may precipitate multiple disclosures by other extended family members.

The community can likewise exacerbate the sexually abused child's plight or serve to alleviate it. The community is a broad group of individuals and agencies, including family, friends, school, church, community groups, law enforcement, child protection, and medical personnel. It is common for a sexually abused child to first test the disclosure of abuse by telling someone in the community prior to sharing it with a family member. Community supports can be invaluable to the child in facilitating recovery.

The importance of cross-cultural variables has been increasingly evident as an issue in the delivery of mental health services (Taylor Gibbs et al, 1989). Different ethnic and cultural groups have different views and attitudes regarding sexual abuse. This may be evident in parental response to a child's disclosure or to medical evidence of child sexual abuse. The medical professional should be alert to the fact that some parents may have an "unhelpful attitude" toward the child. This negative attitude on the part of the parents may be complicated by other issues, such as their own abuse histories, and other social stresses, such as poverty, unemployment, and difficult adult relationships. The degree to which there may be cross-cultural differences influencing the child's response to sexual abuse has not been fully investigated. However, most clinicians would concur that ethnicity in and of itself is not a salient factor in determining impact, compared to variables such as those delineated earlier. While there has not been extensive research into this issue, one particular body of research bears mentioning, the normative research on the *Child Sexual Behavior Inventory* (Friedrich, 1997). An interesting pattern emerged in this regard: low income was related to reduced reporting of all behavior problems, including sexual behaviors, but ethnicity was significantly related once income level was controlled for statistically. This lends further support to the position that ethnicity itself is not a factor in the impact on the child. Nevertheless, it is important for the medical professional to provide culturally sensitive medical services, utilizing an appropriate interpreter when necessary, and understanding as much about the patient's cultural background as possible.

Passage of Time

The final component of the model highlights the passage of time. This concept is key to children, who are continually developing and changing. The model highlights the importance of the continuum of pre-trauma, trauma, and post-abuse. For example, regressed behavior in a very young abused child may be expected, and even common, but it is much more serious when it occurs in an adolescent. Delayed effects may show up only as the child moves through time. For example, agitation following abuse that manifests as inattentiveness becomes important as the child enters school. Anxiety associated with sexual intimacy or body image distrubances may become clinical issues only when the child moves into adolescence or young adulthood. Parenting problems that reflect the victim's lack of support at the time of the abuse may show up only when the victim become a parent. As a pediatrician, when the parent asks if the child is "damaged", it is important to provide an answer that is both sensitive and reflective of the entire developmental continuum.

In summary, the *Comprehensive Model of Trauma Impact* addresses four major areas: nature of trauma, child's functioning and development, systemic contexts, and passage of time. Each of these areas identifies a number of interactive variables that impact upon the child and so mediate the child's adjustment to the trauma of sexual abuse. This model can serve as useful organizational format with which to consider variables that have had and will have an impact on the child.

DISCLOSURE

The child's capacity to disclose is thought to be determined by a number of factors. Among these are the nature of the abuse, the impact of the abuse upon the child, parental support, and family and community supports. In the initial disclosure, most sexually abused children tell only a small part of the abuse history. If the initial disclosure is received in a supportive manner, the child may go on to disclose additional details. If, however, the disclosure is met with anger and retaliation, it is very common for the child to retract the disclosure and adamantly deny it. Retraction is an easily understood phenomenon when one considers the price that many children pay for having disclosed. The child may be rejected by the parent(s), siblings, and extended family; the abuser may be jailed; and the child may be subjected to lengthy interrogations, court appearances, and placement in foster homes. The child is convinced quickly that if the story is retracted, life will return to "normal." Sadly, for some children, retraction does return their lives to "normal," and they are forced to deal with the abuse in silence.

As sexual abuse charges become increasingly litigious, the accuracy of the child's disclosure has become a central concern. New research on children's memory and their ability to accurately report when questioned about events has been very helpful to those practitioners who work with victims. Research focused on the issues of recall and suggestibility of the child has shown that children ages three and under are more vulnerable than adults to misleading questioning, but the accuracy of older children relative to adults, is good. (Goodman et al, 1987; Goodman, 1984) It has also been demonstrated that younger children are more susceptible when it comes to recall of the salient aspects of the event, such as who, what, and where (Friedrich, 1990). Cognitive interviewing, a strategy wherein the child is taught how to be accurate and detailed in recall, is also a promising development (Saywitz and Elliott, in press).

CONCLUSION

The impact of sexual abuse on the victim is well understood. Researchers have begun to investigate the impact on parents and caregivers. A number of researchers have documented that some parents and caregivers experience secondary victimization with symptoms of PTSD (Friedrich, 1995; Manion et al, 1996). This vicarious traumatization in a parent may seriously effect their parenting, even more so if they are struggling with unresolved abuse. The practitioner must be sensitive to the parent's simulatneous need to cope with the trauma associated with being the parent of a child-victim. Providing support to the parent is critical to providing a healthy family environment for the child.

In addition to the pragmatics of assessing salient variables that influence the child, the medical professional must also deal with personal feelings about sexual abuse, the nature of which is such that it may trigger a broad range of uncomfortable, and often unfamiliar, feelings. In response to this the medical professional may want to push away these feelings and deny them. In the process, it is possible that the child will be pushed away and required to deny her or his abuse. The medical professional must resist the temptation to oversimplify the child's symptoms of distress and complex history as a means of quelling her or his own feeling of discomfort and confusion about how to deal with the problem. Medical professionals are encouraged to seek out other colleagues with whom they can process their feelings about sexual abuse. In so doing, they can deal more effectively with patients who present with a history of sexual abuse. A particularly helpful and comprehensive volume on the topic of vicarious traumatization is *Trauma and the Therapist* (Pearlman and Saakvitne (1995). In it the authors argue persuasively that it is critical for professionals to "stay psychologically healthy," particularly when working with victims of trauma. The oath to do no harm sadly can all too easily be broken if the practitioner is not aware of how personal feelings and issues may compromise the ability to provide competent care to a child sexual abuse victim and her or his family. Working as part of a multi-disciplinary team and avoiding solo practice in this area is one very pragmatic component of ensuring psychological health.

Each sexually abused child has a unique set of symptoms, together with a unique life story and context, which in most cases is quite painful. The medical professional must be alert to symptoms indicative of abuse and, most importantly, be willing to listen to child's story. To be able to do this for the child, vicarious traumatization must be acknowledged and processed in order to be involved in this type of work.

REFERENCES

Bagley, C and L Young. Depression, self-esteem, and suicial behavior as sequels of sexual abuse in childhood: Research and therapy. In M Rothery and

G Cameron (Eds.), *Child Maltreatment: Expanding Our Concept of Healing* (pp. 183–209). Erlbaum: Hillsdale, NJ, 1989.

Beitchman, JH, KJ Zucker, JE Hood, GA daCosta, and D Akman. A review of the short-term effects of child sexual abuse. *Child Abuse and Neglect*, 1991;15:537–556.

Belsky, J. Child maltreatment: An ecological integration. *American Psychologist*, 1980;35:320–335.

Belsky, J. Etiology of child maltreatment: A developmental-ecological analysis. *Psychological Bulletin*, 1993;114:413–434.

Committee on Sexual Offenses Against Children and Youth. *Sexual Offenses Against Children in Canada Summary*. Supply and Services Canada: Ottawa, ONT, 1984.

Conte JR and JR Schuerman. The effects of sexual abuse on children: A multidimensional view. In: Wyatt GE, GJ Powell (Eds.) *Lasting Effects of Child Sexual Abuse*. Sage Publications: Newbury Park, CA, 1988.

De Bellis, MD, L Lefter, PK Trickett, and FW Putnam. Urinary catecholamine excretion in sexually abused girls. *Journal of the American Academy of Child and Adolescent Psychiatry*, 1994;33:320–565.

Deblinger, E, SV McLeer, and D Henry. Cognitive behavioral treatment for sexually abused children suffering post-traumatic stress: Preliminary findings. *Journal of the American Academy of Child & Adolescent Psychiatry*, 1990; 29:747–752.

Finkelhor, D. Impact of child sexual abuse: Review of the research. *Psychological Bulletin*, 1994;99:66–77.

Finkelhor, D, S Araji, L Baron, A Browne, S Doyle Peters, and GE Wyatt. *Sourcebook on Child Sexual Abuse*. Sage Publications: Newbury Park, CA, 1986.

Finkelhor, D. Early and long-term effects of child sexual abuse: An update. *Professional Psychology Research and Practice*, 1990;21:325–330.

Finkelhor, D. *Sexually Victimized Children*. Free Press: New York, 1979.

Finkelhor, D and A. Browne. Initial and long-term effects: A conceptual framework. In: Finkelhor, D, S Araji, L Baron, A Brown, S Doyle Peters, GE and Wyatt (Eds.). *A Sourcebook on Child Sexual Abuse*. Sage Publications: Newbury Park, CA, 1986.

Finkelhor, D. Current information on the scope and nature of child sexual abuse. *Sexual Abuse of Children*, 1994;4 (2):31–53.

Friedrich, WN. *Psychotherapy with Sexually Abused Boys*. Sage: Newbury Park, CA, 1995.

Friedrich, WN. *Child Sexual Behavior Inventory: Professional Manual*. Psychological Assessment Resources: Odessa, FL, 1997.

Friedrich, WN. Behavioral manifestations of child sexual abuse. *Child Abuse and Neglect*, 1998; 22: 523–531.

Friedrich, WN, JL Fisher, R Acton, L Berliner, J Burlter, L Damon, WH Davies, A Gray, and J Wright. Child Sexual Behavior Inventory: Normative, Psychiatric, and Sexual Abuse Comparisons.

Friedrich, WN, L Lengua, J Fisher, WH Davies, W Pithers, and B Trentham. Parent report of PTSD and Dissociation: Normative, Psychiatric and Sexual Abuse Comparisons, under review.

Friedrich, WN. *Psychotherapy of Sexually Abused Children and their Families*. Norton: New York, 1990.

Gomes-Schwartz, B, J Horowitz, and A. Cardarelli. *Child Sexual Abuse: The Initial Effects*. Sage Publications: Newbury Park, CA, 1990.

Gibbs, JT, LN Huang, and Associates. *Children of Color*. and Jossey-Bass: San Francisco, CA, 1989.

Goodman, GS, C Aman and J Hirschman. Child sexual and physical abuse: Children's testimony. In: Ceci, SJ, MP Toglia, DF Ross, (Eds). *Children's Eyewitness Memory*. Springer-Verlag: New York, 1987.

Goodman, GS. The child witness: conclusions and future directions for research and legal practice. *Journal of Social Issues*, 1984; 40:157–175.

Janoff-Bulman, R. *Shattered Assumptions: Towards a New Psychology of Trauma*. Free Press: New York, 1992.

Jensen, JB, JJ Pease R ten Bensel, and BD Garfinkel. Growth hormone response in sexually or physically abused boys. *Journal of the American Academy of Child and Adolescent Psychiatry*, 1991;30:784–790.

Kendall-Tackett, L Meyer Williams, and D Finkelhor. *Psychological Bulletin*, 1993;113 (1): 164–180.

Koverola, C, D Foy, and A Heger. Relationship of post-traumatic stress disorder to child disclosure and medical evidence in sexually abused children. Paper presented at the Sixth Annual Meeting of the Society for Traumatic Stess Studies, New Orleans, Louisiana, 1990.

Koverola, C, A Heger, and C Lytle. Assessment of sexually abused children: a multi-modal approach. Paper presented at the Canadian Psychological Association Meeting, Ottawa, Canada, 1990.

Manion, IG, J McIntyre, P Firestone, M Ligezinska, R Ensom, and G Wells. Secondary traumatization in parents following the disclosure of extrafamilial child sexual abuse: Initial effects. *Child Abuse Neglect*, 1996;11,1095–1109.

Mannarino, AP, JA Cohen, and M Gregor. Emotional and behavioral difficulties in sexually abused girls. *Journal of Interpersonal Violence*, 1989;4,437–451.

McGrath, E, GP Keita, BR Strickland, and NF Russo. *Women and Depression: Risk Factors and Treatment issues*. APA: Washington, DC, 1990.

McLeer SV, E Deblinger, MS Atkins, EB Foa, and DL Ralphe. Post-traumatic stress disorder in sexually abused children. *Journal of the American Academy of Child and Adolescent Psychiatry*, 1988; 27:650–654.

Offord, DR, MH Boyle, and Y Racine. Ontario child health study: Correlates of disorder. *Journal of the American Academy of Child and Adolescent Psychiatry*, 1989;28:856–860.

Pearce, JW and TD Pezzot-Pearce. *Psychotherapy of Abused and Neglected Children*. Guilford: New York, 1997.

Pearlman, L A and KW Saakvitne. *Trauma and the Therapist*. Norton & Company: New York, 1995.

Rossman, R and MS Rosenberg. *Multiple Victimization of Children*. Haworth Press: Binghamtom, New York, 1998.

Saywitz, KJ and D Elliott. *Interviewing Children in the Forensic Context: A Developmental Approach*. APA: Washington, DC, in press.

Swanston HY, JS Tebbutt, BI O'Toole, and RK Oates, Sexually Abused Children 5 Years after Presentation: A Case Control Study. *Pediatrics*, 1997;125:600–608.

Tong, L, K Oates and M McDowell. Personality development following sexual abuse. *Child Abuse and Neglect*, 1987;11:371–383.

Tufts New England Medical Center, Division of Child Psychiatry. Sexually exploited children: Service and research project. *Final Report for the Office of Juvenile Justice and Delinquency Prevention*. U.S. Department of Justice: Washington, DC, 1989.

Trickett, PK and Putnam, FW. The impact of sexual abuse on female development: towards a developmental, psychobiological integration. *Psychological Science*, 1993;4:81–87.

Wolfe VV, C Gentile, and DA Wolfe. The impact of sexual abuse on children: A PTSD formulation. *Behavior Therapy*, 1989;20:215–228.

4

THE MEDICAL INTERVIEW

CAROLYN J. LEVITT

The medical interview has become a critical component of the diagnostic, legal, and remedial aspects of child sexual abuse. Because
specific medical evidence of abuse is often lacking and there are no
eyewitnesses, the child's verbal statements describing abuse and the
questions used to elicit these statements are being carefully scruti-
nized. Although there is no gold standard established, and interviews must adapt to the individuality and variability of children,
there are guides for forensic interviewing to prevent undermining
children's credibility by improper questioning (Sorenson et al,
1997). In many communities the role of the specialized or forensic
interviewer has been established by multidisciplinary child abuse
teams, children's advocacy centers, or interagency agreement.
When special protocols or procedures have been developed, the
medical interview may serve as the forensic interview or as a coordinated component of the child's forensic interview. In a specialized

medical setting where children feel safe and comfortable with intimate discussions, the medical interview provides very specific details from the children regarding what happened to their bodies. The medical professional also is comfortable in this role eliciting a broad medical history including pertinent factors from the past medical history, and family and psychosocial history, including exposure to domestic violence, drugs, and pornography.

Medical interviews for abuse are conducted in a variety of circumstances: when a preliminary finding of sexual abuse has been established and greater substantiation is required; when a child's behavior and or physical symptoms have raised a suspicion that child sexual abuse has occurred, necessitating an inquiry; and, at times, when reports of sexual abuse arise unanticipated during an examination for another presenting complaint. In each of these cases, the ability to protect a child may rest upon the manner, clarity, and authority with which the examiner documents the child's statement, history, and physical finding for abuse.

Some have speculated that the credibility and stature of medical professionals led to their pivotal role in providing the evidentiary basis for legal actions. Medical professionals have an exclusively credible window on the child's experiences, and the very exclusivity of the disclosure or the medical findings necessitates that the examination and interview be rigorous and well documented (Myers, 1986; Levitt, 1986; AAP 1999).

BEGINNING THE INTERVIEW

Methodology in the interview is matched in importance by the medical professional's ability to establish a comfortable, reassuring, and trusting atmosphere for the child. Even though an interviewer or another medical professional may be uncomfortable with the nature of the inquiry, it is critical that this not be conveyed to the child; the child should perceive the medical professional as open and unshaken by any information the child may disclose. As with a classroom teacher, a combination of authority and interest must be conveyed to the child. Children should not be forced or subtly coerced to answer questions by preventing them from seeing their parents or finishing the interview until they have answered the questions.

It is easier to establish a comfortable atmosphere if the child is encouraged to make some decisions and choices early in the encounter. For example, the examiner could ask the child for assistance in selecting soda or juice from the refrigerator or in choosing the materials to be used for the interview. If the child feels that he or she has some measure of control, that child will be more comfortable in the interview setting and separate more easily from the parent(s).

Before beginning the interview, the examiner could ask the child to draw a picture, and then ask questions regarding the picture. An informal, low-risk conversation serves the double purpose of establishing a level of comfort while allowing the examiner to determine the child's developmental level and verbal skills. The examiner should carefully attend to language patterns and limitations, keying later questions to the child's ability to comprehend.

Children should be made to feel that their role in the interview is important. Research supports the theory that young children perform well and are less suggestible when the interviewer is supportive than when the interviewer is aloof or unfriendly (Goodman et al, 1991). Simple compliments that seem natural and well timed, such as "you are doing a good job" provide proper encouragement for the child's attention and cooperation (Myers, 1996). While presenting an open and trusting atmosphere, the examiner must be careful that the child does not mistake an approval of disclosure as inducement to bring forth information.

STANDARDS OF THE INTERVIEW

The highest priority for the examiner should be the patient's safety, comfort, and quality of care. The second priority is establishing a high quality of communication and coordination with investigative officials. A swift response by officials to a positive finding may directly correlate to the level of trust and familiarity between the examining clinic or medical professional and the officials' agencies. It is important that the medical professional be familiar with the nature and scope of possible and likely legal interventions to make appropriate decisions about the timing and nature of reports and other information. This becomes particularly important when a possible abuser has accompanied the child to an interview or when new, critical information is disclosed. A confident medical professional working through a well-established evaluation protocol can provide an effective and timely report, and timeliness is critical. A prompt report can lead to the forensic interview of a child who has fresh complaints, and can offer immediate detailed statements rather than being forced into silence during a time lapse. Tertiary resources that can provide consultation and assistance in establishing a rapid response to an unexpected finding of child maltreatment are available and can be identified in advance (Medical diagnostic child abuse programs in United States and Canada, 1998).

QUESTIONING THE CHILD

As with any medical history, the interviewer's questions should proceed from general to specific. The interviewer must ensure that the child understands each question and can give consistent answers to similar questions posed in different ways. Early questions should be simple and within the child's ability to answer, giving the child a sense of confidence and providing clues about the child's cognitive level and language capabilities. General questions about the child's family, house, school, and friends, such as, "With whom do you like to play?" "Would you like to tell me about your pets?" and "Where do you go to school?" are generally appropriate ones with which to open an interview.

Most children enjoy this portion of the interview. It is non-threatening and shows them at their communicative best. After raising the child's confidence with general, simple questions, the interviewer can remind him or her that it is acceptable to say that "I don't know," or "I don't remember" if he or she does not know an answer. Encouraging the child to make truthful statements and to demonstrate an understanding that not telling the truth is wrong or has bad consequences promotes greater reliability in a child's statements. Preschool children do not respond well when asked if they know the difference between the truth and a lie, but they can demonstrate by their responses to simple questions that they indeed understand what is true and what is a lie, and that you get in trouble for telling a lie (Lyon, 1996). Asking simple questions, such as if the child had spaghetti-O's for breakfast and whether that is the truth or a lie, or if a little toy in the interview room is an elephant, when it really is a mouse, can demonstrate the child's understanding.

Next, the child can be asked about child-care practices and intimate relationships, such as who gives them baths, washes their hair, gives them spankings, kisses, and hugs. Through this process, the interviewer can determine who may have access to the child and the nature of their relationship. Questions such as "Where do you sleep at night," "Who else sleeps in your house?" and "Where do they sleep?" give a view of nighttime access to the child. If the parents are divorced, the questions should relate to the patterns of child care in each home. In all cases, questions should be as open-ended as possible, avoiding those that contain the answer in the question, or those that can be answered in one word or in the affirmative or negative. Focused questions that draw the child's attention to a certain subject should be interspersed with questions that invite narrative descriptions from the child on that subject. With a young child, it is sometimes helpful to have him or her show you or to appear puzzled regarding the information they are providing, asking for their help in understanding to elicit additional information. Appearing naive regarding particular types of sexual acts often illicits startlingly detailed narratives or demonstrations (Levitt, 1986).

The demeanor of the interviewer should be calm and accepting, indicating interest, but not surprise, at the information provided by the child. Despite the offensive content of these disclosures, the interviewer should convince the child that it is okay to tell more. It is important that the child be left with the impression that no matter what is disclosed, the interviewer will not become angry or sad. It is appropriate to provide some support for the difficulty the child is having in disclosing particular aspects of the abuse, acknowledging the emotional state of the child, and providing assurance regarding protection and support in the future.

RELIABILITY AND LEADING THE CHILD

There has been growing concern regarding the potentially coercive or inherently rewarding nature of child abuse interviews. Questions as to the suggestibility of children, particularly very young children, have been raised in clinics and in the courts. The necessity of using questions that do not appear to prompt an answer or lead the child may run directly into conflict with the developmental realities of a young child. Young children spontaneously recall less information than older children and adults when asked open-ended questions. Also, young children are more suggestible than older children (Ceci and Bruck, 1993). Thus, we have the frustrating reality that questions must be carefully posed to be direct, elicit good information, and cue memory without appearing to lead the child into a particular answer. These concerns about suggestibility are not as important with older children who appear to be no more suggestible than adults. The interviewer should be aware that reliability increases with the specificity of the question. Research supports that girls fail to mention genital or anal touch that occurred during their medical examination when asked open-ended questions about what happened. Some did not even admit to the genital or anal exam when questioned directly "Did the doctor touch you here?" In sharp contrast, all girls who had an exam for scoliosis described their exam when asked what happened (Saywitz et al, 1991). Another study found that, of 70 children ages 5–10, only one child disclosed the sexual victimization in response to open-ended questions, and the vast majority who did disclose did so in response to direct inquiry focusing either on the person who abused, the part of the body touched, the circumstances of the abuse, or a prior disclosure the child may have made to someone (DeVoe, 1995). Thus, asking "Did something happen to you?" may be less effective in eliciting specific information than "Did something happen to your bottom?"

Anatomical dolls have been the focus of both study and sharp criticism in recent years with proponents asserting that dolls are a useful tool in eliciting accounts of abuse from children when used in conjunction with specific questions. Research has not supported concerns that the dolls are, at best, leading, and at worst, grossly distorted so as to emphasize genital presentation and promote inaccurate attention to that part of the anatomy (Boat and Everson, 1996; Bays, 1990). Early attempts to use anatomically explicit dolls as a tool for gleaning children's possible abuse from their play have been replaced by a more representational approach to the dolls. It is most useful for the child to use the dolls to demonstrate what happened. Even very sexualized play with the dolls does not form a reliable basis for an interpretation of sexual abuse (APSAC, 1995). When referring to questions about body touch, children younger than four years of age found it easier to use their own bodies than anatomical dolls (Bruck et al, 1995). The practitioner should use dolls with care, and may prefer to use diagrams or a child's own body as a source of illustration. The American Professional Society on the Abuse of Children (APSAC, 1995) has developed practice guidelines for the use of anatomical dolls in child sexual abuse assessments.

CONDUCTING THE INTERVIEW

Interviewing the Child Who Has Disclosed

When the child has been interviewed previously, the interviewer has information from other responsible adults or from the referral source about the nature of the abuse and the identity of the suspected abuser. In these cases, the child is often aware that the interview is related to sexual abuse. If this is verified, the interviewer can acknowledge to the child that something has happened and ask the child to tell about it in the child's own words. With younger children a more direct approach, focusing questions on either the part of the body, the place or circumstances of the abuse, or the possible perpetrator may be necessary to clarify the subject matter to be discussed. At this point, some children may become reticent about continuing the interview because of their own discomfort. At first, questions about where it happened are the easiest to answer. Other children begin to discuss the details spontaneously. A younger child may be quite forthcoming with information, but it may be difficult to interpret what is being said. The interviewer must listen carefully, allowing the child to complete the description without probing, noting issues for later resolution. Some children may give many details about a portion of their experience or provide only a broad summary or information that minimizes the abuse. These children may readily respond to direct questions involving details of the abuse. Some examples of questions are included in Table 4–1.

Older children may feel guilty or ashamed about the abuse and embarrassed about having allowed the abuse to go on without reporting it. The interviewer can often diffuse this sense of responsibility by acknowledging that other young people have expressed difficulty in discussing what has happened to them. In some cases, reluctant children may choose to avoid the details, skirting them in

Table 4–1. Guidelines for Interviewing Children Suspected of Being Sexually Abused

Procedures and Goals	Line of Inquiry
• Initiate inquiry • Obtain information from caretaker/social worker/law enforcement separate from child	• Include past medical, developmental, and behavioral history • Ask about exposure to violence, drugs and pornography
• Interview child alone in a safe environment, comfortable for the child • Establish rapport with child • Can determine child's verbal and cognitive abilities, level of comfort and attention	• What's your name? How old are you? • Where do you live? With whom? • What kind of house? • Do you have any pets? Names? • What school do you go to?
• Ask about daily living and intimate relationships	• Where do you sleep? Where do mommy/daddy sleep? • Who gives you a bath?
• Determine if child knows difference between truth and lies, and remind them to tell the truth	• If I told you that this rabbit was an elephant, what would that be? (truth or lie) • Let's only talk about things that are true, that really happened
• Ask child to identify body parts, including names for genitalia, anus (use a diagram) • Use child's name for body part • Ask about different types of touch • Include kisses, hugs, tickles, spankings, and pinches or bites	• Identify hair, eyes, nose, mouth, belly button, breasts, and private parts • Who gives you kisses? Hugs? Spankings? etc • Show me where the kisses go. Hugs? Spankings? • How do hugs make you feel? Kisses? Spankings?
• Try to determine what happened • Begin with open-ended questions • Need to use more focused questions for younger or reluctant children	• Do you know why you came to see me today? • Did something happen to you? • A focused question is, Have you had a touch on your bottom (use child's name for body part) that hurt or bothered you? • Can you tell me about that?
• If child begins to disclose, ask easier questions first • Work up gradually to the harder details • Ask younger child to show you what happened • Avoid questions that contain the answer	• Where were you when that happened? • Where was Mommy? Daddy? • Who did it? What did he/she do? • How did it make you feel? How did it make your peepee feel? • Did he/she say anything?

Table 4–1. *Continued*

Procedures and Goals	Line of Inquiry
• Avoid questions that can be answered yes or no	• Did you tell anyone? Whom? • What did he/she say when you told?
• Elicit the details of the abuse from the child • Use the diagram to ask about all possible abusive touches • Any other times (places) it happened	• Ask the child specifically about the penis • Who has one? What is it for? What did it look like? • What did you see/feel it do? Where did it go? • Anything come out of it? What? Where did it go? • Who cleaned it up?
• For older child or adolescent, questions can be more specific	• Obtain date and time of assault • Oral, breast, rectal, or genital contact or penetration • Ask about ejaculation and bathing, brushing teeth, urinating, defecating, douching, changing clothes since assault, and saving clothes or bedding • Obtain menstrual history, whether patient is sexually active and/or uses contraceptives • Were any lubricants or a condom used?
• Concluding the interview	• Tell the child he/she did a good job • It was good that he/she told so we can help
• Document—we prefer videotape to capture the child's expression and demonstrations	• Document questions asked and answers given. Try to record exact words, phrases, and emotional reactions
• Explain the examination • Ask the child during the examination to show you what they told you happened • If there was no disclosure, ask if anyone has hurt or touched the genital or anal parts being examined	• Now I'm going to do a check-up • Listen to your heart, lungs, feel your tummy, and look at your private parts to make sure they are OK • Conclude by reassuring child that his/her body is ok, minimize any findings during discussion with child

Some or all questions can be used depending on a child's needs.

Developed by Carolyn Levitt, MD, and Kim Martinez, CPNP, MPH, Midwest Children's Resource Center, St. Paul.

a narrative, and referring only remotely to the abusive incident it-self, or they may point toward parts of their body or nod in response to direct questions. As their level of comfort increases during the interview, more specific information may be forthcoming.

Both in cases where the child is willing to disclose details and when the child is more reluctant, the earliest questions should be the simplest. The child should be asked to try to remember where the incidents first happened, what he or she was wearing, whom the child was with, and where a parent or caretaker was. As the child demonstrates comfort in responding to these questions, the details of the setting, where other family members were at the time of the abuse, what exactly the abuser did, and how the child felt can be elicited. It can be fruitful to ask the child to point to the area where a penis or finger was inserted or to ask for a demonstration of how something occurred. In describing oral penetration, many children open their mouths widely, pointing deeply down the throat to illus-trate the way in which the penetration occurred. One child, demon-strating forced oral contact with his father, crouched slightly, as he would have done in adjusting to the level of his father's penis, while opening his mouth widely.

Further questions should elicit information regarding all forms of sexual contact and the nature of any contact, including penetra-tion, bleeding, and ejaculation. It is critical to elicit details of the sexual abuse, for instance asking if anything came out of a man's penis, or, in incidents involving oral sexual contact, asking the child how the semen tasted and what the child did with it once it was in his or her mouth. The child should be encouraged to describe all of the physical effects of the abuse. The interviewer needs to know if the child was hurt at the time of contact, if there was soreness afterward, and if the child experienced pain or burn-ing upon urination following penetration. If a child has been pene-trated anally, the symptoms following the abuse may relate to defecation. Oral sexual contact may have resulted in gagging, vom-iting, or a sore throat. The child should be allowed and encouraged to use his or her own words, the interviewer later asking for clarifi-cation to confirm what the child has said. Younger children, for instance, often describe ejaculate as "pee." Rather than interrupt-ing the description from the child, the interviewer should later return to the term and ask the child for help in understanding what this "pee" was like, what it felt like if it touched the skin, what color it was, and so on. Details of how the child washed or cleaned up afterward are also important. It is quite usual for children to point to their body parts or indicate by gesturing. The nature of the general gestures should be recorded.

The examiner should not rule out the possibility of establishing corroboration for the sexual abuse and should inquire of the child whether others were present at the time of, immediately prior to, or immediately following the abuse. Occasionally, more than one child is involved in the abuse. If this is the case, the second child should be interviewed separately and the statements compared.

Interviewing the Child When Abuse Is Suspected

Often a child is referred to a medical professional for evaluation after an adult has become concerned that the child has been exposed to an abusive environment or is displaying behavioral or physical indicators that lead to a suspicion of abuse. When this happens, the examiner is presented with a report of symptoms such as onset of enuresis or genital pain or injury and must establish, through careful history taking, the basis for the symptoms.

It is not overly simplistic to liken the medical evaluation of a child suspected to have been victimized with that of a child who may have appendicitis. A detailed history of the symptomatology must be elicited from the parents followed by a careful discussion with the child regarding the history and nature of current symptoms, inquiries as to where there is pain or discomfort, what improves the symptoms, what exacerbates the problem, and how long the symptoms have been present. The examiner should conduct a review of symptoms, asking about a variety of genital, anal, and oral symptoms. This should be followed by a medical exam to establish medical findings.

It is usually helpful to begin interviews with a child by asking why he or she has come to see the doctor. Ask the child, "What did your mommy tell you about coming to see me today?" This allows the child to displace discomfort when describing symptoms by attributing the basis for the visit to a parent. The examiner should help the child become comfortable by diffusing the child's possible sense of isolation and by placing some distance between the child and the topic of sexual abuse. Impersonal attributions such as, "sometimes children who tell us their potties (or another child-led term) hurt" have been touched in a way that made them "feel funny" and "sometimes grown-ups do or say scary things to children," serve to assist children in depersonalizing or universalizing the information they are being asked to share. While moving to a direct line of inquiry, asking a child if anything scary has happened to him or her may elicit a disclosure. The interviewer might ask whether the child knows that these things happen to other children and assure the child that such incidents are not the child's fault. It might be useful to ask the child, "Who could you tell about it?" and "Who else could you tell?"

Some interviewers find that using a "good touch/bad touch" approach is helpful in orienting children to descriptions of bodily experiences, and they use an anatomical diagram of the same gender and age of the child being interviewed as a focal point (Groth and Stevenson, 1984). The child can use the picture as a reference in naming body parts, and then can be asked to point out the parts of their body where they dislike being touched, kissed, or tickled. Some children respond well to the use of colored markers to indicate the spots where each type of touch is not liked. The examiner can easily follow this up by asking if the child has ever been kissed, touched, or tickled in these spots. If the child discloses some details about sexual touching, more details can be elicited from the child by using the techniques described earlier for interviewing a disclosing child.

The examiner can elicit information from the child regarding the child's emotional state during the incident being described. Children can describe not just what happened to them, but all of the things they felt, saw, heard, and learned from a sexual encounter. One four-year-old reported that "a yitto (little) drip of ocean (lotion) came out of his pee-pee." When asked what happened next, she stated, "He said, 'Oh, oh.'" The examiner then asked why he said "oh, oh" and the child responded, "because the ocean (lotion) came out." Often, when asked about how the abuse felt, the child will describe how he or she felt emotionally rather than physically. One four-year-old replied "ugly." When asked to define this more clearly, she grimaced and held her stomach as if she had a stomachache and stated, "I felt ugly inside." She was describing in her own words an emotion that captured the experience.

Interviewing the Child Who Spontaneously Discloses

It is not always the child referred for an interview who presents the greatest challenge to the medical professional, but rather the child who is referred for a physical problem and then, during the course of the examination, reveals that he or she is being sexually abused, often by a known and trusted adult. A professional faced with this type of spontaneous disclosure must focus first upon the child's safety needs and second upon legal reporting requirements that must be fulfilled. It is not unheard of for a child to disclose abuse while the abuser sits in the waiting room. One medical professional received a report of sexual abuse by a father after telling a 13-year-old that her pregnancy test was positive. The medical interviewer, knowing that the girl's father was sitting in the waiting room, sought consultation and called for a police investigator to ensure that the girl's confidentiality would be protected and that no squad would be sent to "tip off" the waiting father. The medical professional was able to use the time following the initial disclosure to elicit significant and detailed information that enabled the arriving investigator to act decisively. The child was well served by the coordination of the system and the pediatrician's careful interview.

Following the Interview

When the interview has been completed, the interviewer can help a child prepare for the physical examination by discussing what will happen and assuring the child that part of the exam is intended to ensure that he or she is "all right," that no part of the body has been harmed. The child can be engaged to help the medical professional examine the parts of his or her body that may have been touched or hurt from the sexual encounter. It is important to avoid medical jargon and to use nonthreatening language to describe findings. Using the term "scratch" instead of "tear," for example, can be reassuring to a child who is uncertain about whether the injury will "heal." All efforts should be extended to ensure that the child is given the opportunity to feel normal.

Documentation

The examiner may videotape the interview. When the interview involves a young child who may gesture or point rather than verbalize, videotape preserves the spontaneity and vivid nature of the child's statements and recollections and may avoid repeated interviews. Videotaping improves the quality of the forensic interview. Whether or not videotape is used, the interviewer should make every effort to record each word, in the language of the child, as part of the medical record. The taped or written record should also include a description of the child's general affect, mood, facial expressions, and demonstration when discussing the abuse. It is most important to get the truest documentation of the child's expressions, for it is the degree to which these are believably and accurately the child's own that later determines admissibility in court.

FUNCTIONING AS PART OF THE SYSTEM

The procedures and practices described in this chapter are intended to assist the medical professional in conducting a thorough interview with a child. However, the examiner who is most effective in interviewing a child regarding sexual abuse is one who is acutely aware of the practices and protocols used in the social services and legal systems within the community. The pattern of practices by other agencies determines whether a child has been interviewed prior to the time the examiner sees the child. The outcome of previous interviews or the nature of the child's responses during those interviews and ongoing concerns about the child are important elements. Furthermore, the expectations of each of these systems as they turn to the medical professional for collaboration or advice must be clear and well-defined. When these elements are in place, the medical professional is in the best position to serve as an effective link in the detection and prevention of child sexual abuse.

REFERENCES

American Academy of Pediatrics Committee on Child Abuse and Neglect. Guidelines for the evaluation of sexual abuse of children. *Pediatrics.* 1999;103: 186–191.

American Professional Society on the Abuse of Children. *Practice Guidelines: Use of Anatomical Dolls in Child Sexual Abuse Assessments.* Chicago, 1995.

Bays, J. (1990). Are the genitalia of anatomical dolls distorted? *Child Abuse and Neglect.* 1990;14:171–175.

Boat, BW and MD Everson. Concerning practice of interviewers when using anatomic dolls in child protective services investigations. *Child Maltreatment.* 1996;1:96–104.

Bruck, M, S Ceci, E Francoeur, and A Renick. Anatomically detailed dolls do not facilitate preschoolers' reports of a pediatric examination involving genital touching. *Journal of Experimental Psychology: Applied.* 1995;1:95–109.

Ceci, S and M Bruck. The suggestibility of the child witness, a historical review and synthesis. *Psychological Bulletin.* 1993;113:403–439.

DeVoe, E. *Final Report: Computer Assisted Interviewing with Children Who May Have Been Sexually Abused.* Unpublished manuscript, School of Social Work, University of Michigan, 1995.

Goodman, GS, BL Bottoms, BM Schwartz-Kenney, and L Rudy. Children's testimony about a stressful event: Improving children's reports. *Jour. of Narrative & Life History.* 1990;I:69–99.

Groth, N and M Stevenson. *Anatomical Drawings for Use in the Investigation and Intervention of Child Sexual Abuse.* Forensic Mental Health Associates, Inc., Newton Center, 1989.

Levitt, CJ. Sexual abuse in children: A compassionate yet thorough approach to evaluation. *Postgrad Medicine.* 1986;80:201–215.

Lyon, TD. Assessing children's competence to take the oath: Research and recommendations. *APSAC Advisor.* 1996;9:1,1–7.

Medical diagnostic child abuse programs in the United States and Canada. In *A Guide to References and Resources in Child Abuse and Neglect.* Jones JG and CJ Levitt, (eds) second ed., pp. 195–245. American Academy of Pediatrics, Elk Grove Village, 1998.

Myers, JEB. The role of the physician in presenting verbal evidence of child abuse. *Journal of Pediatrics.* 1986;109:409–411.

Myers, JEB. Taint hearings to attack investigative interviews: A further assault on children's credibility. *Child Maltreatment.* 1996;1:213–222.

Saywitz, KS, GS Goodman, E Nicholas, and SF Moan. Children's memories of a physical examination involving genital touch: Implications for reports of child sexual abuse. *Journal of Consulting and Clinical Psychology.* 1991;59:682–691.

Sorenson, E, B Bottoms, and A Perona. *Handbook on Intake and Forensic Interviewing in the Children's Advocacy Center Setting.* pp. 25–54. U.S. Dept. of Justice, Washington, D.C., 1997.

5

PHYSICAL EXAMINATION OF THE CHILD AND ADOLESCENT

S. JEAN EMANS

The timing and nature of the physical examination of the sexually abused child or adolescent depend on the presenting complaint, the resources in the community, and the expertise and style of the medical professional caring for the patient. Children and adolescents may present to emergency facilities, physician offices or clinics, or social service or law enforcement agencies. For example, a child may register in an emergency ward because of an acute assault, an acute disclosure, or for medical problems not initially identified as caused by sexual abuse. A child may be brought to a pediatrician's office or other health care facility for a routine examination or for a medical illness, behavioral problem, or physical finding that may prompt a consideration of sexual abuse in the differential diagnosis. Medical complaints include genital, anal, or urethral trauma, bleeding, or discharge; pregnancy (especially in a sexually developed preteen or young teen); dysuria; abdominal pain; headaches; chronic constipation or encopresis; or foreign bodies in the vagina or rectum (AAP, 1991; Hymel and Jenny, 1996; Emans et al, 1998). Behavioral indicators of possible sexual abuse include temper tantrums, sleep disturbance, phobias, self-injury, substance abuse, and school problems (see Chapter 1). A child may make a disclosure to a parent or other adult and be brought to a physician's office or emergency ward for evaluation or a physical examination. If a child's case is being investigated by social service or law enforcement agencies, the child may be brought to a health care provider for a physical assessment (see Chapter 2 for a discussion of children's services and advocacy centers).

Because of the varying presentations of children to emergency wards, ambulatory clinical settings, and agencies, clinicians must be knowledgeable about the appropriate physical examination, even if specialized resources are available in the community. In some cities, specialized centers, either freestanding or in conjunction with a medical center, are available 24 hours a day to respond to the need for disclosure interviews and physical examinations. In many other cities, a specialized team of psychiatric providers, nurses, and physicians evaluate children suspected of having been sexually abused. Many of these teams have high caseloads, so community providers continue to fill an important role in the initial and continuing management of sexually abused children. In many parts of the country, clinicians have identified some resources to aid in evaluation, but they do most of the physical examinations and medical care in their own offices. With advances in understanding normal genital anatomy, many clinicians are comfortable with providing evaluations and care of these children.

The timing of the history and physical examination depends on the urgency for collection of evidence. In most cases of sexual abuse in children, the last episode of abuse occurred weeks to months before the disclosure, so the physical examination can be delayed until a disclosure interview is undertaken. In children presenting with a history of sexual assault or abuse within 72 hours or symptoms of genital discharge, bleeding, or pain, a history and physical examination should be done as expeditiously as possible in order to collect forensic evidence (see Chapter 6). Although investigative interviews should be conducted by a designated agency or individual in the hospital or community to minimize multiple interviews, the clinician performing the physical examination should seek pertinent medical history and ask open-ended questions about the abuse to document what has occurred. For some children, more detailed information may be elicited during the actual physical examination.

Many states and individual hospitals and emergency wards have protocols to increase information collection and to ensure uniform specimens (see Appendices). Practitioners in the community may find these protocols useful to document history and physical findings since sexual abuse cases often do not go to court for months or years and clearly substantiated records are extraordinarily helpful. To do an adequate physical assessment, clinicians should have the following available: a source of magnification such as an otoscope (preferably with a round head for light and a wider field of magnification), a hand lens, or standard or video colposcope; a microscope; and culture media for *Neisseria gonorrhoeae* and *Chlamydia trachomatis*. The colposcope offers the advantage of light, magnification, direct measurement of hymenal orifice dimensions, and photographic capability; colposcopes are used in many centers specializing in child sexual abuse. Colposcopic photographs and video image can be used for teaching residents and practitioners normal and abnormal genital anatomy, can be shared with other experts testifying in sexual abuses cases, and may be helpful in the courtroom to identify abnormal genital findings for the judge and/or jury. However, clinicians should keep in mind that excellent genital examinations can be done using magnification from an otoscope or hand lens, and drawings and descriptions of abnormal findings can be kept in the medical record. The experienced examiner rarely sees additional findings using the colposcope beyond those already documented with the simple magnification techniques of the otoscope.

Normal genital anatomy has been assessed extensively in the past 15 years, with both cross-sectional and longitudinal studies providing the basis for comparisons with genital examinations in sexually abused children (Emans et al, 1987; Herman-Giddeus, 1987; Pokorny and Kozinetz, 1988; McCann et al, 1990; AAP Committee, 1999; Berenson et al, 1992; Jenny et al, 1987; Berenson, 1993; Berenson, 1995; Pokorny, Emans et al, 1994). The American Professional Society on the Abuse of Children (APSAC)

has created through consensus more uniform terminology and definitions of anatomical terms (APSAC, 1995). Most studies have focused on girls, rather than boys because abnormal hymenal and
posterior fourchette findings in girls are more common than anal
findings in girls or boys. Understanding normal anatomic structures
and positions for examination is key to the process of evaluation and
is covered in Chapters 7 and 8 and in the color plates. The clinician
should remember that the examinations of most children with substantiated sexual abuse are normal. The percentage of "normal examinations" has varied from 16 percent to 90 percent, with most
studies reporting 70%–90%, depending on the case mix, the age of
the patients, the definition of "normal" versus abnormal and the examiners (Emans et al, 1987; Adams et al, 1994; Muram, 1988; Muram Rimsza and Niggemann, 1982; Muram et al, 1991; Muram,
1989; Muram and Elias, 1989). Even when the perpetrator gives an
actual description of vaginal penetration, nonspecific or normal
genital findings have been reported in 39% of victims (Muram,
1989). Both perpetrator and victim may believe that vaginal penetration occurred during vulvar coitus. The likelihood of detecting
evidence of penetration, nongenital trauma, or genital trauma increases with age of the patient, in part, because adolescents are
more likely to have been victims of a rape by a stranger or acquaintance. Abnormal examinations are also more likely if bleeding or
pain occurred during the abusive episode. After the physical examination, the clinician should always relay the presence or absence of
findings to the family and child while emphasizing the child's good
health and wholeness.

The three positions commonly used for genital examination of
girls are the supine separation technique, the supine traction technique, and the knee-chest position (Emans et al, 1998; McCann et
al, 1990) (Figs. 5–1, 5–2, 5–3). In the supine separation technique,
the labia are separated with the tips of the fingers in a lateral and
downward position until the vestibule and hymen are exposed. If
the edge of the hymen cannot be seen well in this position, the
supine traction technique is helpful. The examiner grasps the lower
portion of the labia majora between the thumb and index finger and
gently but firmly pulls outward and slightly upward. In the knee-
chest position, the child rests her head on her folded arms, her abdomen is sagging downward, and her knees are bent six to eight
inches apart with her buttocks in the air. The examiner then presses

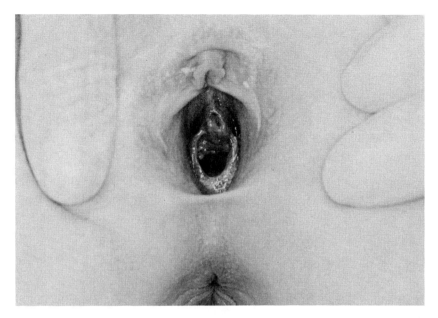

Fig. 5–1. Supine separation technique. (From Emans SJ, Laufer MR, and Goldstein DP. *Pediatric and Adolescent Gynecology*, 4th edition, Philadelphia: Lippincott Raven, 1990. Reprinted by permission of Lippincott Raven.)

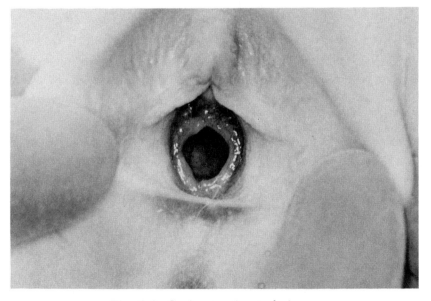

Fig. 5–2. Supine traction technique.

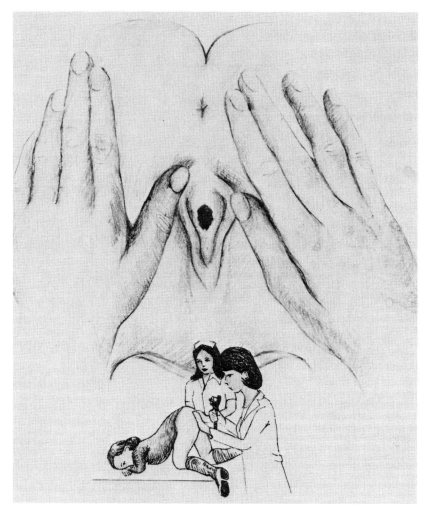

Fig. 5–3. Knee-chest position. (From Emans SJ, Laufer MR, and Goldstein DP. *Pediatric and Adolescent Gynecology*, 4th edition, Philadelphia: Lippincott Raven, 1990. Reprinted by permission of Lippincott Raven.)

a thumb outward on the leading edge of the gluteus maximus. A similar viewing of the lower half of the hymen may be accomplished with the child in the supine position with the knees pulled up onto the abdomen.

An early study by Jenny (1987) confirmed that all girls are born with hymens. Bernson and coworkers (1991) recorded the configuration and findings of over 400 neonates, observing frequent clefts, ridges, bumps, and tags. In a longitudinal study of infants at birth and 1 year of age, Berenson (1993) found that 58% of girls had a normal decrease in hymenal tissue as estrogen levels waned. Fewer girls had an external genital ridge at 1 year than at birth, and most had a crescentic configuration of the hymen. Inferior complete (to the base of the hymen) clefts or notches at 4 to 8 o'clock were not observed at birth or one year-of-age.

The three most common configurations of hymen identified in prepubertal girls are a posterior rim or crescent hymen, an annular hymen, and a redundant hymen (Pokorny and Kozinetz, 1998; McCann et al, 1990; Berenson et al, 1991; Pokorny, 1987). Other less frequent configurations include a sleeve-like hymen with an anterior opening, a microperforate hymen, and an imperforate hymen. In a sample of 93 girls (aged 10 months to 10 years) selected for non-abuse, McCann and colleagues (1990) reported erythema of the vestibule in 56%, periurethral bands in 51%, labial adhesions in 39%, posterior fourchette midline avascular area in 26%, and urethral dilation with labial traction in 15%. Hymenal findings included "mounds" in 34%, notches in 6%, septa in 2.5% and intravaginal ridges in 90%. In a larger study of a triethnic population of 211 girls with a mean age of 21 months, Berenson and colleagues (1992) reported hymenal "mounds" in 7%, hymenal tags in 3%, midline sparing in 4%, vestibular bands in 98%, longitudinal intravaginal ridges in 25%, and external ridges in 15% of girls in whom the anatomy could be visualized. Labial fusion sufficient to obscure the hymen was noted in 5% and partial agglutination in an additional 17%, predominantly in girls under 1 year of age. Hymenal notches extending to the base of the hymen occurred superiorly and laterally, but none were found inferiorly on the lower half of the hymen between the 4 o'clock and 8 o'clock positions. Kellogg and Para (1991) described a normal midline white structure below the hymen, termed the linea vestibularis, in newborns and prepubertal girls.

Signs consistent with acute sexual abuse have included hematomas, abrasions, lacerations of the hymen, perihymen, and posterior fourchette. Signs of previous sexual abuse have included hymenal remnants, scars, and transections. Muram (1988) and Adams (1992, 1997) have suggested classification systems for categories of abuse.

The use of dimensions of the hymenal orifice as an indicator of sexual abuse is controversial. If an enlarged hymenal opening is detected, it is typically accompanied by other changes in the hymen.

Thus, an enlarged opening may be helpful if other signs, symptoms, behavioral indicators, or disclosure are present but should not be used as the sole indicator of a sexual abuse diagnosis. The hymenal orifice can be measured by several techniques. Some colposcopes are fitted with an eyepiece that shows millimeters; the scale is later superimposed on the photograph or a small ruler can be placed within the field of photography. Alternatively, a photograph can be taken immediately following the genital photographs using the same focal setting or a 2 or 5 cm ruler can be held near the perineum to estimate the dimensions. It is essential for the clinician to remember that dimensions are greatly altered by the child's position during the examination (the orifice is generally larger in the knee-chest position), the amount of hymenal tissue present, the degree and length of time of applied traction, and the amount of relaxation, such as a larger diameter with general anesthesia. McCann and coworkers (1990) noted that the knee-chest position consistently produced the largest vertical measurements, while the supine traction position resulted in the largest horizontal transhymenal span. The dimensions are also altered by the type of hymen; a narrow posterior rim hymen has a larger orifice than a redundant hymen. Hymenal dimensions also increase with age. Using the supine traction technique, McCann and colleagues (1990) found a mean horizontal diameter of 5.2 ± 1.4 mm (range 2–8 mm) for girls 2 to $4\frac{11}{12}$ years old and 5.6 ± 1.8 mm (range 1–9 mm) for girls 5 to $7\frac{11}{12}$ years old. Berensen and associates (1992) in measuring only annular and crescentic hymens, reported a mean horizontal diameter of

2.5 ± 0.8 mm (range 1.0–3.5 mm) for   1–12-month-old girls
2.9 ± 1.2 mm (range 1.5–6.5 mm) for 13–24-month-old girls
2.9 ± 1.0 mm (range 1.0–6.5 mm) for 25–48-month-old girls
3.6 ± 1.2 mm (range 2.0–4.8 mm) for 49–81-month-old girls

A gaping opening of 1.2–1.5 cm in a 5-year-old would be distinctly abnormal; however, it should be accompanied by hymenal defect. Clinicians need to remember that orifices with small estimated diameters do not preclude penetration for all the reasons noted above. Additionally, the hymen is somewhat elastic, a property that increases with circulating estrogen.

Normal genital and hymenal findings have also been recently delineated in adolescents. In a study of 300 girls (100 who denied sexual activity and had used only pads, 100 who denied sexual activity and had used tampons, and 100 who had been sexually active), sexually active girls were significantly more likely to have "complete clefts" (transections) between the 2 and 10 o'clock positions. Among non-sexually active girls, only 3% had a "complete cleft" between 4 and 8 o'clock, and only one (0.5%) a "complete cleft" at 6 o'clock. Whether any of the small number of "complete clefts" observed in the non-sexually active group were due to unreported consensual or nonconsensual intercourse is unknown. Tampon use, sports participation, and prior pelvic examinations did not alter genital findings in non-sexually active girls. Median hymenal orifice diameter was greater in the sexually active group than the non-sexually active group, but there was overlap. Exact measurements of the elastic hymen of the adolescent are even more difficult than in prepubertal girls.

As noted in the color plates, a number of medical conditions may present a challenge to the clinician and may be initially diagnosed as sexual abuse (Emans et al, 1998; Bays and Jenny, 1990). These conditions include lichen sclerosus, urethral prolapse, failure of midline fusion (from the anus to the posterior fourchette), localized vulvar pemphigoid, herpes zoster, Crohn's disease, linear IgA dermatosis, allergic contact dermatitis, psoriasis, Ehlers-Danlos syndrome, ulcerating hemangiomas, and accidental genital trauma. Deciding whether genital trauma is accidental or secondary to sexual abuse in the absence of a witnessed fall can be challenging (Bond et al, 1992; Dowd et al, 1994; Pokorny et al, 1992; Hostetler et al, 1994). Straddle injuries typically cause trauma to the soft tissues over the symphysis pubis, the ischiopubic ramus, or adductor longus tendon; accidental injuries are usually unilateral, anterior, and cause damage to the external rather than internal genital structures. Rectovaginal injuries, however, can occur in girls who fall directly onto sharp objects. In a large study on unintentional perineal injury in 56 prepubertal girls, Bond and colleagues (1995) reported that hymenal injury occurred to only one patient. Similarly, in a series of 72 females seen for straddle injuries, Dowd and colleagues (1994) reported that vaginal injury occurred in seven patients and two had hymenal injuries (two had penetrating injuries and two others had fallen on a crossbar or curb). Clearly most transections of the hymen by penetrating injuries are the result of sexual assault.

Although there is some variation in protocols for culturing children and adolescents for sexually transmitted diseases, the trend in the past five years has been toward more selective testing of prepubertal children (CDC, 1998, Ingram et al, 1997; Muram et al, 1996; Sicoli et al, 1995; Siegel et al, 1995; Sirotnak, 1994). Questions that should be asked include the possibility that the suspected offender has, or is at high risk, for a STD, the presence of signs or symptoms of a STD in the child, and the prevalence of STDs in the community. Although STDs can be asymptomatic in prepubertal children and a positive test is helpful in prosecution, the cost of testing all victims, the low risk of infection, and the potential discomfort to the child have resulted in a more selective approach to culturing. Tests for STDs are usually obtained in girls with a history of genital discharge, direct contact with the perpetrator's genitalia, or when the examination reveals genital discharge or trauma or evidence indicating oral, genital, or rectal contact (Hymel and Jenny, 1996; Siegel et al, 1995; Sirotnak, 1994; Sicoli, 1995). Hymel and Jenny (1996) have proposed that STD screening be done at the time of the assault on children who have a history or physical examination indicative of penetrating trauma, have been molested by a perpetrator at high risk of STD, or have a vaginal discharge or history of vaginal discharge. In low risk prepubertal patients, cultures are deferred for two weeks after an acute assault, and the girl is reexamined to see if signs or symptoms have occurred. In Muram's series (39), 1.4 percent (12/865) of prepubertal girls seen within 72 hours of assault were positive for *N. gonorrhoeae*, and all had signs of acute vulvovaginitis. In a series of 2,731 girls (ages 1–12 years) referred to the child sexual abuse team and who had vaginal cultures performed, Ingram and colleagues identified 84 girls with gonococcal infections; 80 had vaginitis, two had a history of vaginal intercourse with a perpetrator with gonorrhea, one had *N. gonorrhoeae* isolated from a urine culture and one had a sister with gonorrhea (1997) (see Chapter 9). Similarly, the number of prepubertal children who have a history of only genital fondling and/or are asymptomatic and have a positive culture for *C. trachomatis* is exceedingly small.

In contrast to the low risk of STDs in prepubertal children, adolescents are at high risk of acquiring STDs, and all should be cultured for *N. gonorrhoeae* and *C. trachomatis* (Committee on Adolescence, 1994; Glaser et al, 1991; Jenny et al, 1990). The risk of acquiring these infections is significant and many adolescents may have pre-existing infections from consensual intercourse (see Chapter 9).

If cultures are obtained in prepubertal children, samples for *N. gonorrhoeae* are obtained from the vagina in girls, the urethra in boys, and the pharynx and rectum in both. Cultures for *C. trachomatis* are usually obtained from the vagina (and rectum if possible) of prepubertal girls, the endocervix of adolescent girls, and the urethra and/or rectum for boys. Nonculture tests for *C. trachomatis* should be avoided because of the possibility of false-positive results. Lesions suggestive of herpes should be cultured, and notation should be made of the presence of *Condyloma acuminatum* (human papillomavirus). At the time of examination of girls, vaginal secretions are usually examined under the microscope for *Trichomonas vaginalis* and *clue cells*. A diagnosis of bacterial vaginosis in the adolescent girl is made by finding increased pH (>4.5), clue cells, a positive whiff test, and absent lactobacilli on wet preparation or gram stain (see Chapter 9). Culture for *Gardnerella vaginalis* is not indicated in children or adolescents. Similarly, tests for HPV are not presently indicated in asymptomatic children and adolescents because of the small number detected (Siegfried et al, 1998).

Similar considerations are applicable for testing for other STDs, including obtaining serologies for syphilis, hepatitis B, and human immunodeficiency virus (HIV). The chances of a positive test are extraordinarily low, but possible, and tests are indicated for acute assaults, oral/genital/rectal contact with high-risk perpetrators, with the occurrence of other sexually transmitted diseases, and with any other concerns from providers, patients, or families (see Chapter 9). Most children are now immunized against hepatitis B, so serologies are not indicated.

In the case of an acute assault on child or adolescent, a wet mount is done to look for sperm (see Chapter 6). Fixed slides should be preserved. Swabs of the vagina, vulva, and any area showing fluorescence with the Wood lamp should be saved for police laboratory tests for acid phosphatase, p-30, and MHS-5, among others.

The anus is inspected with the child in lateral recumbent position or supine (holding knees to the abdomen/chest). The examiner uses gloved hands to gently separate the buttocks and determine the degree of anal dilation. Reflex dilation of the anus may occur in children who have been repeatedly sodomized, but also occurs in normal non-abused children. Acute anal findings include swelling, redness, abrasions, and fissures that usually heal rapidly. If bleeding or trauma is noted, endoscopic examination may be necessary.

With this background in mind, the clinician is prepared to undertake the physical examination of the child or adolescent. The examination should be tailored to the age of the child, the nature of the complaint, and the style of the examining nurse or physician. There is no right way to approach all patients or problems, and a wide variety of techniques and styles are used by the authors of this text. The most important factors in a successful examination are an unhurried approach to the child, an explanation of the examination, and a relaxed examiner. If possible, the young child should be asked to bring a favorite toy or stuffed animal on the day of the examination. The child, and particularly the adolescent, need to know in advance why the appointment has been made and that a special examination is to be done. Caretakers should be informed that most of the examination is inspection and that internal examination is not part of the evaluation of the prepubertal child, so that the child does not feel fearful of the encounter. Caretakers of small children may be advised to wear comfortable slacks/jeans in case assistance is needed, for example, by holding the child on his or her lap.

The examination should be preceded by a history from the caretaker, preferably while the child is occupied in another room. Following this interview, the medical provider should take a brief history from the child (see Chapter 4). Some child abuse experts find that the history from the child is accomplished more easily if the child is alone; others prefer to have a familiar face present. Interviewing with a parent in the room has been used to discredit the history given by the child, particularly in cases involving a child custody dispute. This interview gives the examiner the opportunity to establish rapport with the child and explain the nature of the examination. Some evaluators videotape the interview to document the history given by the child.

The child should be told that he or she is an important part of the team and nothing will be done without his or her approval. The purpose of the examination should be explained, emphasizing that this is a "check-up" and will include a general physical examination and an examination of the genital area or "private parts." Allowing children to say when they are ready for the examination gives them a sense of control. The examiner may even need to leave the room, letting the child know that the exam will occur once the child feels comfortable. Usually within five minutes the child is prepared for a proper external genital examination. Children should be permitted to have a person of their choice in the room during the examination. Speaking to the child out of earshot of the caretaker can help the child make this choice without being pressured by the adult. For the young prepubertal child, the mother (or accompanying adult) generally stays in the room and is enlisted to help with the examination unless she is definitely non-supportive. The older child or adolescent often prefers a nurse to be present.

Before the examination, the child should be told what will take place with a clear emphasis on "looking." Because the reason and nature of the examination were explained in the preliminary conversation with the child, it may or may not be important at this point to restate the fact that it will be necessary to "look at your private parts" or, for example, in the case of a girl with genital pain, "take a look at your vagina where you said it hurt." The conversation can include statements to a girl such as, "I understand that your mother is worried about your vagina" or "about your girl parts" or "Why don't we both look and I'll tell you what I see?" To a boy, the statements might include a "look at his boy parts" or "pee-pee" or "bum." Using the child's terminology is important for preschoolers. The child should be shown the otoscope, hand lens, and/or colposcope and be allowed to touch and look through each before the examination. Children and adolescents can be encouraged to view jewelry and fingers through the magnifying device. Toys can be examined through the colposcope, and the examiner can show that the light changes from green to white to green; the child can then be asked to change the light color as well. If the child seems reluctant to undress, he or she can be allowed to get up on the table and try the various positions while still clothed.

At the time of the examination, invite the child to choose a gown by color, and ask about other options, such as wearing a T-shirt. To increase a child's sense of control, the examiner might pose such questions as, "Did you pick these shoes?", and so forth. Young boys and girls may prefer to leave on a T-shirt and avoid the gown. The examiner then asks the child if he or she needs help to get on the examining table or if using the "big stairs" or a "stool" is preferable. Some clinicians assist the child in undressing, while others leave this task to the caretaker. Sometimes the examination is best accomplished if the child remains clothed, such as a girl remaining in her dress, and the underpants gently removed or pulled aside from the crotch area to allow genital assessment.

Although many examiners start with familiar parts of the physical exam such as palpation of the abdomen and auscultation of the heart, others prefer to start with the genital examination. Doing the general examination first allows the child to become familiar with non-threatening physical contact and establishes the examiner as "doctor" or "nurse." It also allows assessment of the skin for other signs of trauma, bruising, or dermatoses (skin creases and scalp). During the general physical examination, the clinician looks for signs of puberty, adenopathy, and pharyngitis. The inguinal areas are palpated for adenopathy. A gentle, unhurried approach is crucial, especially when caring for young children. If the child becomes tearful or resistant, the exam is no longer possible. During the examination, the examiner should continue to engage the child and supportive adult in a conversation about toys, pets, favorite activities, and so forth. If possible, enlisting the help of the accompanying adult in distracting the child through conversation and word games is worthwhile. Adolescents require a very different approach.

PREPUBERTAL GIRLS

For a young girl, the examiner should focus on external genital anatomy. The emphasis is on "taking a look, not touching the vagina." The child is initially examined either on an examining table or in the caretaker's lap using a frog-leg position (feet together, knees apart); in the older child the stirrups can be used with the knees spread apart. Alternatively, if the child does not wish to be alone on the table, the caretaker can sit semireclined on the pelvic table with feet in the stirrups and the child held on the lap with the child's legs straddled across the caretaker's thighs. The vulva and hymen are examined by separating the labia as noted earlier, using the supine separation and supine traction techniques. The hymenal borders usually can be seen well in these two positions, and the anterior one third of the vagina often can be seen. If the borders can not be seen easily, they can be "floated" up by squirting a small amount of warm saline or water into the vestibule. In other cases, where the examination causes too much discomfort for good visualization, viscous xylocaine can be used as a topical anesthetic. The girl's cooperation can be elicited by having her look at her vulva with a hand-held mirror. A colorful poster can be used to distract the child. Using the light and magnification of an otoscope, a hand lens with an overhead lamp, or colposcope, the examiner can look at vulvar and hymenal anatomy.

In girls with vaginitis or bleeding or in those in whom the edges of the hymenal border cannot be ascertained or show questionable changes, the knee–chest position allows visualization of the stretched hymen (especially the lower half), the vagina, and the cervix. This position is not used routinely by all examiners if sufficient information can be obtained with the patient lying in the supine or with the knees pulled to the chest. The examiner can tell the child that she may have slept in this way as a small child "when you were little," or she might feel that she is "hopping like a bunny." The older prepubertal child is told that because she may "feel embarrassed, a sheet will be placed over your bottom." Some children cannot assume this position because they have been abused in a similar position, and it may remind them of the episode during the assessment. During the examination, the child can be complimented for "holding still," and the caretaker, examiner, aide, and child can carry on a conversation about food or toys she likes or asked riddles. The anus can be examined in the knee-chest position prone or supine.

If available, the colposcope is used directly after genital inspection in the supine position. During the colposcopic examination, the child is again shown the colposcope, and the examiner sits on a stool and asks the patient to notice that the colposcope does not touch her. Most colposcopic examinations are done with the child in the lithotomy position with the use of stirrups or in the frog-leg position. The knee-chest position can also be used. The aide, caretaker, or child gently separates the labia. The child is warned to expect a bright light with the flash. With some colposcopes, the child can actually hold the cable and assist by triggering the camera. Video colposcopes allow dynamic visualization of the hymen and genital areas. If the dimensions of the hymenal orifice are measured, the position used must be noted. Spontaneous statements by the child about the abuse may occur at any time during examination and should be recorded in the child's own words.

Cultures, obtained selectively, and rectal examination, if indicated, are done last. The child is allowed to handle and feel the soft cotton-tipped or Dacron applicators. As alternatives to using the saline-moistened Calgiswab, a small feeding tube attached to a sy-

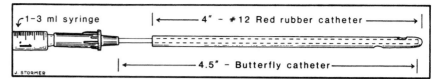

Fig. 5–4. Assembled catheter-within-a-catheter. (From Pokorny and Stomer.[10] Reprinted by permission of the *American Journal of Obstetrics and Gynecology*.)

ringe, a soft plastic eyedropper, or a modified syringe and urethral catheter used to squeeze a small amount of saline into the vagina are additional techniques available for obtaining vaginal cultures. Pokorny and Stormer (1987) have described the following technique for obtaining multiple samples. Insert the proximal four inch end of an intravenous butterfly catheter, with needle cut off, into the distal four inches of a #12 bladder catheter with a syringe attached (Fig. 5–4).* The examiner stands to one side of the reclined patient, gently spreads the labia apart, and quickly slides the catheter into the vagina, similar to catheterizing the bladder. A small amount of sterile (non-bacteriostatic) saline (0.5–1 cc) can be injected into the vagina and aspirated for samples. For the child who will not allow intravaginal cultures, Muram has described a technique of squirting saline into the vagina, holding three swabs just outside the vagina with the labia held gently together, and then asking the child to cough. For *N.gonorrhoeae*, the swab should be plated directly onto media appropriate for culturing, such as Thayer-Martin Jembec or other appropriate transport media. A dacron swab is used to obtain cultures for *C. trachomatis*. Vaginal washes have been used for Chlamydia detection using the polymerase chain reaction (PCR) tests, but more data is needed before these sensitive molecular tests can be used routinely (Embree et al, 1996).

The entire examination usually can be accomplished in one session in the office. Occasionally the patient needs several visits. If examination is urgent because of bleeding or trauma, an examination under anesthesia may be necessary.

---

* Also available as Pediatric Vaginal Aspirator from Cook Ob Gyn (Spencer, IN).

ADOLESCENT GIRLS

The adolescent girl should receive a thorough description of each part of the genital examination in advance, and she should be given a sense of control over the tempo of the examination. She should be told that the examination is important, but that the examiner can stop if the patient wishes and finish at another appointment. Pictures or the plastic Ortho Gyn model can be used to familiarize the adolescent with the type of examination. The adolescent should be allowed to have someone—nurse, friend, or mother—present during the examination if she desires. She is given a gown and sheet and asked to remove her clothes while the clinician is out of the room. A general physical examination is done first to relax the patient. She is told that "it is okay to feel nervous" or "lots of girls feel kind of scared during a first pelvic exam." The clinician should emphasize that the patient will be told everything during the exam.

Expert sexual abuse examiners disagree about the need to use a speculum to obtain samples and cultures in the asymptomatic adolescent with no history of vaginal penetration. At minimum, the external vulva and hymen should be inspected with the patient in lithotomy position, and the edges of the hymen assessed by visual inspection. Evidence of transection of the hymen can be assessed by running a saline moistened cotton-tipped applicator around the hymen. Alternatively, the experienced examiner can inflate the balloon of a 12- or 14- gauge Foley bladder catheter and gently pull back to enhance the assessment of the hymenal edges (Starling and Jenny, 1997). Normal hymens in girls who have never been sexually active are extremely unlikely to have "complete clefts" on the lower half (Emans et al, 1994). Other genital trauma also should be evaluated.

In the adolescent with a history of penetration or evidence of penetration on initial examination of the hymen, a speculum examination can usually be completed atraumatically to obtain endocervical cultures for *N. gonorrhoeae* and *C. trachomatis*, vaginal samples for wet preparations, semen tests in the case of an acute assault (see Chapter 6), and a Pap smear. As further data is obtained on the accuracy of PCR and LCR using urine testing alone, the speculum examination may be less essential in these girls. A one-finger water-moistened gloved vaginal examination (without lubricant) should be done prior to insertion of the speculum to allow the clinician to assess the size of the hymenal opening (and proper speculum size) and the feasibility of a speculum examination. Prior to insertion, the speculum should be warmed and touched to the inner thigh of the patient so that she can feel the quality of the metal or plastic. The smallest useful speculum for the adolescent is the Huffman speculum ($\frac{1}{2} \times 4\frac{1}{4}$ inches); it can usually be inserted without discomfort. In the sexually active adolescent, a larger speculum, the Pederson ($\frac{7}{8} \times 4\frac{1}{2}$ inches), allows improved visualization of the cervix. The clinician should tell the patient, "let me know if something is uncomfortable" and should make sure that the face of the patient is visible. If the patient grimaces or her toes are curling, she should be told what is happening, and the speculum should be adjusted to alleviate discomfort. Bi-manual examination is important in the adolescent to exclude cervical or adnexal tenderness or pregnancy.

A sensitive urine or serum pregnancy test, such as Tandem ICON hCG (Hybritech), should be obtained at the visit and repeated two weeks after the last sexual contact in all pubertal girls. In contrast to selective testing of prepubertal girls for STDs, the examiner should obtain cultures for STDs from all postpubertal girls and treat them for potential acquisition of STDs as outlined in Chapter 9 (Glaser et al, 1991; Jenny et al, 1990).

BOYS

Boys require the same sensitive and age-appropriate examinations as girls. The genital examination should focus on the penis, testes, and particularly the anus, as sodomy is frequently the predominant form of abuse in boys. The external genitalia can be examined with the child lying in supine or standing. When evaluating the anus, the clinician can use any of several positions. The young child may be examined in the supine position immediately following examination of the penis. Older boys are usually more comfortable if the anus is examined while in the left lateral position with either the right knee or both knees pulled up to the chest. Findings of urethral and anal discharge and any evidence of *Condyloma acuminatum* (human papillomavirus infection) should be recorded. Anal findings may include scars, sphincter tears, and distortion of the anus.

FOLLOW-UP

After the examination, the child or adolescent should be asked to dress in private, and the findings and implications should be discussed in another room. Reassurance is an important part of the examiner's role. With some children, and certainly with all adolescents, the medical-legal results should be discussed with the patient as well as with the accompanying adult. It is sometimes inappropriate to discuss the findings with the adult and child or adolescent together, especially when the adult is not supportive. Whether or not the results are discussed with the child, all statements should emphasize good health and intactness, such as, to a boy, "I want to make sure that you understand that your rectum looks normal and healthy," or to a girl, "I want to make sure that you understand that your vagina is healthy." Even if findings are present, children can usually be reassured that they will heal nicely and that, as their body matures, future physicians will be unlikely to notice any alteration caused by the abuse. Parents should be reminded that small children may have behavioral outbursts or difficulty sleeping the night after the examination because the clinic visit may bring back memories of previous genital contact and the child may wish to talk about them.

Antibiotics to cover *N. gonorrhoeae*, *C. trachomatis*, *Trichomonas*, and incubating syphilis are primarily given to acute assault victims and adolescents. Recommendations for prophylaxis to lessen the risk of acquiring HIV are under consideration and are available in many centers (Katz and Gerberding, 1997) (see Chapter 9). Prepubertal children are treated on the basis of symptoms and culture results. Follow-up blood tests for syphilis and HIV infection are outlined in Chapter 9. Hormone therapy to prevent pregnancy should be offered to pubertal girls seen within 72 hours of a rape, such as emergency contraception with two tablets of ethinyl estradiol 50 µg/norgestrel 0.5 mg taken within 72 hours of the rape, two additional tablets taken 12 hours later OR levonorgestrel 0.75 mg taken within 72 hours of the rape and repeated 12 hours later (Emans et al, 1998; Taskforce, 1988). Stool softeners or phenazopyridine may be indicated; tetanus toxoid should be given along the guidelines of the American Academy of Pediatrics. Hepatitis B immunization should be initiated if not previously completed. A repeat sensitive pregnancy test should be done two weeks after the last sexual contact. Healing of genital and anal injuries usually occurs very rapidly and residua may not be present if several days or weeks have passed (McCann et al, 1992; Finkel, 1989). Since the most important sequelae of sexual abuse are psychological, long-term support for the patient and her or his family are essential (Shrier et al, 1998; Nagy et al, 1995; Hibbard et al, 1990).

The medical report should be carefully written, preferably typed, and should include a brief history, physical findings, and overall assessment. For example, when the finding is that of a "normal genital examination," the examiner may wish to note that this "does not rule out a prior history of sexual abuse." A report of non-specific findings, such as erythema, vaginal discharge, or labial fusion, should note that these are abnormalities that may occur in a number of conditions, including sexual abuse. Specific findings, for example, a recent or healed laceration of the hymen or vagina, teeth marks, a sexually transmitted disease, or semen, should be clearly indicated. Although specific findings are more common in those girls for whom the perpetrator has acknowledged penetration, even this group may not have specific findings.

Records should be kept in compliance with state statutes because children and families may decide years later to press for prosecution of a perpetrator. Accurate observations and drawings or photographs are invaluable aids to the clinician called to testify on behalf of a child.

REFERENCES

AAP Committee on Child Abuse and Neglect. Guidelines for the evaluation of sexual abuse of children. Pediatrics. 1991;87:254–260.

Adams, JA. Sexual abuse and adolescents. *Pediatr Annals*. 1997;26:299–304.

Adams, JA, K Harper, S Knudson. A proposed system for classification of anogenital findings in children with suspected sexual abuse. *Adolesc Pediatr Gynecol*. 1992;5:73–75.

Adams, JA, K Harper, S Knudson, et al. Examination finding in legally confirmed child sexual abuse: It's normal to be normal. *Pediatrics*. 1994;94:310–317.

APSAC. Terminology Subcommittee of the American Professional Society on Abuse of Children Taskforce on Medical Evaluation of Suspected Sexual Abuse (APSAC). Practice Guidelines: Descriptive Terminology in child sexual abuse medical evaluation. 1995;1–8.

Bays, J, and C Jenny. Genital and anal conditions confused with child sexual abuse trauma. *AJDC*. 1990;144:1319–1322.

Berenson, AB. Appearance of the hymen at birth and one year of age: A longitudinal study. *Pediatrics*. 1993;91:820–825.

AAP Committee on Child Abuse and Neglect. Guidelines for the evaluation of sexual abuse of children. *Pediatrics.* 1999;103:180–191.

Berenson, AB. A longitudinal study of hymenal morphology in the first 3 years of life. *Pediatrics.* 1995;95:490–496.

Berenson, AB, AH Heger, JM Hayes, RK Bailey, SJ Emans. Appearance of the hymen in prepubertal girls. *Pediatrics.* 1992;89:387–394.

Bond, GR, MD Dowd, I Landsman, and M Rimsza. Unintentional perineal injury in prepubescent girls: A multicenter, prospective report of 56 girls. *Pediatrics.* 1995;95:628–631.

CDC. 1998 Guidelines for treatment of sexually transmitted diseases. *MMWR.* 1998;47 (RR-1):108–114.

Committee on Adolescence. Sexual assault and the adolescent. *Pediatrics.* 1994;94:761–765.

Dowd, MD, L Fitzmaurice, J Knapp, et al. The interpretation of urogenital finding in children with straddle injuries. *J Pediatr Surg.* 1994;27:7–10.

Emans, SJ, MR Laufer, DP Goldstein. *Pediatric and Adolescent Gynecology*, 4th ed. Philadelphia: Lippincott-Raven 1998.

Emans, SJ, ER Wood, N Flagg, A. Freeman. Genital findings in sexually abused, symptomatic, and asymptomatic girls. *Pediatrics.* 1987;79:778–785.

Emans, SJ, ER Wood, EN Allred, and E Grace. Hymenal findings in adolescent women: Impact of tampon use and consensual sexual activity. *J Pediatr.* 1994; 125:153–160.

Embree, JE, D Lindsay, T Williams, et al. Acceptability and usefulness of vaginal washes in premenarcheal girls as a diagnostic procedure for sexually transmitted diseases. *Pediatr Infect Dis J.* 1996;15:662–7.

Finkel, MA. Anogenital trauma in sexually abused children. *Pediatrics.* 1989; 84:317–322.

Glaser, JB, J Schachter, S Benes, M Cummings, et al. Sexually transmitted diseases in postpubertal female rape victims. *J infect Dis.* 1991;164:726–730.

Hermans-Giddens, ME, TE Forthingham. Prepubertal female genitalia: Examination for evidence for sexual abuse. *Pediatrics.* 1987;80:203–208.

Hibbard, RA, GM Ingersoll, and DP Orr. Behavioral risk, emotional risk, and child abuse among adolescents in nonclinical settings. *Pediatrics.* 1990;86: 896–901.

Hostetler, BR, D Muram, CE Jones. Sharp penetrating injuries to the hymen. *J Adolesc Pediatr Gynecol.* 1994;7(2)94–96.

Hymel, KP, C Jenny. Child sexual abuse. *Pediatr in Rev.* 1996;17:236–249.

Ingram, DL, D Everett, AR Flick, et al. Vaginal gonococcal cultures in sexual abuse evaluations: Evaluation of selective criteria for pre-teenaged girls. *Pediatrics.* 1997;99(6). (www.pediatrics.org/cgi/content/full/99/6/e8)

Jenny, C, TM Hooton, BA Browers, MK Copass, and JN Krieger. Sexually transmitted diseases in victims of rape. *N Engl J Med.* 1990;322:712–716.

Jenny, C, MLD Kuhns, and F Arakawa. Hymens in newborn female infants. *Pediatrics.* 1987;80:399–400.

Katz, MH and JL Gerberding. Postexposure treatment of people exposed to the human immunodeficiency virus through sexual contact or injection-drug use. *N Engl J Med.* 1997;336:1097–8.

Kellogg, ND and JM Parra. Linea vestibularis: A previously undescribed normal genital structure in female neonates. *Pediatrics.* 1991;87:926–929.

McCann, J, J Voris, M Simon, et al. Perianal findings in prepubertal children selected for nonabuse: A descriptive study. *Child Abuse Negl.* 1989;13:179–193.

McCann, J, J Voris, M Simon, and R, Wells. Comparison of genital examination techniques in prepubertal girls. *Pediatrics.* 1990;85:182–187.

McCann, J, J Voris, and M Simon. Genital injuries from sexual abuse: A longitudinal study. *Pediatrics.* 1992;89:307–317.

McCann J, R Wells, M Simon, J Voris. Genital findings in prepubertal girls selected for non-abuse: A descriptive study. *Pediatrics.* 1990;86:428–439.

Muram, D. Classification of genital findings in prepubertal girls who are victims of sexual abuse. *Adolesc Pediatr Gynecol.* 1988;1:151.

Muram, D. Child sexual abuse-genital tract findings in prepubertal girls. I. The unaided medical examination. *Am J Obstet Gynecol.* 1989;160:328–33.

Muram, D. Child sexual abuse: Relationship between genital findings and sexual acts. *Child Abuse Neglect.* 1989;13:211–216.

Muram, D, and S Elias. Child sexual abuse-genital tract findings in prepubertal girls. II. Comparison of colposcopic and unaided examinations. *Am J Obstet Gynecol.* 1989;160:333–335.

Muram, D, PM Speck, and SS Gold. Genital abnormalities in female siblings and friends of child victims of sexual abuse. *Child Abuse Neglect.* 1991;15:105–10.

Muram, D, PM Speck, and M Dockter. Child sexual abuse examination: Is there a need for routine screening for *N. gonorrhoeae*? *J Pediatr Adolesc Gynecol.* 1996; 9:79–80.

Nagy, S, R, DiClemente, and AG Adcock. Adverse factors associated with forced sex among southern adolescent girls. *Pediatrics.* 1995;96:944–946.

Pokorny, SF. Configuration of the prepubertal hymen. *Am J Obstet Gynecol.* 1987;157:950–956.

Pokorny, SF, and LVN Stormer. Atraumatic removal of secretions from the prebertal vagina. *Am J Obstet Gynecol.* 1987;156:581–582.

Pokorny, SF, and CA Kozinetz. Configuration and other anatomic details of the prepubertal hymen. *Adolesc Pediatr Gynecol.* 1988;1:97–103.

Pokorny, SF, W Pokorny, and W Kramer. Acute genital injury in the prepubertal girl. *Am J Obstet Gynecol.* 1992;166:1461–6.

Rimsza, ME, and Niggemann EA. Medical evaluation of sexually abused children: A review of 311 cases. *Pediatrics.* 1982;69:8–14.

Shrier, LA, JD Pierce, SJ Emans, and RH DuRant. Gender differences in risk behaviors associated with forced or pressured sex. *Archiv Pediatr Adolesc Med.* 1998;152:57–63.

Sicoli, RA, JD Losek, JM Hudlett, and D Smith. Indications for *Neisseria gonorrhoeae* cultures in children with suspected sexual abuse. *Archives Pediatr Adolesc Med.* 1995;149:86–89.

Siegel, RM, CJ Schubert, PA Myers, et al. The prevalence of sexually transmitted diseases in children and adolescent evaluated for sexual abuse in Cincinnati: Rationale for limited STD testing in pepubertal girls. *Pediatrics.* 1995;96: 1090–1094.

Siegfried, E, J Rasnick-Conley, S Cook et al. Human papillomavirus screening in pediatric victims of sexual abuse. *Pediatrics.* 1998;101:43–47.

Sirotnak, AP. Testing sexually abused children for sexually transmitted diseases: Who to test, when to test, and why. *Pediatric Annals.* 1994;23:370–374.

Starling, C, and C Jenny. Forensic examination of the adolescent female genitalia: The Foley Catheter technique. *Archiv Pediatr Adolesc Med.* 1997;151:102–103.

Taskforce on Postovulatory Methods of Fertility Regulation. Randomised controlled trial of levonorgestrel versus the Yuzpe regimen of combined oral contraceptives for emergency contraception. Lancet 1998;352:428–433.

6

FORENSIC EXAMINATION: THE ROLE OF THE PHYSICIAN AS "MEDICAL DETECTIVE"

CAROLE JENNY

When examining and treating sexual assault victims, the physician is not only responsible for the welfare of the patient but also becomes an investigator gathering evidence of a crime. This requires special skills and an awareness of one's obligations to the criminal justice system (Rogers, 1996).

The tasks of the forensic examination include documenting physical findings; collecting evidence for law enforcement agencies and forensic laboratories; meeting the legal requirements for the collection, storage, and transfer of the evidence collected; and creating a complete and accurate medical record that can be presented in a court of law.

A forensic medical examination can be time-consuming and stressful to the patient. The victim will have had an extremely difficult and sometimes violent or terrifying experience and is likely to find the examination intrusive. Children are even less able than adults to tolerate medical examination and testing after being victimized. The needs of the patient must be weighed against the needs of the criminal justice system. Patients should be treated thoughtfully and gently, with procedures carefully explained. Privacy should be protected, and the patient should be given as much control over the examination situation as possible.

Patients have the right to refuse examination or evidence collection procedures, but usually they are anxious to cooperate if the purpose is explained to them. Sedation or anesthesia may be necessary, in which cases proper consents should be obtained. Such actions are more likely to be needed when examining small children or developmentally disabled adults immediately after assault.

WHEN IS A FORENSIC EXAM INDICATED?

The procedures for evidence collection should be done as soon as possible after sexual assault. The timing of the examination is based on the likelihood of recovering evidence of assault, especially sperm and biochemical evidence (Allard, 1997). Sperm has been shown to persist in the vagina after intercourse for up to 17 days (Sharpe, 1963). Acid phosphatase has been recovered for up to 5 days (Davies and Wilson, 1974). The possibility of recovering evidence decreases quickly, and it is unlikely to occur after a few days (Davies and Wilson, 1974; Duenhoelter et al, 1978). A reasonable compromise is to perform a forensic examination if the patient presents within 72 hours of the assault.

A forensic examination for sexual assault should be considered for any unconscious patient presenting with unexplained injury. Important evidence could be lost before the patient is able to relate what happened.

The most difficult decision is whether or not to do a full forensic examination on a preverbal child who may or may not have been assaulted. The possible benefit of recovering evidence in a case where acute assault is suspected but not proven has to be weighed against the effect of subjecting the child to the examination. Children evaluated for non-specific complaints such as genital irritation or rash are not likely to be found to be victims of abuse or assault (Kellogg et al, 1998). The clinician's best judgment determines when the examination is indicated.

MAINTAINING THE CHAIN OF CUSTODY OF EVIDENCE: LEGAL REQUIREMENTS FOR STORAGE AND TRANSFER OF EVIDENCE

Facilities Needed for Forensic Examinations

The samples collected from sexual assault victims to be presented as evidence must be protected from contamination, degradation, and tampering (Lee et al, 1998). Everyone involved in the collection and processing of the materials must be identified. Evidence should be stored in cabinets, refrigerators, and freezers under lock and key. Access to storage areas should be limited. In emergency rooms, one person, usually the head nurse, holds custody of the keys. A log documenting access to the locked storage areas is critical. When evidence is transferred to law enforcement officers, release forms must be signed.

These requirements make it very difficult to perform forensic examinations or store evidence in a clinic or physician's office. Most forensic examinations are done in hospital emergency rooms. If a facility does not have appropriate storage areas, the sexual assault patient should be referred.

Special freezers that maintain constant temperatures below $-10°$ C are needed for optimal preservation of biological evidence such as specimens for deoxyribonucleic acid (DNA) typing. Household freezers may cause repeated thawing and freezing and degrade specimens. When specimens are not immediately transferred to the police, "self-defrosting" household freezers should not be used for the storage of evidence.

Use of Protocols

Forensic examinations should be done according to a specific protocol. In some jurisdictions, the protocol is provided by law enforcement agencies. California, for example, mandates collection of sexual assault evidence using a kit containing specific storage containers for samples and a detailed medical record. In other states, each hospital maintains its own protocol and storage materials.

Ideally, protocols are updated frequently to reflect new knowledge in forensic science and medicine. Hospital-based protocols are more flexible in this regard, while legally mandated protocols provide for more uniformity among institutions within a jurisdiction. Examples of several protocols are provided in the appendices.

Using a protocol protects the integrity of evidence. It can eliminate the need for hospital personnel to testify at each trial about how the evidence was collected and maintained. It guards against errors of omission in the evidence collection process.

Specimen Labeling

All specimens should be put in sealed envelopes, bags, or containers with a proper label including the name of the patient, source of the specimen, and date and time of collection. The person witnessing the collection of the specimen and the person who secures and seals the package should sign the package across the seal. To avoid contamination, envelopes should be sealed using a moist cotton swab and water rather than licked.

PHYSICAL EXAMINATION

The General Physical

The shoes and clothing worn by the victim during the assault are collected for analysis. Tissue paper is placed over stains, which are folded to the inside. The patient is asked to undress over two pieces of heavy paper. The top sheet of paper is saved to look for hairs, fibers, or other materials that might identify the assailant or the location of the crime (Paul, 1977).

If the victim scratched the assailant, material from underneath the fingernails is collected. This can be done by scraping the nails with a cuticle stick and/or closely clipping and saving the fingernails.

The victim's pubic hair is then combed over a piece of paper using a comb containing cotton between the teeth to dislodge stray hairs. Pubic hair transfer occurs in approximately 17 percent of sexual encounters involving intercourse (Exline et al, 1998). The comb is folded into the paper and both are saved for hair analysis.

When examining a sexual assault victim, the medical professional should do a careful and complete physical examination, looking for evidence of recent or past injury. The patient's history should be considered, for example, if he or she reports being strangled, the neck should be examined for redness or swelling. If a child has been lifted up or restrained by the trunk, the axillae should be checked for redness or bruising. If the legs have been forced apart, bruising or abrasions may appear on the inside of the thighs. If a hand was placed over the victim's mouth, the inside of the lips and gums should be examined for bleeding or bruising. In the case of oral assault, the examiner should look for petechiae on the palate and gums or swelling of the tongue. Ligature marks on wrists or ankles may be observed (Kanda et al, 1985).

Lesions, including bite marks, should be carefully measured (Butler, 1973). The color of bruises should be noted (Schwartz and Ricci, 1996). Bruises evolve through a series of color changes from dark red to blue or black to green to yellow, although the sequence is variable. The length of time for healing is also extremely variable and determining the age of bruises is an inexact process (Schwartz and Ricci, 1996). Yellow coloration, generally thought to indicate old bruises, can appear as soon as eighteen hours after the injury (Langlois and Gresham, 1991). The evolution of colors occurs more quickly in the genital area than in other tissues because of the good blood supply to the tissues. Bruises may not appear until 24 hours after injury and may require 1 to 4 weeks to heal completely.

While examining the patient, the medical professional should search for trace evidence. Stray hairs, sand, dirt, grass, or lint found on the patient's body should be saved for analysis by the forensic laboratory (Taupin, 1996).

Any injuries should be photographed with a good quality camera (APSAC, 1995). A ruler placed in the field provides a size reference. This is especially important when photographing bite marks. The photos can be compared with dental impressions obtained from the alleged assailant (Furness, 1981). If a ruler is unavailable, a coin can be placed next to the lesion to be photographed as a size standard. A standard color bar in the photograph is also helpful.

Some injuries may not be obvious at the initial examination.

Bruises or bite marks may appear the following day. Reexamination may be needed to document the lesions.

Any areas of the body where semen might be found should be scanned using an ultraviolet lamp in a darkened room. Semen fluoresces a blue-green to orange color at 400 to 480 nanomicrons (Sensabaugh, 1977). Other oily substances such as creams and lotions will also fluoresce, as will urine (Gabby et al, 1992). Any fluorescent areas should be swabbed with two saline-moistened cotton swabs and processed as described in the section about genetic markers.

Hairs can be clipped and plucked from the victim to be compared with loose hairs recovered from the victim's body and from the crime scene. If this is done, a variety of hairs from different regions of the patient's scalp should be obtained. In addition, hairs are cut and plucked from the pubic and anal regions, as well as from the chest and beard, where applicable (Bisbing, 1982). Plucking can be intrusive and traumatic to the victim (Martin et al, 1985), but is the preferred method because the hair root can be analyzed.

GENITAL AND ANAL EXAMINATIONS

The same principles used in the general examination apply to the genital and anal examinations. Three tasks are accomplished in the examination of the assaulted orifices—documenting and treating injuries or other pathological conditions, testing for sexually transmitted diseases, and collecting samples for forensic evidence.

After observing and photographing external lesions, staining the perineum and posterior fourchette with toluidine blue dye can increase the recognition of minor tissue injuries. This dye detects the disruption of the superficial epithelial layers of skin cells by pyknotic staining of the nucleated cells in the dermis. Superficial abrasions not previously visualized may then be seen (McCauley et al, 1986).

Using the colposcope to examine genital and anal trauma has been shown to significantly increase the rate of detection of traumatic lesions (Slaughter and Brown, 1992; Lenahan et al, 1998). A colposcope equipped with a photographic or video camera can provide better documentation of injuries.

The techniques of genital and anal examinations are described in Chapter 5.

Collection of Forensic Specimens

At least two swabs should be taken whenever forensic specimens are obtained. One can be used by the prosecution, and one can be saved for independent analysis by the defense. Forensic specimens should be obtained from any assaulted orifice.

When swabbing the mouth, the medical professional should swab behind the tonsillar pillars, between the lips and the gums, and under the tongue. When a vaginal speculum examination can be done, swabs should be obtained from both the vaginal vault and cervical os. In younger children, swabs or washes should be obtained from the vagina. A vaginal wash with normal saline may be a more efficient way to recover sperm and male DNA, but may dilute other semen markers.

Any bite marks should be swabbed immediately after the bite marks are photographed with swabs moistened with sterile saline. These swabs can be analyzed for genetic markers, which can aid in identifying the assailant (Sweet et al, 1997; Gaensslen, 1983).

Swabs should be completely dried before storage to protect genetic markers. Specially made swab dryers increase the efficiency of this process. The specimens can be locked in the dryer to avoid contamination while drying.

TYPES OF FORENSIC ANALYSIS

Evidence of the Presence of Semen

Spermatozoa. The presence of spermatozoa in samples taken from the vagina, rectum, or oropharynx proves sexual contact. Motile sperm can be found in the endocervix up to 6 days after intercourse in adults (Nicholson, 1965). In vaginal samples, motile sperm commonly are not found after a few hours (Soules et al, 1978). Nonmotile sperm persist for up to 17 days (Sharpe, 1963). The recovery from forensic specimens depends on several factors as follows:

1. The body cavity from which the sperm is obtained. Semen is not likely to be detected in the mouth after a few hours (Enos and Beyer, 1978). It is removed quickly by the cleansing action of saliva and by bacterial degradation. Semen persists in the vagina longer than in the rectum.

2. The activity of the victim after the assault. Physical activity such as running or walking can decrease the length of time sperm can be recovered, as can activities such as defecating, douching, urinating, spitting, or brushing teeth. Sperm can be recovered longer from dead bodies (Wilson, 1974).

3. Physical and chemical characteristics of the environment, such as pH and temperature. If the victim uses chemical spermicides before or after the assault, sperm may be rapidly destroyed.

4. Biological characteristics, such as the presence of bacteria, enzymes, and anti-sperm antibodies, or the stage of the menstrual cycle of the female (Morrison, 1972).

5. Sperm cannot be recovered if the assailant is azospermic, successfully vasectomized, or impotent.

Tests for the presence of sperm include saline wet mounts done by the clinician at the time of the examination, permanent smears such as Pap smears, and the collection of sperm from dried swabs, stains, or saline washes. Saline wet mounts are the only way to determine the presence of motile sperm.

Acid Phosphatase. Prostatic acid phosphatase belongs to the family of enzymes that liberates inorganic phosphate from phosphoric esters. It is found in large amounts in prostatic secretions (Kind, 1964). A small amount of acid phosphatase has been found in the vaginal secretions of adult females. Levels of vaginal acid phosphatase associated with coitus have been statistically characterized (Findley, 1977). Vaginal acid phosphatase levels in normal, nonabused children have not been determined.

Significant levels of acid phosphatase cannot be found 12 hours after intercourse in 50% of vaginal swabs (Sensabaugh, 1979). It can persist much longer in dried semen stains (Kaye, 1951). Acid phosphatase can be found in semen after vasectomy.

p30 Protein. p30 protein is a semen-specific glycoprotein of prostatic origin. It is not found in vaginal fluid in the absence of semen (Sensabaugh, 1978). It is detected by an enzyme-linked immunosorbent assay (ELISA). The mean time to loss of detection in vaginal fluid is 27 hours after intercourse (Graves et al, 1985). Measuring p30 protein levels is a more sensitive and specific method of semen detection than acid phosphatase testing. p30 protein is found in the semen of vasectomized men.

Seminal Vesicle-Specific Protein. A monoclonal antibody (MHS-5) has been developed for use in an ELISA to recognize a protein secretory product of the human seminal vesicle epithelium (Herr et al, 1986). The protein is found in semen, but not in other human body fluids. It can be detected on dried semen stains kept at room temperature for up to 6 months. The ELISA assay can detect as little as 300 ng/ml of seminal fluid. This is approximately a 1: 75,000 dilution of seminal fluid (Herr and Woodward, 1986). The assay has been shown to be highly sensitive and specific for semen (Keil et al, 1996).

Gender Determination of Forensic Samples. Identification of Y chromosomes in forensic samples can be accomplished by polymerase chain reaction (PCR) amplification of gender-specific portions of DNA (Pouchkarov, 1998).

Evidence Identifying Characteristics of Assailants

Hair. Many different characteristics of hair are examined in the forensic laboratory including color, reflectivity, diameter, spatial configuration, pigment type, cuticle, and scale pattern (Shaffer, 1982). Although specific identification of the assailant cannot be made with hair analysis, the hair analysis can "rule in" or "rule out" specific individuals as suspects. Population studies of hair characteristics have been done to estimate frequencies of hair types among racial groups (Gaudette, 1976; Gaudette and Keeping, 1974). More recently, isolation and characterization of mitochondrial DNA found in hair shafts has been used for forensic identification. Polymerase chain reaction (PCR) methods allow for valid identification of single hairs (Wilson et al, 1995).

Genetic Markers in Blood, Saliva, and Semen. Genetic markers are used to identify samples obtained in sexual assault cases. ABO blood group antigens are most commonly used. The frequency of these markers in the population has been determined (Gaensslen, 1983). Saliva samples can be tested to determine whether or not a person is a secretor of these antigens. Secretor status and ABO antigen type from alleged offenders can be compared with ABO test results from forensic samples such as vaginal swabs, semen stains from the victim's body or clothing, or swabs obtained from bite marks on the victim's body. Depending on the results, suspects can be "ruled in" or "ruled out" in many cases. If no blood group antigens are found in forensic samples, or if the ABO group and secretor status of the victim and alleged assailant are the same, the data is not useful (Sensabaugh et al, 1985). Conventional immunologic methods of testing for ABO blood groups have been augmented by PCR-based methods for ABO genotyping (Herrin, 1996). These methods have been shown to be quick and reliable, and are less likely to be affected by bacterial contamination and environmental degredation (Ladd et al, 1996).

Other polymorphic protein enzymes can be analyzed in forensic laboratories to increase the discrimination power of samples. The most commonly used markers are the enzymes phosphoglucomutase (PGM) and peptidase A (Pep A). The ten phenotypes of PGM and three phenotypes of Pep A allow a considerable variety of semen samples to be identified. When variations of PGM, Pep A, and ABO are considered together, 40 different combinations can be identified, often ruling out 90% of the population as contributors of the semen (Sensabaugh et al, 1985).

The genetic markers are quickly lost in vaginal secretions after intercourse, usually after six hours (Price et al, 1976; Parkin, 1981). The markers persist much longer in semen stains. Careful collection of the victim's stained clothing in the emergency room can increase the likelihood of obtaining useful information in the forensic laboratory.

DNA Typing. The most specific form of forensic evidence is DNA typing. DNA is the genetic material found on chromosomes responsible for inheritance. DNA in each individual is unique, except for identical twins, who share the same genetic material.

Researchers have identified regions of human DNA that are extremely variable between individuals (*hypervariable minisatellites* or *restriction fragment length polymorphisms*) (Jeffreys et al, 1985; Nakamura et al, 1987). By analyzing DNA from samples of blood or semen, very specific identification of forensic samples can be made (Jeffreys et al, 1985; Giusti et al, 1986; Kanter et al, 1986).

DNA typing is potentially more useful than other forensic tests because of its specificity. In principle, one individual can be distinguished statistically by DNA type from all others, except an identical twin, in the population provided that enough genetically variable sites are analyzed (NRC, 1992). DNA is a long, stable molecule, biochemically more stable than protein molecules. It is more likely to resist environmental degradation than protein genetic markers. Spermatozoa are rich in DNA, making them an excellent source of genetic information about assailants.

Polymerase chain reaction (PCR) methods can identify DNA in extremely small samples (Higuchi et al, 1988). Results can be obtained faster using PCR methods than with Southern blotting. Since PCR targets small segments of DNA, degraded samples are more likely to be analyzable (Lee et al, 1994).

DNA typing is now commonly used in forensic casework (Lewis et al, 1990; Ruano et al, 1992; Nelson et al, 1996; Lorente, 1997; Gross et al, 1997). DNA typing evidence has been presented in courts of law in every state in the nation (Lee et al, 1994). Appellate courts have ruled on its acceptability as evidence (Beeler and Wiebe, 1988). The scientific basis of the technology has been found to be credible, but the use of the technology in individual laboratories is being questioned (Thompson and Ford, 1989). Cases have also been questioned because of inadequate collection and storage of materials (Lee et al, 1988). Stringent quality control and uniform methods are needed to ensure the acceptance of DNA evidence by courts.

The discrimination power of DNA analysis makes the clinician's job more important. Collection and preservation of the highest-quality evidence samples can lead to a specific identification of the source of a forensic sample.

THE MEDICAL CHART

The medical chart in sexual assault cases must be prepared thoughtfully, especially since it can become evidence in a court of law. Documenting the history and physical examination findings provides helpful information for the police, prosecutors, and defense attorneys. Handwriting should be legible, and a detailed and accurate history should be recorded. The mental status of the patient and all physical examination findings should be described carefully. Drawings and photographs should be included, as needed. All procedures and tests should be documented. Often, a specific form is used to ensure completeness of the record. The more detailed the chart, the easier it is for the physician to remember the case accurately if called to be a witness months, or years, in the future.

Access to the chart should be limited to protect the patient's privacy and prevent altering or tampering with the report. The chart should be signed by the medical staff participating in the patient's care.

SUMMARY

Recognizing that the welfare of the patient is always the first responsibility of the physician, although forensic examinations can be stressful, patients often benefit from careful collection of evidence and documentation of injury. Their assailants are more likely to be brought to justice, and they and others may be protected against future crimes. Everyone is served well by careful collection of evidence—the sexual assault victim, the person accused of crime, the criminal justice system, and society as a whole.

REFERENCES

Allard, JE. The collection of data from findings in cases of sexual assault and the significance of spermatozoa on vaginal, anal and oral swabs. Science and Justice. 1997;37:99–108.

APSAC. Photodocumentation Subcommittee of the American Professional Society's Task Force on Medical Evaluation of Suspected Child Abuse. *Practice Guidelines: Photographic Documentation of Child Abuse.* American Professional Society on the Abuse of Children, Chicago, IL, 1995.

Beeler, L, and WR Wiebe. DNA identification tests and the courts. *Washington Law Rev.* 1988;63:903–955.

Bisbing, RE. The forensic identification and association of human hair. In: Saferstein, R, ed. *Forensic Science Handbook.* Englewood Cliffs, NJ: Prentice-Hall; 1982.

Butler, OH. The value of bite mark evidence. *Int J Forensic Dent.* 1973;1:23–24.

Davies, A, and E Wilson. The persistence of seminal constituents in the human vagina. *Forensic Sci.* 1974;3:45–55.

Duenhoelter, JH, IC Stone, R Santos-Ramos, and DE Scott. Detections of seminal fluid constituents after alleged sexual assault. *J Forensic Sci.* 1978; 23:824–829.

Enos, WF, and JC Beyer. Spermatozoa in the anal canal and rectum and in the oral cavity of female rape victims. *J Forensic Sci.* 1978;23:231–233.

Exline, DL, FP Smith, and SG Drexler. Frequency of pubic hair transfer during sexual intercourse. *J Forensic Sci.* 1998;43:505–508.

Findley, TP. Quantitaton of vaginal acid phosphatase and its relationship to time of coitus. *Am J Clin Pathol*. 1977;68:238–242.

Furness, J. A general review of bitemark evidence. *Am J Forensic Med Pathol*. 1981;2:49–52.

Gabby, T, MA Winkleby, T Boyce, DL Fisher, A Lancaster, and GF Sensabaugh. Sexual abuse of children: The detection of semen on skin. *Am J Dis Child*. 1992;146:700–703.

Gaensslen, RE. *Sourcebook in Forensic Serology, Immunology, and Biochemistry*. Washington, DC: U.S. Government Printing Office 1983:183–190.

Gaensslen, RE. *Sourcebook in Forensic Serology, Immunology, and Biochemistry*. Washington, DC: U.S. Government Printing Office, 1983:322–328.

Gaudette, BD. Probabilities and human pubic hair comparisons. *J Forensic Sci*. 1976;21:514.

Gaudette, BC, and ES Keeping. An attempt at determining probabilities in human scalp hair comparison. *J Forensic Sci*. 1974;19:599.

Giusti, A, M Baird, S Pasquate, I Balazs, and J Glassberg. Application of deoxyribonucleic acid (DNA) polymorphisms to the analysis of DNA recovered from sperm. *J Forensic Sci*. 1986;31:409–417.

Graves, HC, GF Sensabaugh, and ET Blake. Postcoital detection of a male-specific semen protein by ELISA: Application to rape investigation. *N Engl J Med*. 1985;312:338–343.

Gross, AM, G Carmody, and RA Guerrieri. Validation studies for the genetic typing of the D1S80 locus for implementation into forensic casework. *J Forensic Sci*. 1997;42:1140–1146.

Herr, JC, TA Summers, RS McGee, WM Sutherland, M Sigman, and RJ Evans. Characterization of monoclonal antibody to a conserved epitope on human seminal vesicle-specific peptides: A novel probe/marker system for semen identification. *Biol Reprod*. 1986;35:773–784.

Herr, JC, and MP Woodward. An enzyme linked immunosorbent assay (ELISA) for human semen identification based on a biotinylated monoclonal antibody to a seminal vesicle-specific antigen. *J Forensic Sci*. 1986;32:346–356.

Herrin, G Jr. A simplified amplification procedure for two regions of the glycosyl transferace (ABO blood group) gene. *J Forensic Sci*. 1996;41:138–141.

Higuchi, R, CH von Beroldingen, GF Sensabaugh, and HA Erlick. DNA typing from single hairs. *Nature*. 1988;332:543–546.

Jeffreys, AJ, JFY Brookfield, and R Semeonoff. Forensic application of DNA fingerprints. *Nature*. 1985;318:577–579.

Jeffreys, AJ, V Wilson, and SL Thein. Hypervariable 'minisatellite' regions in human DNA. *Nature*. 1985;314:67–73.

Kanda, M, JN Thomas, and DW Lloyd. The role of forensic evidence in child abuse and neglect. *Am J Forensic Med Pathol*. 1985;6:7–15.

Kanter, E, M Baird, R Shaler, and I Balazs. Analysis of restriction fragment length polymorphisms in DNA recovered from dried bloodstains. *J Forensic Sci*. 1986;31:403–408.

Kaye, S. The acid phosphatase test for seminal strains. A study of the reliability of aged stains. *J Crim Law Criminol*. 1951;41:834–835.

Keil, W, J Bachus, and HD Troger. Evaluaion of MHS-5 in detecting seminal fluid in vaginal swabs. *Int J Legal Med*. 1996;108:186–190.

Kellogg, ND, JM Parra, and S Menard. Children with anogenital symptoms and signs referred for sexual abuse evaluations. *Arch Pediatr Adolesc Med*. 1998; 152:634–641.

Kind, SS. The acid phosphatase test. *Methods Forensic Sci.* 1964;4:267–288.

Ladd, C, MT Bourke, CA Scherczinger, EM Pagliaro, RE Gaensslen, and HC Lee. A PCR-based strategy for ABO genotype determination. *J Forensic Sci.* 1996;41:134–137.

Langlois, NEI, and GA Gresham. The ageing of bruises: A review and study of the colour changes with time. *Forensic Sci Int.* 1991;50:227–238.

Lee, HC, C Ladd, MT Bourke, E Pagliaro, and F Tirnady. DNA typing in forensic science. I. Theory and background. *Am J Forensic Med Pathol.* 1994; 15:769–782.

Lee, HC, C Ladd, CA Scherczinger, and MT Bourke. Forensic applications of DNA typing. Part 2: Collection and preservation of DNA evidence. *Am J Forensic Med Pathol.* 1998;19:10–18.

Lenahan, LC, A Ernst, and B Johnson. Colposcopy in evalution of the adult sexual asault victim. *Am J Emergency Med.* 1998;16:183–184.

Lewis, ME, RE Kouri, D Latorra, KM Berka, HC Lee, and RE Gaensslen. Restriction fragment length polymorphism DNA analysis by the FBI Laboratory protocol using a simple, convenient hardware system. *J Forensic Sci.* 1990; 35:1186–1190.

Lorente, M, JA Lorente, JC Alvarez, B Budlowe, MR Wilson, and E Villanueva. Sequential multiplex amplification: Utility in forensic casework with minimal amounts of DNA and partially degraded samples. *J Forensic Sci.* 1997; 42:923–925.

Martin, PY, D DiNitto, S Maxwell, and DB Norton. Controversies surrounding the rape kit exam in the 1980s: Issues and alternatives. *Crime Delinquency.* 1985;31:223–246.

McCauley, J, RL Gorman, and G Guzinski. Toluidine blue in the detection of perineal laceration in pediatric and adolescent sexual abuse victims. *Pediatrics.* 1986;78:1039–1043.

Morrison, AI. Persistence of spermatozoa in the vagina and cervix. *Br J Vener Dis.* 1972;48:141–143.

Nakamura, Y, M Leppart, P O'Connell, R Wolff, T Holm, M Culver, et al. Variable number of tandem repeat (VNTR) markers for human gene mapping. *Science.* 1987;235:1616–1622.

Nelson, MS, EA Benzinger, MJ Budzynski, MT Boodee, A Matthews, E Buel, MB Schwartz, C von Beroldingven, RL Wampler, TM Coons, et al. Validation of probe EFD52 (D17S26) for forensic DNA analysis. *J Forensic Sci.* 1996; 41:557–568.

Nicholson, R. Vitality of spermatozoa in the endocervical canal. *Fertil Steril.* 1965; 16:758–764.

NRC Committee on DNA Technology in Forensic Science, National Research Council: *DNA Technology in Forensic Science.* National Academy Press, Washington, DC, 1992.

Parkin, B. The evidential value of peptidase A as a semen typing system. *J Forensic Sci.* 1981;26:398–404.

Paul, DM. The medical examination in sexual offenses against children. *Med Sci Law.* 1977;17:251–258.

Pouchkarev, VP, EF Shved, and PI Novikov. Sex determination of forensic samples by polymerase chain reaction of the amelogen gene and analysis by capillary electrophoresis with polymeratrix. *Electrophoresis.* 1998;19:76–79.

Price, CJ, A Davies, and BG Wraxall. The typing of phosphoglucomutase in vaginal material and semen. *J Forensic Sci Soc.* 1976;16:29–42.

Rogers, D. Physical aspects of alleged sexual assaults. *Med Sci Law.* 1996;36: 117–122.

Ruano, G, EM Pagliaro, TR Schwartz, K Lamy, D Messian, RE Gaensslen, and HC Lee. Heat-soaked PCR: An efficient method for DNA amplification with applications to forensic analysis. *Biotechniques.* 1992;13:266–274.

Schwartz, AJ, and LR Ricci. How accurately can bruises be aged in abused children? Literature review and syntheses. *Pediatrics.* 1996;97:254–257.

Sensabaugh, GF. Identification and individualization of semen in the investigation of rape. *Final report,* grant 74-NI-99-0041, National Institute of Law Enforcement and Criminal Justice, Law Enforcement Assistance Administration, U.S. Department of Justice; 1977.

Sensabaugh, GF. Isolation and characterization of a semen specific protein from human seminal plasma: A potential marker for semen identification. *J Forensic Sci.* 1978;23:106–115.

Sensabaugh, GF. The quantitative acid phosphatase test. *J Forensic Sci.* 1979; 24:346–365.

Sensabaugh, GF, J Bashinski, and ET Blake. The laboratory's role in investigating rape. *Diagn Med.* 1985;1–6.

Shaffer, SA. A protocol for the examination of hair evidence. *Microscope.* 1982; 30:151–161.

Sharpe, N. The significance of spermatozoa in sexual offenses. *Can Med Assoc J.* 1963;89:513–514.

Slaughter, L, and CRV Brown. Colposcopy to establish physical findings in rape victims. *Am J Obstet Gynecol.* 1992;166:83–86.

Soules, MR, AA Rollard, KM Brown, et al. The forensic evaluation of evidence in alleged rape. *Am J Obstet Gynecol .* 1978;130:142–147.

Sweet D, JA Lorente, A Valenzuela, M Lorente, and E Villanueva. PCR-based DNA typing of saliva stains recovered from human skin. *J Forensic Sci.* 1997;42:447–451.

Taupin, JM. Hair and fiber transfer in an abduction case—Evidence from different levels of tract evidence transfer. *Journal of Forensic Sciences.* 1996;41:697–699.

Thompson, WC, and S Ford. DNA typing: acceptance and weight of the new genetic identification tests. *Virginia Law Rev.* 1989;75:45–108.

Wilson, EF. Sperm's morphological survival after 16 days in the vagina of a dead body. *J Forensic Sci.* 1974;19:561–564.

Wilson, MR, JA DiZinno, D Polanskey, J Replogle, and B Budlowle. Validation of mitochondrial DNA sequencing for forensic casework analysis. *Int J Legal Med.* 1995;108:68–74.

7

ANATOMY

EMBRYOLOGY OF THE GENITAL TRACT

DAVID MURAM

Sexual differentiation is dependent on the genetic make-up of the developing embryo. In general, when a Y chromosome is present sexual differentiation proceeds along male lines, whereas in the absence of a Y chromosome the embryo develops to become a female. A structural gene, the testis-determining factor encoded on the sex-determining region of the Y chromosome (SRY) controls the differentiation of the primitive gonad into a testis (Page et al, 1987; Sinclair et al, 1990; Berta et al, 1990). The SRY protein activates transcription of genes on the sex chromosomes and autosomes that collectively control normal sexual differentiation (Page et al, 1987; Harley et al, 1992; Dubin and Ostrer, 1994). In those having the SRY gene, the undifferentiated gonad becomes a testis, while in those not having the gene, the undifferentiated gonad develops into an ovary. In addition, other genes located on various autosomes affect sexual differentiation (Moore and Grumbach, 1992).

The human embryo develops along female lines unless testicular development is actively induced. An ovary is formed even if only one X chromosome is present. Germ cells exist in 45, X human fetuses. But if two intact X chromosomes are not present, 45, X ovarian follicles usually degenerate by birth. The second X chromosome appears to be responsible for ovarian maintenance rather than ovarian differentiation. Analysis of individuals with terminal deletions of the X chromosome has shown that ovarian-maintenance determinants are present on both the X short arm and the X long arm. Each arm probably has at least two regions of importance for ovarian development. In addition to the sex chromosomes, there are autosomal loci that are essential for normal ovarian development.

GONADS AND DUCTS

In the presomite embryo, male and female alike, primordial sex cells can be recognized near the yolk sac, caudal to the embryonic disk. The tail-fold formation carries the primordial sex cells into the wall of the hindgut where they migrate via the dorsal mesentery to lie in and beneath the epithelium that covers the mesonephric ridge. The overlying epithelium proliferates and then bulges into the coelomic cavity as a genital ridge. The basement membrane disappears, and ill-defined cellular cords penetrate the underlying mesenchyme. These sex cords carry the primordial sex cells with them. Until this stage the male and female gonads are histologically indifferent (Fig. 7–1).

The male gonad is first recognizable as such at 6–8 weeks when mesenchyme spreads beneath the surface epithelium and between the sex cords as the future tunica albuginea and its septa. The primitive sex cords form a series of well-defined cell cords, the testis cords, that communicate with each other. Toward the hilus of the testis, the cords break into a network of small cell strands that later form the tubules of the rete testis. As development of the testis continues, the testis cords lose contact with the surface epithelium, and by the end of the seventh week the cords are separated from it by the tunica albuginea. The surface epithelium finally disappears, and the tunica albuginea then forms the capsule of the testis.

In the female, differentiation of the gonads occurs later than the male, at about 8–10 weeks. The tunica albuginea and the septa do

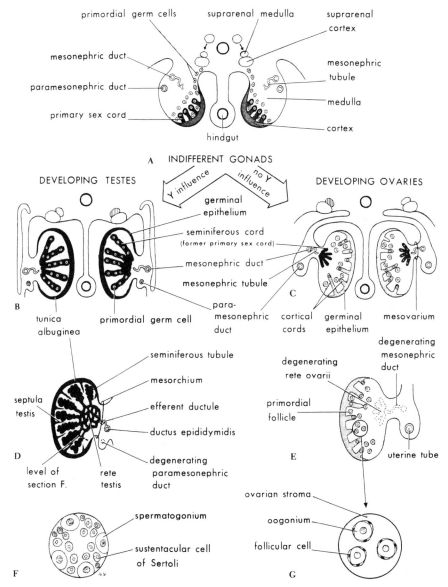

Fig. 7–1. Development of the male and female gonads. (From Moore KL. *The Developing Human: Clinically Oriented Embryology*, 3rd ed. Philadelphia: W. B. Saunders, 1982. Reprinted by permission of W. B. Saunders.)

not form. The sex cords converge to form a primitive rete, but they are not isolated from the coelomic epithelium. Within the cords, primordial follicles form. The surface epithelium surrounds the primordial sex cells and forms a capsule of flattened pregranulosa cells. Mesenchyme then invades the gonad and breaks up the sex cords providing the ovarian stroma. The primordial follicles become isolated within the ovarian stroma. The time sequence of the main events in sexual differentiation is highlighted in Table 7–1.

Once gonadal development is established, differentiation of the internal and the external genitalia proceeds predictably. In the presence of a testis, the ducts and external genitalia develop along male lines, while in the absence of a testis the development proceeds along female lines. The testicular stroma contains two distinct cell lines, Sertoli and Leydig cells. Both Leydig and Sertoli cells function in dissociation from testicular morphogenesis. These two cells secrete hormones that direct subsequent genital differentiation along male lines. Fetal Leydig cells produce an androgen, probably testosterone, that stabilizes Wolffian ducts and permits differentiation of the vas deferens, epididymis, and seminal vesicles (Figs. 7–2 and 7–3). Testosterone is converted by a 5 alpha reductase to dihydrotestosterone (DHT), which virilizes the external genitalia. Fetal Sertoli cells produce a different hormone, a glycoprotein called the anti-Müllerian hormone (AMH). The gene controlling AMH production has been isolated and localized to chromosome 19 (Cates et al, 1986). In the absence of AMH, the internal genitalia develop along female lines, the Müllerian ducts develop into the uterus and Fallopian tubes, and the Wolffian ducts regress. In the absence of testosterone and DHT, the external genitalia develop along female lines (Figs. 7–2 and 7–3).

In a male fetus, the AMH is responsible for regression of the Müllerian duct, the analgen of uterus, the Fallopian tubes, and the

Table 7–1. Sexual Differentiation

Timing	Event
6–8 weeks	Testicular differentiation
	Indifferent external genitalia
	Müllerian duct regression
9 weeks	External genitalia begin to appear gender specific
	Mesonephric ducts fuse & join vaginal plate
	Ovarian differentiation
	Vaginal development begins
9–12 weeks	Uterine development
12 weeks	Ovaries descend below pelvic brim
15 weeks	Vaginal development completed

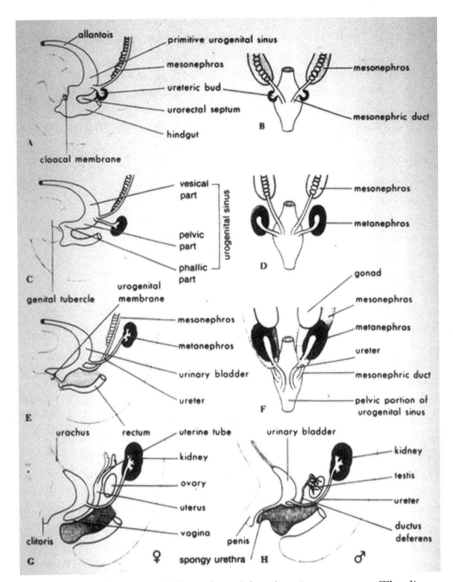

Fig. 7–2. Development of the male and female urinary systems. The diagrams show the cloaca dividing into the urogenital sinus and rectum, the absorption of the mesonephric ducts, and the development of the urinary tract. A is a lateral view of the caudal half of a 5-week-old embryo; B, D, and F are dorsal views; C, E, G, and H are lateral views. (From Moore KL. *The Developing Hunan: Clinically Oriented Embryology*, 3rd ed. Philadelphia: W. B. Saunders, 1982. Reprinted by permission of W. B. Saunders.)

upper two-thirds of the vagina. In female fetuses, AMH causes a decrease in aromatase activity in granulosa cells of the ovary. The human AMH gene consists of five exons: 412, 124, 108, 160, and 856

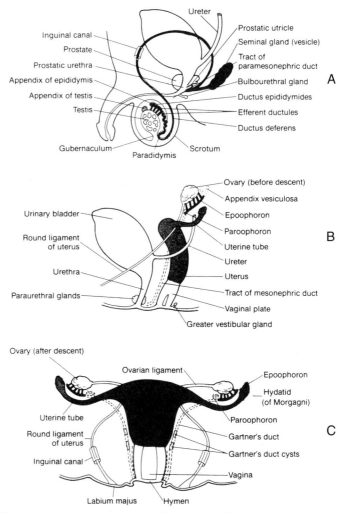

Fig. 7–3. Development of the male (A) and female (B, C) reproductive systems from the primitive genital ducts. Vestigial structures are shown. B is a female fetus at 12 weeks; C is a newborn female. (From Moore, KL. *The Developing Human: Clinically Oriented Embryology*. Philadelphia: W. B. Saunders, 1973. Reprinted by permission of W. B. Saunders.)

bp in length, and is localized near the tip of chromosome 19 in sub-bands 13.2 to 13.3 (Cates et al, 1986; Cohen-Haguenauer et al, 1987).

In the absence of AMH, regression of the Müllerian ducts fails to occur giving rise to the persistent Müllerian duct syndrome (PMDS) that occurs in subjects with a karyotype 46,XY and a male phenotype. PMDS is characterized by the presence of uterus and tubes in otherwise normally masculinized 46,XY males. Patients are normally virilized, and testicular production of testosterone is normal. Both testes may be cryptorchid; alternatively, one testicle may be descended into the inguinal canal or scrotum together with the Müllerian derivatives, a condition known as uterine inguinal hernia syndrome. The condition is an autosomal recessive disorder due to defects of synthesis of the AMH, or to receptor defects that interfere with the action of the hormone. The type of defect can be predicted from the serum levels of AMH. These are very low or undetectable in patients with AMH mutations and are at the upper limit of normal in those with receptor mutations. Only a few patients affected by PMDS may show progressive degeneration of testicular tissue and, eventually, agonadism (Jarminska-Jackowiak et al, 1995; Imbeaud et al, 1995).

THE EXTERNAL GENITALIA

After the tail-fold formation, the cloacal membrane lies in a depression between the umbilicus and the primitive streak from which the proliferating mesoderm extends in all directions. Two major extensions flank the cloacal membrane and raise lateral swellings on either side of it. In addition, the proliferating mesoderm forms the genital tubercle cranial to the cloacal membrane. The genital tubercle elongates as a phallus, and the urogenital sinus extends into its base. As the epithelium of the urogenital sinus proliferates, it forms the urethral plate, which grows toward the tip of the phallus.

The cloacal depression extends to the caudal aspect of the phallus as a urethral groove surrounded by a pair of genital folds. These folds are distinct from the lateral swellings. The floor of the urethral groove is in contact with the urethral plate, and as the urorectal septum reaches it, the cloacal membrane breaks down. The breakdown extends into the floor of the urethral groove, deepens it, and exposes the urethral plate. The leading edge of the urorectal septum is then covered by an ingrowth of tissues from either side. As a result, the genital folds now meet immediately in front of the anus. The lateral swellings are subdivided into genital and anal parts. The anal swellings gradually encircle the anal canal (Fig. 7–4).

In the absence of androgenic stimulation, the neck of the prim-

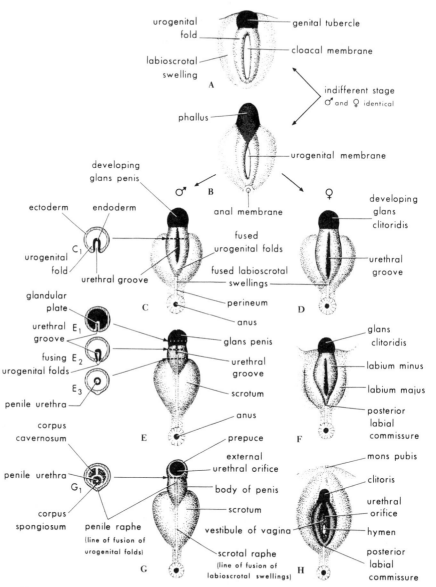

Fig. 7–4. Development of the external genitalia at 4–7 weeks (A, B); male development at 9 (C), 11 (E), and 12 (G) weeks with schematic transverse sections (C_1, E_1–E_3, G_1); female development at 9 (D), 11 (F), and 12 (H) weeks. (From Moore KL. *The Developing Human: Clinically Oriented Embryology;* 3rd ed. Philadelphia: W. B. Saunders, 1982. Reprinted by permission of W. B. Saunders.)

itive bladder elongates to form the urethra. The urogenital sinus becomes shallower and forms the vestibule. The Müllerian tubercle (future vaginal orifice) and the urethra approach the surface. The genital folds become the labia minora, the genital swellings become the labia majora, and the phallus forms the clitoris. The paraurethral ducts, as well as the vestibular and urethral glands, arise as diverticula of the urogenital sinus.

Under the influence of androgens, the neck of the primitive bladder forms the prostatic urethra. Smooth muscle differentiates from the surrounding mesenchyme. The urogenital sinus forms the remainder of the prostatic urethra, as well as the membranous urethra. The genital folds close over the phallic part of the urogenital sinus and the urethral groove. As a result, the urogenital orifice migrates along the ventral aspects of the phallus. The genital swellings fuse together to form the scrotum. Fusion of the genital folds results in the formation of a spongy urethra. Meanwhile, the phallus has enlarged to become the penis, and ectoderm has grown in from its glans to reach the urethral plate. As the breakdown process extends along the urethral groove, the urethral meatus now opens in the ventral aspect of the glans (Figs. 7–2 and 7–4).

GONADAL DESCENT

The caudal end of the developing gonad remains in continuity with the mesonephric ridge. Near the crossing of the Müllerian and Wolffian ducts, the mesonephric ridge is connected to the inguinal region by a peritoneal fold. A column of mesenchyme, the gubernaculum, differentiates within this fold and links the gonad to the genital swelling. The abdominal muscles subsequently develop around the gubernaculum and form the inguinal canal. The gonads undergo a relative shift caudally because of the degeneration of the mesonephros, restraint by the gubernaculum, and rapid growth of the abdominal wall. The gonad thus descends caudally, but retains its neurovascular supply from a higher level. It projects into the inguinal fossa of peritoneum from which a diverticulum—the processus vaginalis—extends down the inguinal canal ventral to the gubernaculum. In the female, the gubernaculum becomes secondarily attached to the cornua of the uterus and forms the ovarian ligament proximal to it and the round ligament distal to it. The processus vaginalis normally is obliterated before birth. The ovary remains in the false pelvis until puberty when it descends with the true pelvis.

Clarnette and colleagues (1997) have suggested that gonadal descent occurs in two stages. The first stage of descent to the inguinal region is controlled by AMH, the second stage, or inguino-scrotal phase of descent, is androgen-dependent. They suggested that the position of the gonad, the nature of the gubernaculum, and cranial suspensory ligament can provide valuable information regarding the mechanisms controlling the final position of the gonads. In the persistent Müllerian duct syndrome, the gubernaculum is "feminized," resulting in a testis in the position normally occupied by an ovary, or an abnormally mobile testis that can prolapse into the inguinal region. In patients with androgen insensitivity, the testis is often located in the inguinal region, indicating that the first phase of descent is normal but that inguinoscrotal descent has failed to occur. The ovaries maintain their normal position in patients with congenital adrenal hyperplasia indicating that androgen alone does not affect gonadal descent.

ANATOMIC AND PHYSIOLOGIC CHANGES

DAVID MURAM

During the first few weeks of life maternal hormones affect the newborn infant for perhaps a month, rarely longer. These hormones, transferred across the placenta, stimulate the hormone-sensitive tissues of the newborn. Breast budding is the most obvious sign of such stimulation, and at times the breasts produce small amount of fluid that may be seen escaping from the nipple. Such breast enlargement is transient and requires no treatment.

FEMALE DEVELOPMENT

Maternal estrogens also stimulate the female external genitalia. The effects of maternal hormones are particularly evident on the hymen, which is thick and turgid. The labia majora and labia minora are prominent, enlarged, and thick. The clitoris is turgid, but not enlarged. Vaginal discharge is often seen escaping from the vaginal orifice; it is composed of mucus produced by the cervical glands mixed with exfoliated vaginal cells. The internal genital organs are similarly affected. The vaginal epithelium is mature and contains glycogen. Lactobacilli are present in the vagina early in infancy, and the vaginal secretions are acidic. The uterus is enlarged, but is composed mainly of cervix (the cervix:corpus ratio at birth is 3:1). The vagina is 4 cm long, and, at the apex, the cervix is clearly visible with a reddened zone of "physiological eversion" caused by protrusion of the columnar epithelium through the external cervical os. Occasionally, declining estrogen levels after birth cause shedding of the stimulated endometrial lining, and vaginal bleeding occurs. This bleeding stops within 7–10 days of life. The ovaries are abdominal organs in childhood and are not palpable on pelvic or rectal examination.

In the first few months of life, the infant's hypothalamic-pituitary-gonadal axis can be quite active with production of gonadal estrogens and persistence of thelarche. As the system becomes fully suppressed by age 2–4 years, the external genitalia assume a different appearance, typical of the prepubescent child. The labia majora are flat, and the labia minora are thin. There is minimal separation between the labia majora and minora. The clitoris, no longer turgid, is hidden in the small cleft of the vulva. The mucous membranes of the introitus and vagina are thin, pink, and atrophic. On cross section they may be only two or three cell layers thick. The mucosal surfaces appear redder than the vaginal epithelium of a woman in the reproductive years because the blood vessels underneath the thin mucosa are closer to the surface. The thin vaginal lining has relatively few rugae, and, therefore, the distensibility is very limited. These atrophic tissues have little resistance to trauma and infection. The secretions are neutral or slightly alkaline and contain mixed bacteria flora. The cervix is no longer distinct, but flush with the vaginal vault. Occasionally, it is difficult to see.

Marshall and Tanner (1969) described the temporal sequence of pubertal development and the various stages of secondary sexual features. Socioeconomic conditions, nutritional status, and general health and well being influence the age of onset and the progression of pubertal development. Genetic factors also affect the age of puberty, as demonstrated by the similar age of menarche in members of an ethnic population and in mother–daughter pairs. Secondary sexual development occurs earlier in black females compared with white females in the United States. Other factors also affect the age of puberty, such as chronic disease, malnutrition, strenuous physical activity, and obesity.

As the hypothalamic–pituitary–gonadal axis becomes active in late childhood (age 7–11 years), the external genitalia begin to show early signs of estrogen stimulation; the mons thickens, the labia majora fill out, the labia minora become rounded, and the hymen becomes thicker. The hymeneal orifice increases in size. The vagina elongates (8 cm) and the mucosa is thicker. In addition to the basal cells, exfoliative cytology may show some parabasal cells and, occasionally, superficial cells. The corpus uteri grows as well and is now as large as the cervix (cervix:corpus ratio is 1:1).

During early puberty (age 9–13 years), the external genitalia assume an adult appearance. Thickening of the hymen and dulling of the surface of the vaginal mucosa from its prepubertal reddish appearance occurs as a result of estrogen stimulation. The major vestibular (Bartholin's) glands begin to produce mucus just prior to menarche. The vagina reaches its adult length (10–12 cm), the mucosa becomes thick and moist, the vaginal secretions are acidic, and lactobacilli reappear. Secretion of clear or whitish discharge increases in the months before menarche. With the development of vaginal fornices, the cervix separates from the vault. Uterine growth is pronounced, but it mainly affects the corpus, which is now twice as large as the cervix. The ovaries descend into the true pelvic cavity. The vaginal pH decreases and lactobacilli reappear.

Secondary sex characteristics often develop rapidly during the late childhood period. The standards proposed by Tanner (1969) have been universally accepted as an objective method to describe the maturation of secondary sexual characteristics. Estrogens control breast development, while the growth of pubic and axillary hair is primarily under the influence of androgens. Classification of the stages of breast development depends on specific characteristics common to all females. It does not include size or inherent shape of the breasts, which are determined by genetic and nutritional factors.

There is no discernible breast tissue in prepubertal girls (Tanner stage 1). Breast development begins with an increase in the pigmentation and diameter of the areola and the development of a small amount of breast tissue (Tanner stage 2). Further growth of the breast and the areola occurs in stage 3. In many girls, as the breast continues to grow, there is secondary mounding of the areola above the plane of the breast (Tanner stage 4). The final stage (Tanner stage 5) is reached with further growth of the breast and recession of the areola into the general contour of the breast.

Classification of the stages of pubic hair development also follows the standards proposed by Tanner. In prepubertal girls only vellus hair is found over the pubic area (Tanner stage 1). In stage 2, there is sparse, long, pigmented, slightly curly hair over the mons and labia majora. In stage 3 there is an increase in the quantity of coarse, pigmented, curly hair, while in stage 4 this coarse hair fully covers the pubic symphysis. Finally, in stage 5, the coarse pigmented hair covers the entire pubic area and extends to the medial surface of the thighs.

The body habitus becomes rounded, especially in the shoulders and hips. Accelerated somatic growth (adolescent growth spurt) occurs along with breast development and sexual hair growth.

MALE DEVELOPMENT

In normal male term infants, testosterone secreted by the Leydig cells and converted to dihydrotestosterone is responsible for the differentiation of male external genitalia. Mean stretched penile length is 3.5 ± cm for a full-term newborn and 3.9 ± 0.8 cm for infants from 0 to 5 months old. The testes are normally descended into the rugated scrotum at birth, with only 2.7 percent of full-term males and 27 percent of premature infants having cryptorchidism. The hypothalamic-pituitary-gonadal axis is active for several months after birth until suppression occurs; the system is not reawakened until puberty.

Puberty in boys begins between 9.5 and 13.5 years. The mean age of onset of puberty for boys as defined by enlargement of testes is 11.6 ± 1.1 years, and the mean age for spermarche is between 13.5 and 14.5 years. The average duration of puberty for boys is 3 years, with a range of 2 to 5 years. The first sign is enlargement of the testes followed by the appearance of pubic hair and growth of the phallus. The pubertal height spurt occurs at an average age of 14 years for boys. During this spurt, males gain 10.3 ± 1.54 cm/year and reach a final mean adult height of 177 cm at 18 years. Mean body fat increases from 4.3 to 11.2 percent by late puberty and is distributed primarily in the truncal area.

In prepubertal boys, the testicular size is less than 2.2 cm and the phallus is immature (Tanner stage 1). The initial manifestation of pubertal development is enlargement of the testes elongate to 2.2–3.0 cm, with enlargement, thinning, and reddening of the scrotal skin. There is also slight enlargement of the phallus (Tanner stage 2). In stage 3, the testes increase in size (3.1–4.0 cm), with further enlargement of the scrotum and phallus. In stage 4, the testicular size is 4.1–4.9 cm., and there is further growth and darkening of the scrotum. During this stage, there is significant phallic growth, both in length and width, and an increase in the size of the glans. Finally, in stage 5, the appearance is that of adult male genitalia; the testes are larger than 5 cm in length; the scrotum is pigmented; and adult phallus size is attained.

ANATOMICAL TERMS OF FEMALE EXTERNAL GENITALIA

SUSAN POKORNY

Physicians performing genital assessments on young females must use proper anatomical terms (Fig. 7–5). The most consistently present landmark is the prominent clitoris, which frequently looks hypertrophic because of the lack of development of other structures and the lack of subcutaneous fat in most young girls. The next structures most easily identified are the labia minora. These two narrow ridges converge in the midline under the prepuce or clitoral hood. They form the anterior lateral margins and the anterior apex of the vulvar vault or vestibule. Bilateral lines drawn posteriorly from the caudal tips of the labia minora and converging medially to meet in the midline at the posterior fourchette constitute the posterior lateral margins and posterior aspect of the vestibule. These lines have been referred to as Hart's lines.

Occasionally, vulvar and/or labial agglutination is so extensive that the only easily identifiable structure is the clitoris. In rare situations the clitoris can also be covered completely by agglutinated skin folds; more frequently, the prepuce can be so agglutinated that it cannot be retracted sufficiently to expose the underlying glans clitoris. The mons and labia majora are not developed in the young child; they are the mounds of tissue anterior and lateral to, respectively, the vestibule and the marginal structures of the vestibule mentioned above.

Within the vestibule the two most important structures are the urethra and the vaginal orifice. Both of these structures have a broad range of normal variation with the site of greatest variability being in the suburethral area and in the anterior periurethral area of the vagina where it is not uncommon to see a variety of mucosal mounds and ridges. The urethra itself can be a pinhole opening or a patulous structure. When the latter becomes congested, necrotic, and inflamed, it is called urethral prolapse. Lateral to the urethra are the Skene's periurethral glands. The crypts and mucosal bands associated with these glands can be quite prominent.

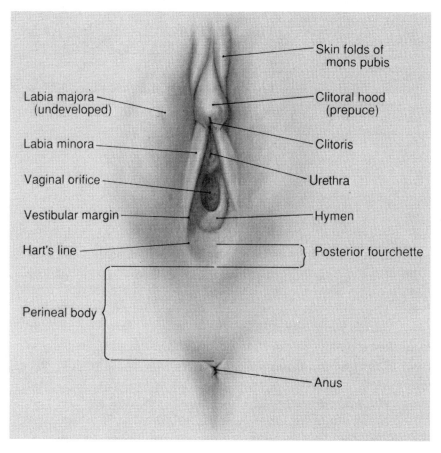

Labia majora
(undeveloped)

Labia minora

Vaginal orifice

Vestibular margin

Hart's line

Perineal body

Skin folds of
mons pubis

Clitoral hood
(prepuce)

Clitoris

Urethra

Hymen

Posterior fourchette

Anus

Fig. 7–5. The prepubertal vulva.

The vaginal orifice is surrounded by a collar or skirt of tissue called the hymen. Terminology has developed so that the hymen is described in a clock-like fashion, with the 12 o'clock position being the suburethral area and the 6 o'clock position being toward the rectum when the patient is in a supine position. The hymen, like the rest of the genital structures, is under the influence of hormones. In the unestrogenized state of the prepubertal years, variations in its configuration are most marked.

Hymenal tissue can be totally absent in the suburethral area from approximately the 10 or 11 o'clock position clockwise to approximately the 1 or 2 o'clock position. The skirt of tissue extending posteriorly can be long or short, creating a high or low posterior rim of tissue, respectively. This configuration of the hymen also has been described as a thick or thin crescent-shaped hymen.

Another common hymen configuration occurs when the skirt of tissue completely circumscribes the vaginal orifice. This hymen has been called annular or circumferential. Frequently there is a cleft in the hymenal skirt of tissue at the 11 o'clock, 12 o'clock, or 1 o'clock position, and the orifice is anteriorly placed.

Estrogen makes the hymenal tissue more redundant, so that it folds on itself, the margins become scalloped, and it protrudes as a prominent turtleneck collar of tissue. This hymenal configuration is also seen with variations in the unestrogenized child and is called fimbriated or denticular hymen. Breaks, tears, or other abnormalities can easily be missed in this type of hymen unless specifically looked for by exploring the margins of the hymenal skirt with a cotton-tipped swab and/or rubber catheter.

The mucosa lining the vulvar vault or vestibule, lateral and posterior to the vaginal orifice and hymen, should be smooth without folds or crypts. The area where acute vulvar trauma is frequently apparent is on the posterior fourchette, that aspect of the vulva between the vaginal margin and the perineal body. The latter is the muscular and fibrous skin-covered bridge of tissue between the vulvar vault and vestibule and the rectum.

REFERENCES

EMBRYOLOGY OF THE GENITAL TRACT

Berta, P, JR Hawkins, AH Sinclair, A Taylor, BL Griffiths, PN Goodfellow, and M Fellous. Genetic evidence equating SRY and the testis-determining factor. *Nature*. 1990;348:448–450.

Cates, RL, RJ Mattaliano, C Hession, R Tizard, NM Farber, A Cheung, EG Ninfa, AZ Frey, DJ Gash, EP Chow, et al. Isolation of the bovine and human genes for Müllerian inhibiting substance and expression of the human gene in animal cells. *Cell*. 1986;45:685–698.

Clarnette, TD, Y Sugita, and JM Hutson. Genital anomalies in human and animal models reveal the mechanisms and hormones governing testicular descent. *Br J Urol*. 1997; 79(1):99–11.

Cohen-Haguenauer, O, JY Picard, MG Mattei, S Serero, VC Nguyen, MF de Tand, D Guerrier, MC Hors-Cayla, N Josso, and J. Frezal Mapping of the gene for anti-Müllerian hormone to the short arm of human chromosome 19. *Cytogenet Cell Genet*. 1987;44:2–6.

Dubin, RA, and H Ostrer. SRY is a transcriptional activator. *Mol Endocrinol*. 8:1994;1182–1192.

Harley, VR, DI Jackson, PJ Hextall, JR Hawkins, GD Berkovitz, S Sockanathan, R Lovell-Badge, and PN Goodfellow. DNA binding activity of recombinant SRY from normal males and XY females. *Science*. 1992;255:453–456.

Imbeaud S, R Rey, P Berta, JL Chaussain, JM Wit, RH Lustig, MA De Vroede, JY Picard, and N Josso. Testicular degeneration in three patients with the persistent Müllerian duct syndrome. *Eur J Pediatr.* 1995; 154(3):187–90.

Jarminska-Jackowiak, T, A Warenik-Szymankiewicz, and WH Trzeciak. Anti-Müllerian hormone. Structure and role in sexual differentiation. *Ginekol Pol.* 1995; 66(1):51–8.

Moore, CC, and MM Grumbach. Sex determination and gonadogenesis: A transcription cascade of sex chromosome and autosome genes. *Semin Perinatol.* 1992;16:266–278.

Page, DC, R Mosher, EM Simpson, EM Fisher, G Mardon, J Pollack, B McGillvray, A de la Chapelle and LG Brown. The sex-determining region of the human Y chromosome encodes a finger protein. *Cell.* 1987;5:1091–1104.

Sinclair, AH, P Berta, MS Palmer, JR Hawkins, BL Griffiths, MJ Smith, JW Foster, AM Frischauf, R Lovell-Badge, and PN Goodfellow. A gene from the human sex-determining region encodes a protein with homology to a conserved DNA-binding motif. *Nature.* 1990;346:240–244.

Further Reading

Behringer, RR. The in vivo roles of Müllerian-inhibiting substance. *Curr Top Dev Biol.* 1994;29:171–187.

Behringer, RR, MJ Finegold, and RL Cate. Müllerian inhibiting substance function during mammalian sexual development. *Cell.* 1994;79:415–425.

Bogan, JS, and D Page. Ovary? Testis? — A mammalian dilemma. *Cell.* 1994;76: 603–607.

Emans, SJ, MR Laufer, and DP Goldstein. *Pediatr Adolesc Gynecol.* 4th Ed. Lippincott-Raven: Philadelphia, PA, 1998.

Graves, JA. The evolution of mammalian sex chromosomes and the origin of sex determining genes. *Phil Trans R Soc Ser B Biol Sci.* 1995;350: 305.

Gubbay, J, J Collignon, P Koopman, B Capel, A Economou, A Munsterberg, N Vivian, P Goodfellow, and R Lovell-Badge. A gene mapping to the sex-determining region of the mouse Y chromosome is a member of a novel family of embryonically expressed genes. *Nature.* 1990;346(6281):245–50.

Haqq, CM, CY King, E Ukiyama, S Falsafi, TN Haqq, PK Donahoe, and MA Weiss. Molecular basis of mammalian sexual determination: activation of Müllerian inhibiting substance gene expression by SRY. *Science.* 1994; 266(5190):1494–500.

Koopman, P, J Gubbay, N Vivian, P Goodfellow, and R Lovell-Badge. Male development of chromosomally female mice transgenic for SRY. *Nature.* 1991; 351:117–121.

Larsen, WJ. *Essentials of Human Embryology.* Churchill Livingstone: New York, 1998.

McElreavey, K, E Vilain, N Abbas, I Herskowitz, and M Fellous. A regulatory cascade hypothesis for mammalian sex determination: SRY represses a negative regulator of male development. *Proc Natl Acad Sci USA.* 1993;90(8):3368–72.

Moore, KL. *The Developing Human: Clinically Oriented Embryology.* 3rd Ed. W.B. Saunders: Philadelphia; 1982.

Richards, JS, SL Fitzpatrick, JW Clemens, JK Morris, T Alliston, and J Sirois, Ovarian cell differentiation: A cascade of multiple hormones, cellular signals, and regulated genes. *Recent Prog. Horm. Res.* 1995:223–54,50.

Ryner, LC, and A Swain. Sex in the 90s. *Cell.* 1995;81:483–493.

Sanfilippo, J, D Muram, P Lee, and JC Dewhurst. *Pediatr Adolesc Gynecol.* W. B. Saunders Co.: Philadelphia, 1994.

Satoh, M. Histogenesis and organogenesis of the gonad in human embryos. *J. Anat.* 1991;177:85–107.

ANATOMICAL AND PHYSIOLOGIC CHANGES

Herman-Giddens, ME, EJ Slora, RC Wasserman, CJ Bourdony, MV Bhapkar, GG Koch, and CM Hasemeier. Secondary sexual characteristics and menses in young girls seen in office practice: A study from the Pediatric. Research in Office Settings network. *Pediatrics.* 1997; 99:505–512.

Marshall, WA, and JM Tanner. Variations in pattern of pubertal changes in girls. *Arch Dis Child.* 1969;44:291–303.

Further Reading

Apter, D. Development of the hypothalamic-pituitary-ovarian axis. *Ann NY Acad Sci.* 1997;816:9–21.

Arslanian, S, C Suprasongsin, SC Kalhan, AL Drash, R Brna, and JE Janosky. Plasma in children: Relationship to puberty, gender, body composition, insulin sensitivity, and energy expenditure: *Metab Clin Exp.* 1998;47:309–12.

Brzezinski, A. Melatonin in humans. *N Engl J Med.* 1997;336:186–95.

Kiess, W, WF Blum, and ML Aubert. Leptin, puberty and reproductive function: Lessons from animal studies and observations in humans. *Eur J Endocrinol.* 1998;138:26–9.

Kulin, HE, JW Finkelstein, MR D'Arcangelo, EJ Susman, V Chinchilli, S Unselman, J Schwab, L Demers, and G Lookingbill. Diversity of pubertal testosterone changes in boys with constitutional delay in growth and/or adolescence. *J Pediatr Endocrinol Metab.* 1997;10:395–400.

Liu, YX, F Jalil, and J Karlberg. Risk factors for impaired length growth in early life viewed in terms of the infancy-childhood-puberty (ICP) growth model. *Acta Paediatr.* 1998;87:237–43.

Lunenfeld, B, and V Insler. An overview of obesity during puberty, adolescence, and reproduction. *Arch Gynecol Obstet.* 1997;261:31–4.

Mantzoros, CS, JS Flier, and AD Rogol. A longitudinal assessment of hormonal and physical alterations during normal puberty in boys: V. Rising leptin levels may signal the onset of puberty. *J Clin Endocrinol Metab.* 1997;82:1066–70.

Robinson, P. Puberty—am I normal? *Pediatr Ann.* 1997;26(2 Suppl):S133–6.

Roemmich, JN, PA Clark. V Mai, SS Berr, A Weltman, JD Veldhuis, and AD Rogol. Alterations in growth and body composition during puberty: III. Influence of maturation, gender, body composition, fat distribution, aerobic fitness, and energy expenditure on nocturnal growth hormone release. *J Clin Endocrinol Metab.* 1998;83:1440–7.

Roemmich, JN, PA Clark, A Weltman, and AD Rogol. Alterations in growth and body composition during puberty: I. Comparing multicompartment body composition models. *J Appl Physiol.* 1997;83:927–35.

Rotteveel, J, C de Ridder, E Schoute, and HA Delemarre-van de Waal. Androstenedione, dehydroepiandrosterone sulfate, and estradiol levels throughout female puberty: Relation to height velocity. *Horm Res.* 1997;48:263–7.

Sharara, FI, and LC Giudice. Role of growth hormone in ovarian physiology and onset of puberty. *J Soc Gynecol Invest.* 1997;4:2–7.

Toublanc, JE. Modifications of growth hormone secretion during female puberty. *Ann NY Acad Sci.* 1997;816:60–75.

ANATOMICAL TERMS OF FEMALE EXTERNAL GENITALIA

Further Reading

Kaufman RH, Friedrich EG Jr, Gardner HL. Anatomy of the vulva and vagina. In: Kaufman RH, Friedrich EG Jr, Gardner HL, eds. *Benign Diseases of the Vulva and Vagina.* 3rd ed. Chicago: Year Book Medical Publishers, 1989.

Mahran M, Saleh AM. The microscopic anatomy of the hymen. *Anat Rec* 1964;149:313–318.

Pokorny SF. Configuration of the prepubertal hymen. *Am J Obstet Gymecol* 1987;157:950–956.

8

PHOTOGRAPHIC ATLAS

This new edition includes new and original plates arranged in sections that illustrate normal anatomy, developmental changes, changes with examination techniques, and nonspecific findings or medical conditions that might be confused with sexual abuse. The sections on anal findings and STDs have been expanded, and a new section on adolescents has been added. In addition, the color atlas includes follow-up examinations of acute injuries from diagnosis through to healing. These longitudinal presentations provide insight into the process of genital healing, which may be extrapolated, to some extent, to interpretation of medical findings in patients evaluated weeks, months, or even years after abuse.

NORMAL GENITALIA

The appearance of the hymen and changes in size of hymenal opening depend on inborn anatomical variations, the size and age of the child, stage of development, and changes in examination technique. Basic differences in morphology are best demonstrated by evaluation of the post-infancy, prepubertal hymen. During this period the hymen is free of any estrogen effects and has the appearance of a smooth, thin membrane. Most prepubertal hymens can be described as crescentic (posterior rim). These hymens attach ventrally at the 10–11 o'clock position and from the 1–2 o'clock position, and in some cases have redundant hymenal tissue surrounding the urethra. The annular hymen is less common and is characterized by tissue surrounding a central opening. Occasionally hymens may be redundant and/or fimbriated, sleeve-like with a ruffled or fringed edge, or appear to have a vertical opening. Other types of hymen include septate hymen (less than 5 percent), cribriform hymen, microperforate hymen, and imperforate hymen.

Developmental changes in the hymen depend on the effects of estrogens. In the newborn, maternal estrogens cause the hymen to appear thickened, sleeve-like, fimbriated, or redundant. The hymenal configuration in the newborn is usually annular, but as estrogen levels wane hymenal tissue appears to diminish ventrally, and most hymens become crescentic. In addition, the hymen becomes thin, translucent, and "scanty." As a girl approaches puberty, the hymen once again assumes a redundant, fimbriated, or rolled appearance. These hymens can have the appearance of a sleeve with a "cuff" of hymenal tissue that can appear "rolled" or "ruffled".

EXAMINATION POSITIONS AND TECHNIQUES

Both the examiner's technique and the position of the patient affect the evaluation of the hymen and introitus. Labial separation and traction are used to visualize the hymen in the supine position. Examination may include the use of water, viscous xylocaine, cotton-tipped applicators, or Foley catheter to evaluate the integrity of the hymenal tissues. In cases in which the posterior rim of the hymen is not easily visualized in the supine position, the child may be placed in the knee-chest position.

CONGENITAL VARIANTS

Anomalies of the genitalia can be divided into two major categories—those that suggest sexual ambiguity (intersex problems), and those that do not. Ambiguous genitalia denote a partial or incomplete virilization of the external genitalia. Ambiguous genitalia may be seen in genetic females who were virilized in utero, in undervirilized males, or in true hermaphrodites.

The hymenal orifice may vary in diameter from very small to very large. There may be one or more small orifices. A thick median ridge separating two lateral hymenal orifices may suggest a septate vagina. The hymenal diaphragm may be a thin membrane or a thickened and fibrous one forming a firm partition. An imperforate hymen forms a solid membrane without an aperture. Occasionally, what initially appears to be an imperforate hymen is found to have one or more tiny openings, a microperforate hymen.

NONSPECIFIC CHANGES

In addition to these normal hymenal variations, there are a number of non-specific changes. For example, mounds are frequently found in association with intravaginal ridges or folds that extend onto the vaginal surface of the hymen and beyond the hymenal rim. The examiner may observe notches and mounds representing congenital remnants. An external hymenal ridge at 6-o'clock is common in newborns. Complete notches or clefts are common in the ventral 180 degrees (between 9-o'clock and 3-o'clock), with the majority occurring at the 12-o'clock position. Complete clefts have not been documented in the lower (dorsal) half of the hymen in prepubertal girls. A small percentage of non-sexually active adolescent girls may have complete notches or clefts in the dorsal portion of the hymen between 3-o'clock and 9-o'clock. Periurethral support bands, or ligaments, appear as symmetrical bands of tissue just lateral to the urethra or attached from the base of the hymen to the vestibular walls. Other hymenal variants include vitiligo, ridges, tags, changes in vascularity, erythema, cysts, and polyps.

ANATOMIC VARIATIONS AND MEDICAL CONDITIONS: DIAGNOSTIC CHALLENGES

As already noted, there are a number of anatomical variations or medical conditions that may be misinterpreted by an inexperienced examiner. These include failure of midline fusion, erythema typical of the non-estrogenized hymen, nonspecific vulvar ulcerations, contact dermatitis, and hemangiomas. Exposed intravaginal rugae may protrude above the hymeneal edge (a mound) and be confused with a healed transection. Labial fusion is quite common in the pre-pubescent female and may occur with or after vulvar irritation. With labial fusion, anatomic landmarks are obscured, and the line of fusion may break down during normal activity or as a result of straddle injury. This is commonly reported as "blood in the underwear." Urethral prolapse may also present with "vaginal bleeding," and the protruding tissue may be mistaken for a swollen hymen. Lichen sclerosus may cause vulvar bleeding, and the examiner may be concerned that such lesions represent genital trauma. Some of the more common conditions that cause genital bleeding are listed in Table 8–1.

Table 8–1. GENITAL BLEEDING

Trauma

    Accidental injury
    Sexual assault

Vulvovaginitis

    Shigella
    B-Streptococcus
    Pinworms

Labial fusion/adhesions

Foreign body

Neonatal maternal estrogen withdrawal

Tags and or polyps

Lichen sclerosus

Condyloma acuminata

Tumor

Precocious puberty

Hemangiomas

Blood dyscrasias

Urinary tract infection

Urethral prolapse

Periurethral cysts

ACUTE GENITAL TRAUMA—ACCIDENTAL

Accidental injuries can closely mimic the injuries of sexual assault. In all cases of genital trauma, the history provided by the child is vital to a correct diagnosis. In girls, accidental injuries usually cause trauma to the vulva, perineum, or labia, sparing the hymen, which is an internal structure. However, hymenal damage does occur in rare cases of accidental penetrating trauma. A straddle injury caused by falling on a curb-like edge or gymnastic equipment may cause damage to the posterior fourchette. The presence of a hymenal laceration should alert the clinician to the possibility of sexual abuse or accidental penetration injury (nail, pencil, or picket fence). Examination under anesthesia is often necessary to evaluate the extent of injuries and to facilitate the repair of introital and hymenal tissues. Straddle injuries in boys can result in significant abrasions and bruising of the scrotum and penis.

FEMALE GENITAL MUTILATION

The term female genital mutilation (FMG) refers to the excision of the clitoris and parts of the labia majora and minora. This procedure, previously termed "female circumcision," is a common practice in Africa, the Middle East, and Southeast Asia. The procedure significantly alters the appearance of the vulva; "membrane" made of labial remnants sutured in the midline obscures the normal anatomic landmarks.

ACUTE GENITAL TRAUMA—SEXUAL ABUSE

It is important to remember that in most sexual abuse cases there is no evidence of painful, forced trauma. However, in those cases in which the victim is examined shortly after the assault, abrasions, lacerations, and bruising may be noted. The genitalia heal rapidly and may appear normal after a short time period.

Prospective, longitudinal research into the healing patterns of injuries of the vagina and anus has provided knowledge of how some injuries can heal completely while others leave pathognomonic signs of penetrating trauma. In most cases of sexual abuse of the prepubescent there is no penetration of the vagina with injury to the hymen. In cases of fondling, simulated intercourse, or penetration to the level of the hymen, there may be acute abrasions or bruising of the vestibular mucosa that heal completely within days. However, penetrating vaginal injuries cause hymenal transections. Through and through hymenal disruptions do not heal spontaneously and often result in a persistent, transection or cleft that extends to the base of the hymen. In contrast, partial transections of the vestibular hymenal mucosa may heal spontaneously.

SEXUAL ABUSE—DELAYED DISCLOSURE

What we termed "chronic changes" in the previous edition are better described as medical findings associated with healed genital trauma. Since most children delay disclosure, medical professionals are typically asked to evaluate a child long after any injuries should have healed. However, as noted previously, when there has been significant trauma associated with vaginal penetration, healed disruptions of the posterior fourchette, vestibular mucosa, hymen, and anus may be found.

NORMAL ANI AND NONSPECIFIC CHANGES

Position, technique, and cooperation from the child assist in the evaluation of the anus. Supine, prone, and left-lateral positions are used. With any of these positions, the anal and perianal soft tissues can be examined and the sphincter tone evaluated. A venous plexus surrounds the perianal area. These veins can become prominent during the examination and be misdiagnosed as bruising. Skinfolds and tags, venous lakes, erythema, and other nonspecific variations are frequently noted. Redundant folds of tissue at the 12-o'clock and 6-o'clock positions are often seen.

Anal tone is dependent on both involuntary and voluntary control. Relaxed anal tone can be secondary to the presence of feces in the rectal ampulla. However, "reflex anal dilatation" may occur in any patient with lateral traction. Excessive anal dilatation is seen in some patients with specific gastrointestinal diseases, such as Hirschsprung's disease, but also may be due to chronic anal abuse.

Infections, infestations, and poor hygiene can be present with nonspecific anal changes like erythema, hyperpigmentation, cellulitis, and pinworms. Lichen sclerosus also can involve the peri-anal area. Superficial anal fissures occur in children with constipation, as well as in some children who have been anally penetrated. Rectal prolapse is another anoraly seen in children with rectal pathology, as well as following anal abuse.

Tags may develop as fissures or lacerations heal, and can be located anywhere around the anal opening.

ANAL TRAUMA AND HEALING

Most victims of anal trauma remain free of any medical findings. However, penetrating anal trauma can result in abrasions, fissures, lacerations, bruising, and edema. Most acute findings heal within a matter of days to weeks. Rare cases in which there has been serious tissue damage or tears through the external sphincter may heal with scarring. Anal tone may be acutely altered, but usually resolves over time. Only those anal injuries with serious deep-tissue damage heal with scarring. Simple fissures and lacerations heal quickly and completely, although occasionally superficial injuries may form a skin tag.

ADOLESCENTS

Estrogen effects provide some protection to the genitalia from injury during intercourse or sexual assault. Estrogenized tissues are thick, moist, and elastic. During penetration, the hymen can stretch and escape trauma. It is not uncommon, therefore, for many victims of sexual assault to present without evidence of acute or old injuries, yet some minor injuries are frequently seen immediately after an assault. It is imperative to document such findings because these injuries heal within a few days, and on a follow-up examination the genitalia appear normal.

Because of the effects of estrogen and the anatomy of the redundant or fimbriated hymen, the adolescent may have a normal-appearing introitus and hymen after healing. This is particularly true when the penetration has resulted in only partial tears of the hymen. Such tears heal and later may appear as clefts or notches indistinguishable from normal adolescent anatomy.

Many adolescents participate in an ongoing consensual sexual relationship. It is impossible to distinguish a healed tear that occurred following consensual intercourse from a tear caused in an assault.

SEXUALLY TRANSMITTED DISEASES

The evaluation for sexually transmitted disease (STD) in the child or adolescent is a major focus of the medical examination for alleged sexual abuse. Most survey studies estimate the incidence of STDs in sexually abused children to be one to five percent. STDs are discussed in greater detail in Chapter 9.

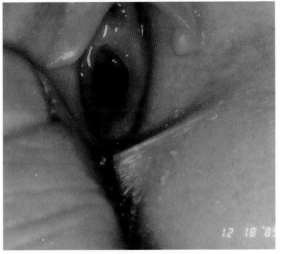

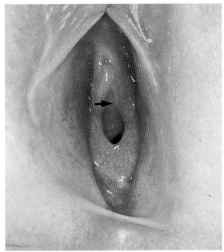

Annular hymen. Thin, wispy annular hymen in a 3-year-old. Hymen is translucent with smooth, symmetrical hymenal opening. (Levitt)

Annular hymen with cleft at the 12-o'clock position. A 10-year-old with a history of vulvovaginitis. Note normal annular symmetrical hymen with a cleft at the 12-o'clock position. (Pokorny)

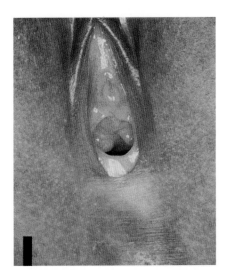

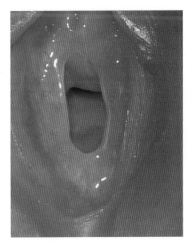

Annular hymen. A five-year-old treated 2 months earlier for vulvovaginitis with a positive *Neisseria gonorrhoeae* culture. Note normal-appearing annular hymen with smooth, symmetrical edges. With relaxation, normal vaginal rugae are easily visualized. (Pokorny)

Annular hymen in a 9-year-old. A 9-year-old with an oval-shaped annular hymen. A measuring device is useful in determining accurate hymenal opening diameters.

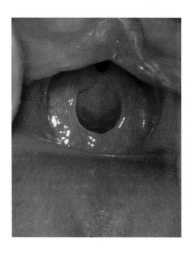

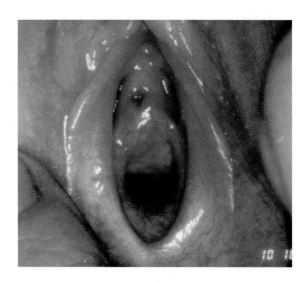

Crescentic hymen. A 4-year-old with a crescentic hymen. Note that in the crescentic hymen there is an absence of tissue ventrally.

Crescentic hymen. A thin, wispy crescent-shaped hymen in a 3-year-old. Note the asymmetry caused by traction to one side. (Levitt)

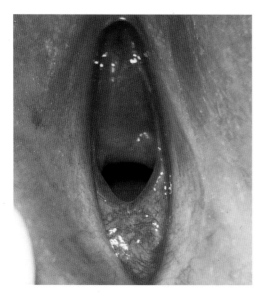

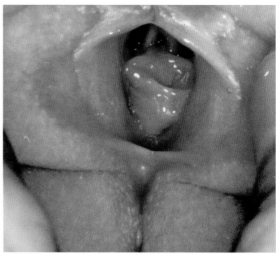

Crescentic hymen. An 8-year-old with a smooth-edged crescentic hymen.

Redundant hymen. A redundant, sleevelike hymen in a 3-year-old. Note symmetry of hymenal opening and vascularity. Urethra and support bands seen ventrally. Note small anterior labial fusion. (Levitt)

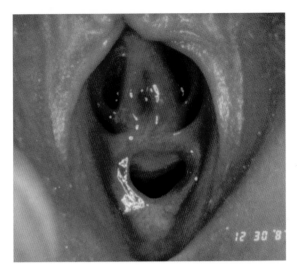

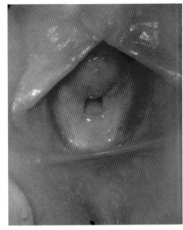

Urethral support ligaments. Normal bands of tissue in the periurethral area demonstrated in a 6-year-old girl. The hymen is normal crescentic with a smooth edge and lacy vascularity. (Levitt)

Crescentic hymen. A 4-year-old with a smooth-edged crescentic hymen. Prominent redundant tissue centrally obscures urethra.

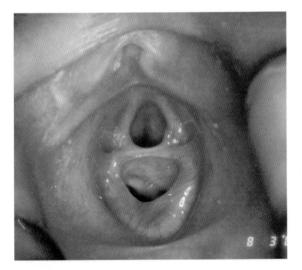

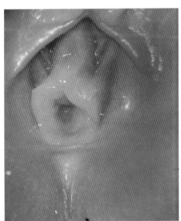

Patulous urethra. Patulous urethra in a 4-year-old. Normal-appearing annular hymen with smooth, velamentous edge; symmetrical with lacy vascular pattern. Note the prominent periurethral support ligaments and symmetrical fossae ventrally. Intravaginal rugae can be easily seen. (Levitt)

Redundant hymen. A 2-year-old with a fimbriated, redundant hymen that appears sleevelike and symmetrical with normal vascular pattern. Note the prominent periurethral support ligaments (bands).

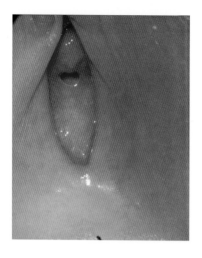

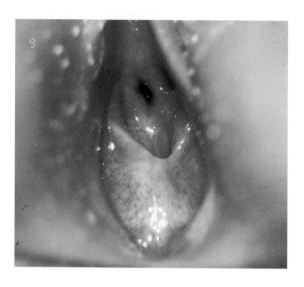

Anterior opening. A 3-year-old with a small (2 mm) anterior opening in a crescentic hymen. Hymenal edges are smooth and translucent, appearing with lacy, symmetrical vascular pattern.

Crescentic hymen. A 7-year-old with a crescentic hymen and a ventral/vertical opening.

DEVELOPMENTAL CHANGES

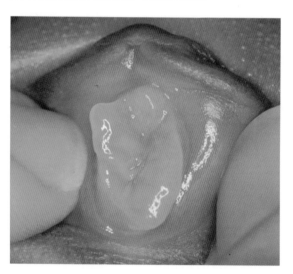

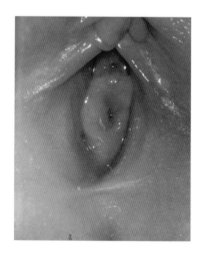

Normal hymen in the first year of life. An 8-month-old with a sleevelike annular hymen. The hymen appears redundant and thickened, suggesting hormonal influence. The edge of hymen is smooth and nondisrupted with normal vascular pattern.

Normal newborn. Thick, boggy redundant hymen found in the newborn. Note the longitudinal intravaginal ridges that extend to the edge of the hymen. (From Berensen A, Heger A, Andrews S. Appearance of the hymen in newborns. *Pediatrics* 1991;87:458–64. Reprinted by permission.)

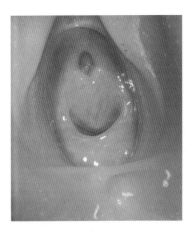

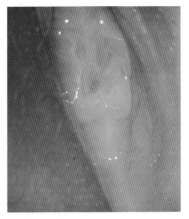

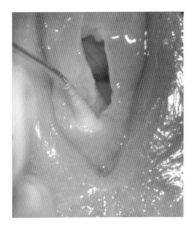

Crescentic hymen in a 6-year-old. A "scanty" crescentic hymen with a diameter of 5 mm. Note the attachment of crescentic hymen at the 1-o'clock and 11-o'clock positions.

Estrogen effects of puberty. A 13-year-old with estrogen effects causing thickening of the hymen. The hymen is a sleeve-like structure, and the ruffling or fringed edges are common in adolescence.

A normal adolescent. The smooth-edged, estrogenized hymen of early adolescence. The cotton swab demonstrates a technique for evaluating a fimbriated hymen for the presence of disruptions or transections.

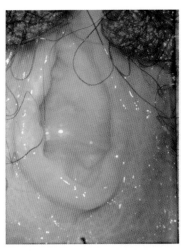

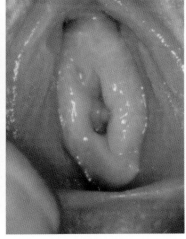

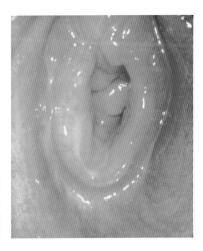

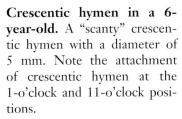

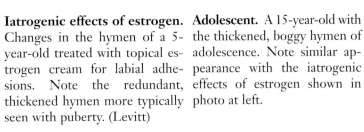

Sexually active teenager. A 16-year-old engaged in consensual sexual activities. Note the thickened, stretched hymen, and Tanner V pubic hair. The posterior fourchette is free of any posttraumatic changes.

Iatrogenic effects of estrogen. Changes in the hymen of a 5-year-old treated with topical estrogen cream for labial adhesions. Note the redundant, thickened hymen more typically seen with puberty. (Levitt)

Adolescent. A 15-year-old with the thickened, boggy hymen of adolescence. Note similar appearance with the iatrogenic effects of estrogen shown in photo at left.

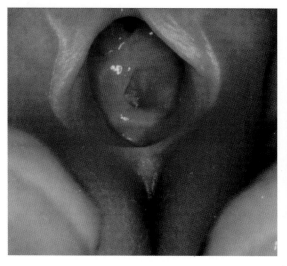

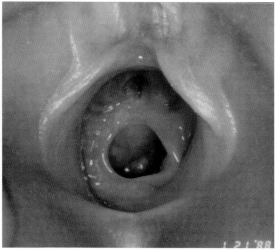

Hymenal changes with relaxation. Left: Hymen of a 3-year-old, appearing more thickened or redundant before she is totally relaxed. Hymenal diameter also appears smaller. **Right:** With relaxation, the hymen appears thinned out and has a larger opening as the vaginal vault opens with complete relaxation. The hymenal edge appears to be smooth and symmetrical with some slight redundancy remaining at the 4-o'clock to 5-o'clock position (**right panel**). (Levitt)

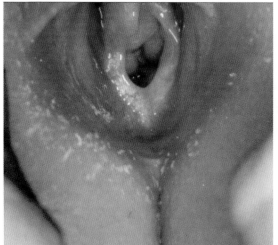

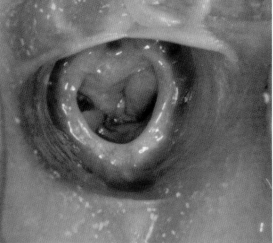

Hymenal changes with traction. The hymen of a 4-year-old with an apparent cleft at the 1-o'clock position. With traction and relaxation, the hymen is drawn open and the cleft is no longer apparent. (Levitt)

Hymenal changes with traction. Normal crescentic hymen with smooth, symmetrical edges, lacy vascularity, and good intravaginal visualization. Note how traction changes the size of the hymenal opening. (Levitt)

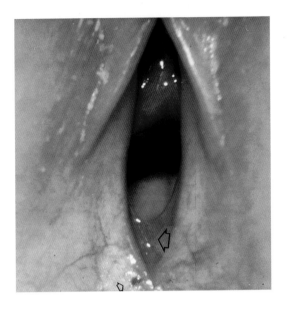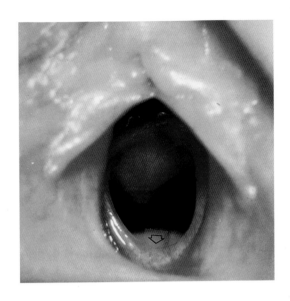

Traction and changes in the hymen. An 8-year-old with a normal crescentic hymen. **Left:** With labial traction ventrally and toward the examiner, note the depth of the hymen apparent at 6-o'clock (large arrow) **Right:** With a slight increase in traction and the addition of more dorsal traction, the depth of hymen appears to be diminished (large arrow). (The small arrow points to slight breakdown of labial fusion during the examination.

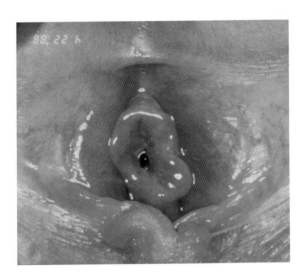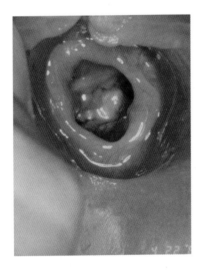

Need for improved visualization. A 6-year-old with a history of sexual abuse by her father. The purulent vaginal discharge interferes with visualization (see next illustration).

Improved intravaginal visualization with traction. With traction, the child from the preceding illustration was found to have an intravaginal foreign body (yellow tack), which was removed under anesthesia. The hymen is annular and redundant, without evidence of trauma. (Levitt)

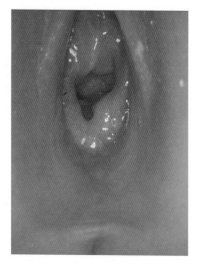 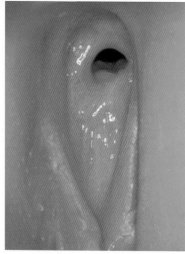

Normal examination in a competitive gymnast. Left: Supine position: Crescentic hymen with mound of tissue between the 3-o'clock and 6-o'clock positions. Note small diameter, smooth edges, and symmetrical vascularity **Right:** Prone position (knee-chest): Mound of tissue disappears, as gravity pulls smooth edge of the hymen ventrally. (Stewart)

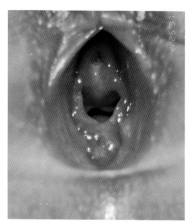 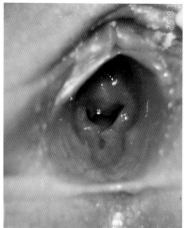 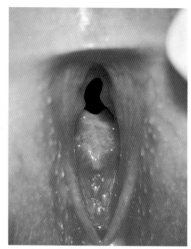

Traction, water, and prone position. Left: A 3-year-old with a crescentic hymen and normal erythema, but with an apparent "fold" of the hymen at 6-o'clock. **Center:** The hymen with the patient in the supine position after the hymen was "floated" with water. **Right:** Note the symmetrical hymenal tags or mounds at 4-o'clock and 8-o'clock that persist with the patient in the prone position.

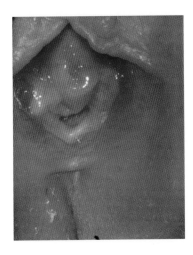
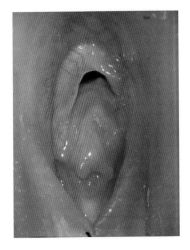
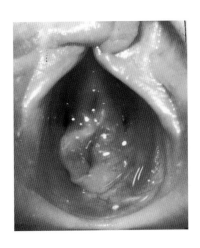

Changes in hymenal morphology with a change in position. Left: Supine position with hymenal irregularities noted in the posterior 180°. Note redundant tissue surrounding the urethra. **Right:** Prone/knee-chest position allowing for visualization of the posterior 180°. The hymen now appears to be crescentic, with a smooth symmetrical edge, normal notching at the 1-o'clock and 11-o'clock positions (supine), and persistence of the periurethral redundant tissue.

Using water to "float" the hymen with the patient lying supine. A 2-year-old with redundant hymen. Hymenal edges are easily evaluated with the addition of water.

CONGENITAL VARIANTS AND MALFORMATIONS

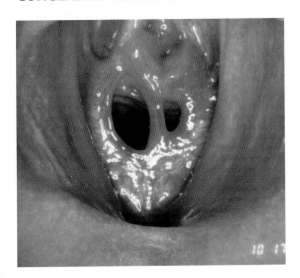
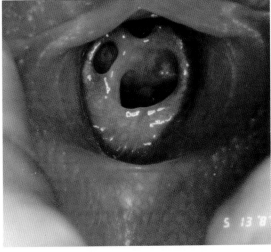

Septate hymen. Septate hymen with midline septum in a 10-year-old. This septum was not readily recognized until the vaginal vault was completely relaxed and gaping open. Note the prominent support ligaments and smooth-edged hymen, glistening mucous membranes, and lacy vascularity. (Levitt)

Septate hymen. Septate hymen in a 6-year-old, with eccentrically placed septum. The hymen remains smooth edged and translucent. The urethra appears enlarged but is normal. (Levitt)

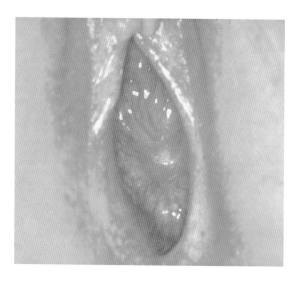

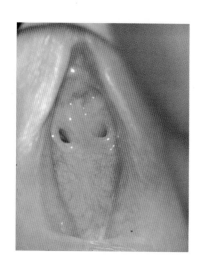

Imperforate hymen. A 4-year-old with imperforate hymen and normal vagina and uterus. (Stewart)

Double microperforate hymen. A 5-year-old with two microperforate hymenal openings ventrally.

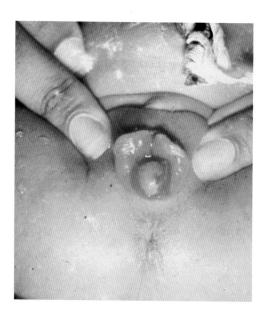

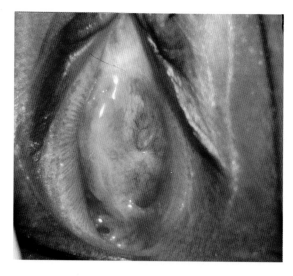

A newborn infant with an imperforate hymen. A large mucocolpos distends the vagina causing the hymenal membrane to bulge outward. (Dr. S. Koronas)

Vaginal agenesis. A 9-year-old with vaginal agenesis. While the appearance is similar to imperforate hymen, pelvic ultrasound shows absence of vagina and uterus.

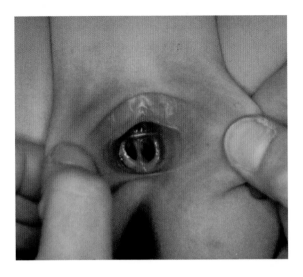

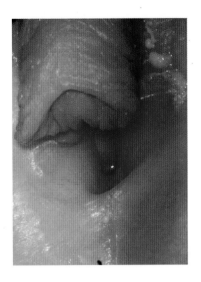

Duplication of the vagina. A 3-year-old with duplication of the vagina noted during an evaluation for vaginitis. She was found to have a double cervix and uteri. (From Emans SJ, Goldstein DP. *Pediatric and Adolescent Gynecology.* 3rd ed. Boston: Little, Brown, 1990. Reprinted by permission.)

Ambiguous genitalia. A 2½-year-old with congenital adrenal hyperplasia and secondary virilization and clitoral hypertrophy.

NONSPECIFIC CHANGES

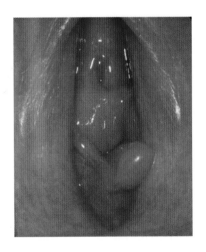

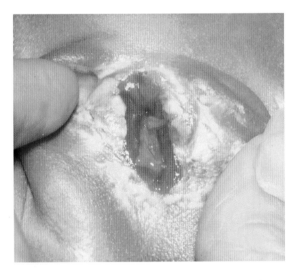

Hymenal tag. An 8-year-old with a 2-year history of genital fondling. Plate shows polypoid hymenal tag at the 5-o'clock to 6-o'clock position. (Stewart)

Hymenal tags. Hymen in newborn with tags at the 12-o'clock position and the 6-o'clock to 7-o'clock positions. Maternal estrogen effects cause this thickening and redundancy in the newborn hymen. (Jenny)

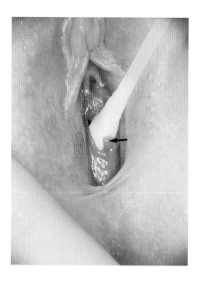

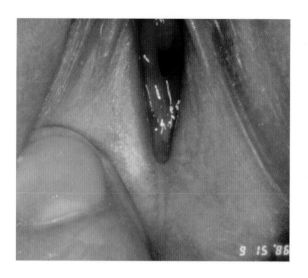

Hymenal tag. Hymenal tag (arrow) found during examination under anesthesia of an 8-year-old child with a year-long history of mucoid vaginal discharge. The tag is similar in appearance to the hymen. (Pokorny)

Median raphe (posterior fourchette). Midline sparing of vascularity extending from posterior fourchette in a 6-year-old. This can be misinterpreted as a scar. Crescentic hymen with smooth, symmetrical edges and lacy vascularity. (Levitt)

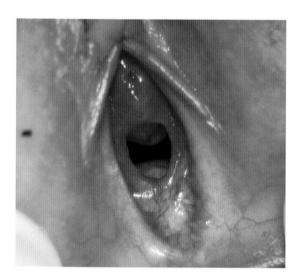

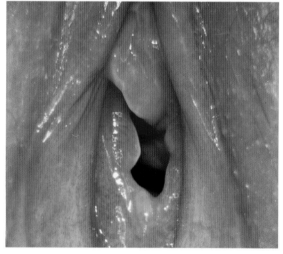

A 6-year-old with the normal "erythema" of latency age, associated with the irregular vascular pattern of the hymen and fossa navicularis.

An early pubescent 11-year-old with irregular hymenal edge. Under the effects of estrogens, the ventral peri-urethral tissue is enhanced, thus reforming the annular hymen of adolescence.

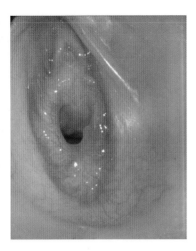

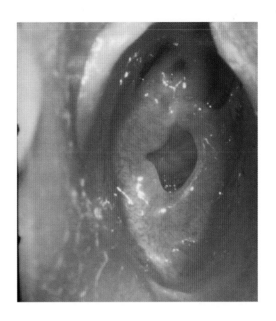

Hymenal mound. A 3-year-old referred for evaluation of possible abnormal examination. The crescentic hymen is normal with a mound at the 5-o'clock position. Mound appears to be a normal variant with continuation or normal lacy vascularity and a smooth translucent edge. The introital vascular pattern is even and symmetrical.

Normal hymen with notch. Smooth-edged, almost annular hymen with symmetrical vascularity. The notch/cleft at the 9-o'clock position is smooth with translucent edges and normal vascular pattern. Periurethral support ligaments seen laterally to urethra. 3-year-old.

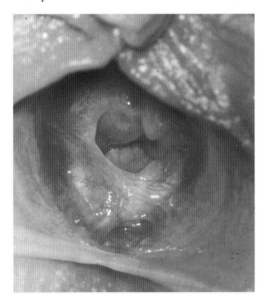

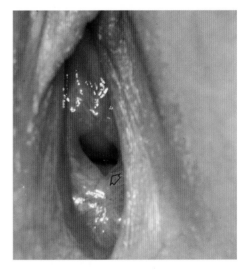

Peri-hymenal bands with notch. A 2-year-old with a notch at 3-o'clock and bands at the hymenal base at 4- 5- and 7-o'clock.

Notch at 6-o'clock. Slight notch or angularity of normal hymen in an 8-year-old.

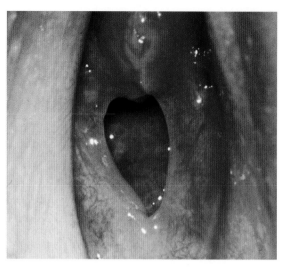

Nonspecific vascular changes. A 10-year-old with angularity at 6-o'clock and nonspecific vascular changes of the hymen and fossa navicularis.

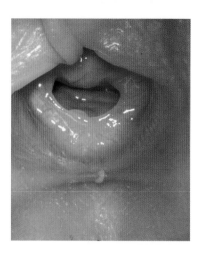

Normal hymen with mound. A 5-year-old with a normal crescentic hymen and exposed rugae or longitudinal intravaginal ridge (LIR) at the 7-o'clock position which should not be mistaken for a healed transection. Normal-appearing hymen in front of ridge.

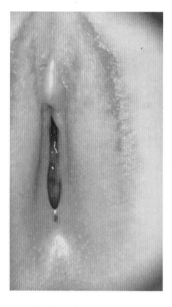

Candida vulvitis with friability of posterior fourchette. A 3½-year-old evaluated for vulvitis and history of sexual abuse. Note general thinning or pallor of the genital area and irritation laterally. Posterior fourchette with friability. (Pokorny)

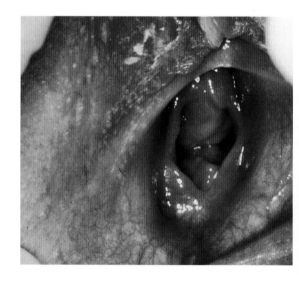

Longitudinal intravaginal ridge (LIR). A 5-year-old with normal erythema and prominent LIR at 5-o'clock, which protrudes above the hymenal edge as a mound.

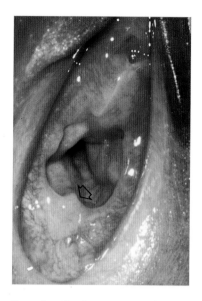

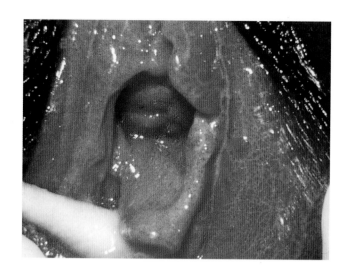

Longitudinal intravaginal ridge (LIR). A prominent ridge with extension onto the hymenal edge in a 9-year-old. Note color changes from the pale v-shaped area (arrow), corresponding to the base of the intravaginal LIR, to the reddened peri-hymenal vestibular mucosa.

Longitudinal intravaginal ridge (LIR) in an adolescent. LIR exposed with use of a cotton-tipped applicator in a 15-year-old. Note elastic hymen of puberty.

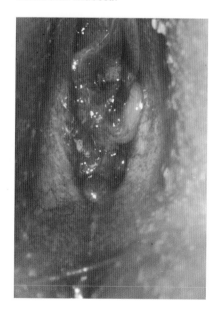

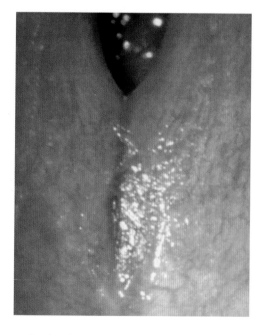

Subcutaneous mounds. Non-specific subcutaneous mounding of the posterior fourchette in a 6-year-old.

Labial adhesion. Partial labial adhesions in a 4-year-old. (From Emans SJ, Goldstein DP. *Pediatric and Adolescent Gynecology.* 3rd ed. Boston: Little, Brown, 1990. Reprinted by permission.)

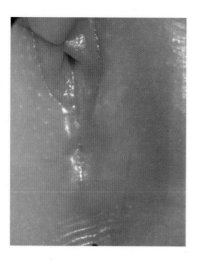

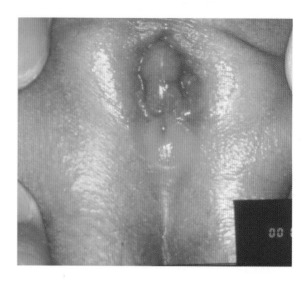

Labial adhesion. 2-year-old referred for evaluation of "imperforate hymen." Labial adhesion leaves only a small opening ventrally.

Complete labial adhesion. With urinary retention.

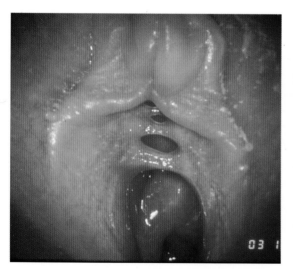

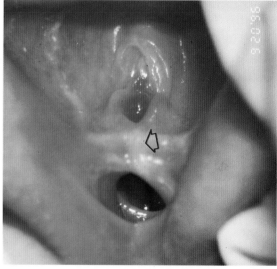

Incomplete vulvar (vestibular) adhesions. Partially formed adhesions ventrally. (Jenny)

Labial fusion. Almost complete labial fusion in a 3-year-old treated with estrogen cream, with resultant estrogenization of the hymen.

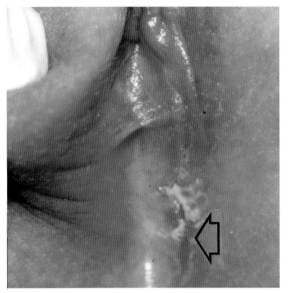

Labial fusion release. Partial release of the labial fusion shown in the preceding illustration.

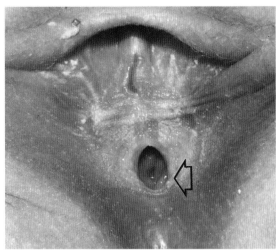

Ventral labial fusion. Labial fusion (arrow) in a 2-year-old with a normal crescentic hymen.

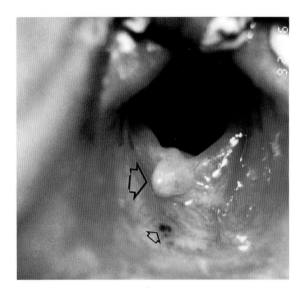

Hymenal tag. A 5-year-old with a hymenal tag at 6-o'clock (large arrow) and a pigmented nevus (small arrow).

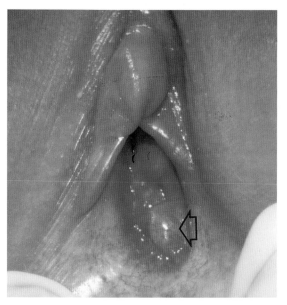
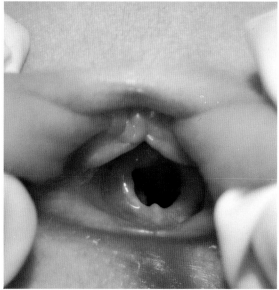

External ridge. A 3-year-old with persistence of the external ridge at 6-o'clock. (Arrow) Note how appearance changes from examination by separation (**left panel**), as compared to examination by traction (**right panel**).

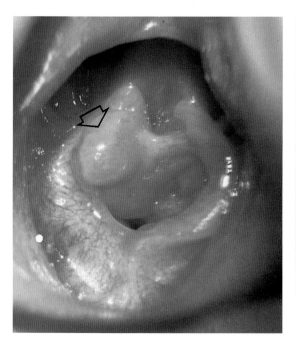
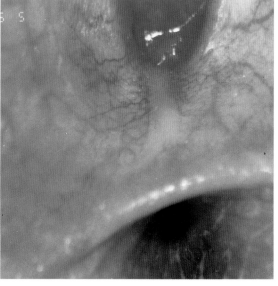

Hymenal polyp and "rolled" edge. A 6-year-old with a hymenal polyp (arrow) and redundant, "rolled" edge between 1-o'clock and 4-o'clock. This edge can easily be moved away from vestibule by changes in traction or the use of water.

Midline sparing. Prominent midline vascular sparing of the posterior fourchette.

ANATOMIC VARIATIONS AND MEDICAL CONDITIONS: DIAGNOSTIC CHALLENGES

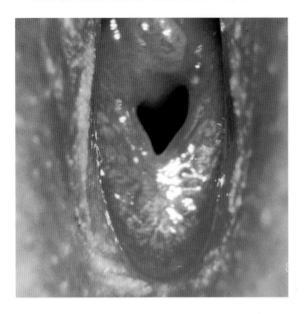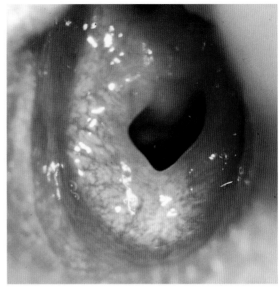

Traction, V-shaped notch. A normal crescentic hymen in 7-year-old, with angularity or V-shaped notch at 6-o'clock (**left panel**), which disappears with traction (**right panel**).

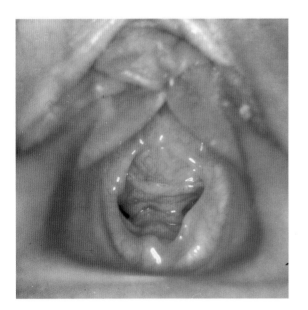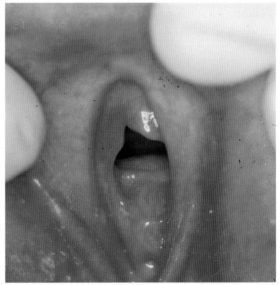

Position, V-shaped notch. A 2-year-old with longitudinal intravaginal ridges and mounds at 6-o'clock and 8-o'clock in the supine position (**left panel**), which become more prominent in the prone position (**right panel**). Note normal appearance of the hymen and significant depth of hymenal tissue at 6-o'clock. The presence of two adjacent LIR with a depression between them might be misinterpreted as a post-traumatic change.

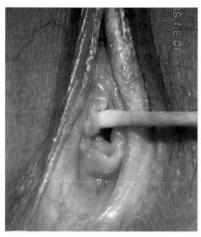

Persistence of notch. A 13-year-old referred for possible sexual abuse when a notch was observed at the 9-o'clock position.

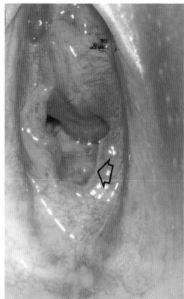
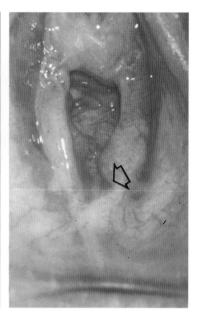

"Concavity" at 6-o'clock compared with post-traumatic transection. Left: A normal crescentic hymen with LIR and associated mounds at both the 3-o'clock and 4-o'clock positions and the 7-o'clock and 8-o'clock positions, and the "valley" in-between. (arrow) **Right:** A completely healed transection of the hymen at 6-o'clock (arrow).

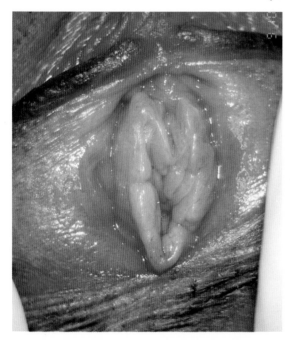
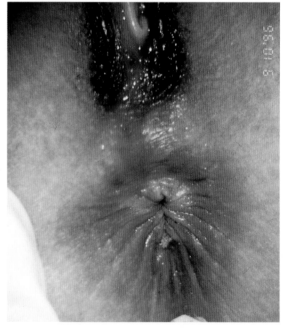

Vaginal bleeding in a 3-year-old. This patient, who presented to a community emergency department with a history of periodic bleeding over 6 months, was referred to the medical center for evaluation of possible sexual abuse. Physical examination showed thelarche, hymenal changes, and labial hyperpigmentation (**left panel**). Anus appears normal (**right panel**).
Final diagnosis: Estrogen-producing ovarian tumor.

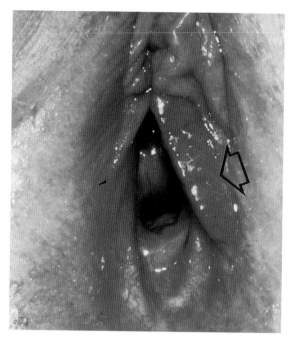

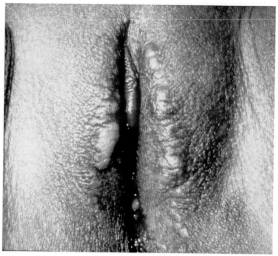

Hyperkeratosis of labia majora. A 3-year-old with a 6-month history of vaginal discharge; a foreign body (pecan shell) was found in the vagina. Biopsy showed hyperkeratosis. (Pokorny)

Hemangioma of the labia minora. A 5-year-old presented with a complaint of "blood in underwear" after an accidental fall. Hemangioma of the left labia minora (arrow). Normal crescentic hymen with slight redundancy to the left.

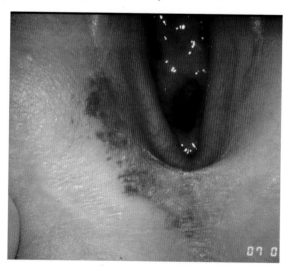

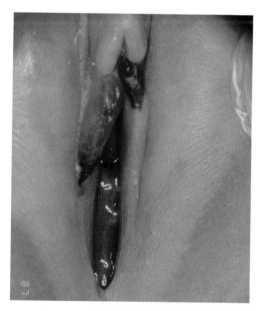

Lichen sclerosus. Lichen sclerosus of vulvar skin. Note sharp demarcation between normal and affected skin as well as cutaneous hemorrhages. Normal annular hymen. (From Jenny C, Kirby P, Fuquay D. Genital lichen sclerosus mistaken for child sexual abuse. *Pediatrics* 1981;83:597–99.)

Lichen sclerosus. Lichen sclerosus with subepithelial hemorrhages of the labia and margin of white epithelium in a 10½-year-old. (Pokorny)

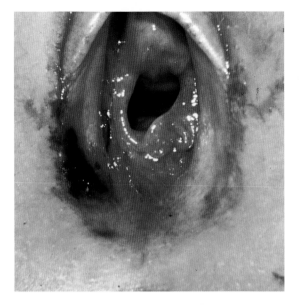

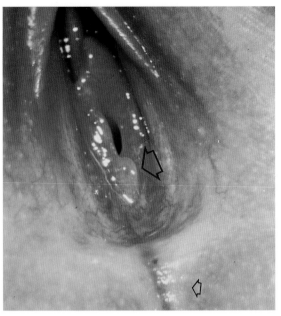

Lichen sclerosus. Previously undiagnosed lichen sclerosus in 7-year-old who presented to a pediatrician with a complaint of "itching and blood in underwear."

Lichen sclerosus. A 4-year-old referred for possible child sexual abuse. History from the mother of chronic "rubbing or masturbation." Typical atrophic appearance of lichen sclerosus (small arrow) and incidental finding of hymenal cyst (large arrow).

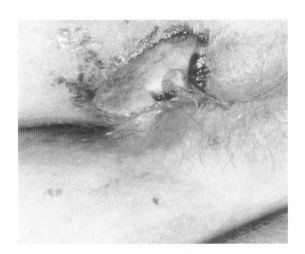

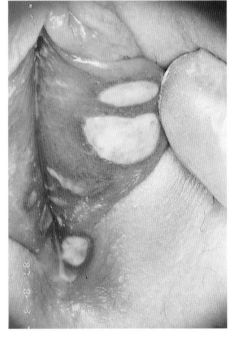

Behçet's disease. An 11-year-old with a chronic labial ulcer. All infectious etiologies must be ruled out to establish the diagnosis.

Behçet's disease. This 12-year-old had mouth ulcers, a vesicular skin rash, and vulvar ulcers, which resolved spontaneously. (Pokorny)

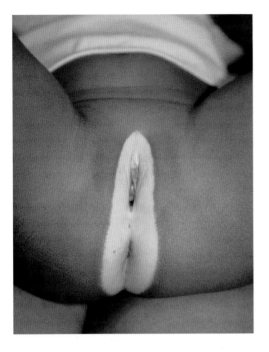

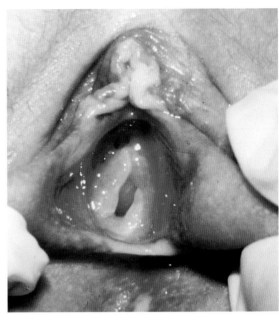

Vitiligo. A 4-year-old with vitiligo.

Vitiligo. A 9-year-old with vitiligo of the labia minora and perineum. The hymen appears normal with slightly scalloped edges.

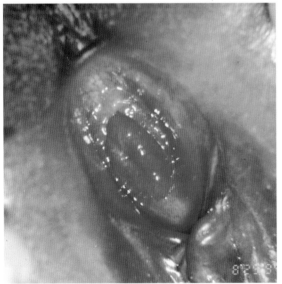

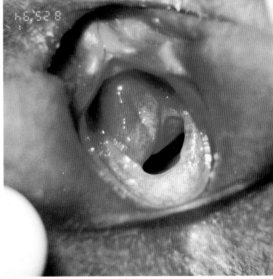

Urethral prolapse. A 5-year-old who presented to the emergency department of a community hospital with complaint of bloody discharge. Children's Service was notified, and the child was brought immediately to the medical center for evaluation of possible sexual abuse. **Left:** Urethral prolapse was misdiagnosed as traumatized hymen. **Right:** With labial traction, the normal crescentic hymen is apparent below the level of prolapse.

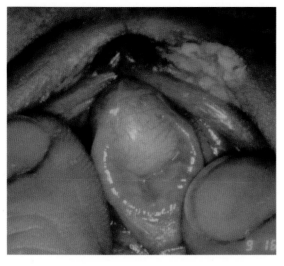

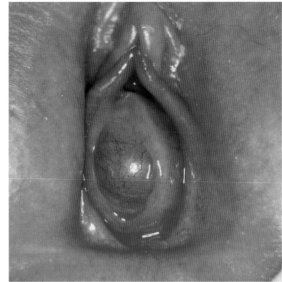

Cyst. Suburethral, intravaginal asymptomatic cystic mass. (Levitt)

Intravaginal cystic polyp. A newborn referred by the emergency department for evaluation of possible imperforate hymen. A fluid-filled cystic mass was later removed from the vagina.

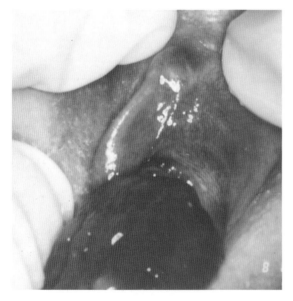

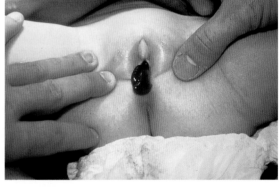

Rhabdomyosarcoma. A newborn with a mass protruding from the vagina. (Levitt)

Sarcoma botryoides. A 20-month-old girl with a 3-day history of bloody vaginal discharge. On examination, a large hemmorhagic mass was seen protruding from the vagina.

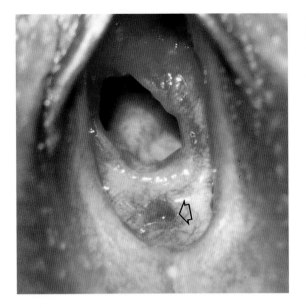

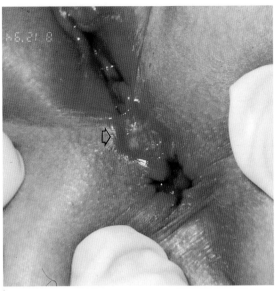

Congenital pit. Blind pouch or pit (arrow) at the base of annular hymen in a 9-year-old.

Perineum: failure of midline fusion. A 3-year-old referred for possible acute sexual assault after a pediatrician noted a midline defect. The failed fusion extends from the anal verge to the base of the hymen.

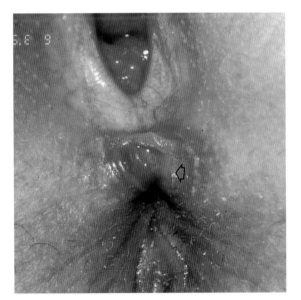

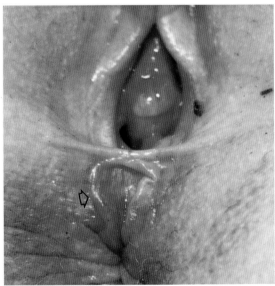

Failure of midline fusion. A 4-year-old raised in an orphanage. **Left:** Initial examination after referral from a pediatrician for possible anal laceration. **Right:** One year later; defect remains unchanged, confirming the diagnosis of congenital failure of midline fusion.

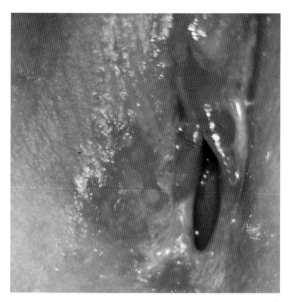

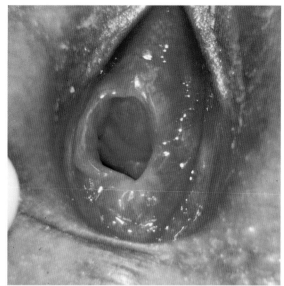

Vulvar ulcers (nonspecific). A 6-year-old with persistent dysuria and bloody "discharge." **Left:** Nonspecific vulvar ulcers of both the labia minora and majora. All cultures were negative and there were no lesions in the oral cavity. **Right:** Follow-up one month later with gradual improvement. Complete resolution after three months.

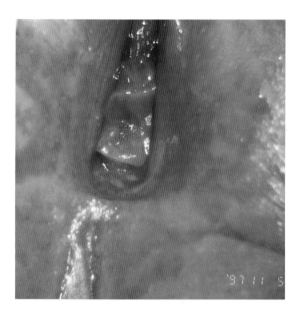

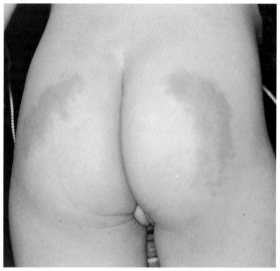

Genital streptococcal cellulitits. A 5-year-old with a history of recent throat infection, dysuria, and "blood in underwear". Examination showed cellulitis caused by Group B streptococcus.

Allergic dermatitis. Circumferential erythema of the buttocks in a 2-year-old with allergy to toilet seat disinfectant.

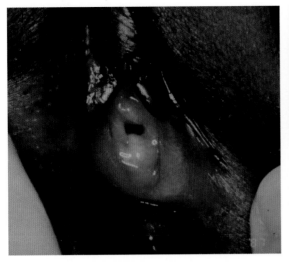

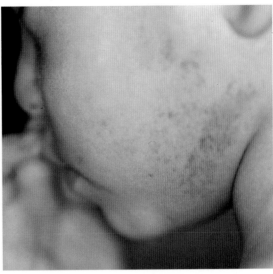

Labial abrasions with straddle injury. A 6-year-old seen 12 hours after straddle injury on bicycle. Note bilateral abrasions at the base of the labia minora (arrows) and nontraumatized hymen. The external ridge of hymen at the 6-o'clock position is a normal variant that can persist from birth. (Pokorny)

Physical abuse. A 2-year-old boy referred for possible sexual abuse associated with physical abuse. Note recent facial bruising. (See the two illustrations below.)

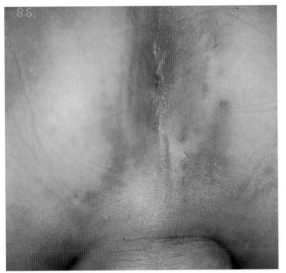

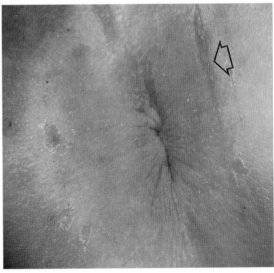

Sexual abuse. The same 2-year-old boy referred for sexual abuse coupled with physical abuse had genital bruising (**left panel**) of a different age than the facial bruising shown in the above illustration. The bruising was associated with perianal abrasions (**right panel** arrow). Not diagnostic of sexual abuse.

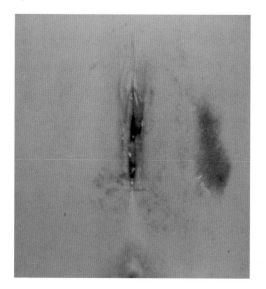
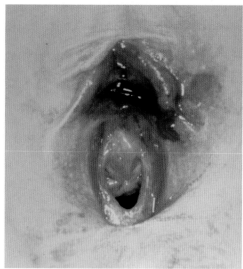

Accidental injury. **Left**: A 7-year-old seen for bleeding after a straddle injury. Note the ecchymosis on the left labia below the clitoris and inner thigh. **Right:** With labial traction, note the edema of the left labia minora, small laceration with bleeding, and the normal hymenal ring (crescentic with smooth symmetrical edge). (From Emans SJ, Goldstein DP. *Pediatric and Adolescent Gynecology.* 3rd ed. Boston: Little, Brown, 1990. Reprinted by permission.)

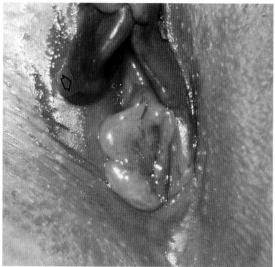
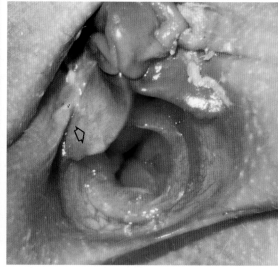

Straddle injury. A 3-year-old: **Left:** Acute injury to the labia minora (arrow) following a straddle injury sustained on a playground. **Right:** After healing: note the old injury site (arrow). The hymen appears normal, redundant, with a notch at 9-o'clock and mobile "rolled" edges.

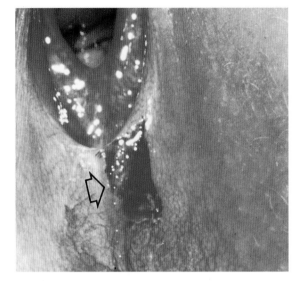

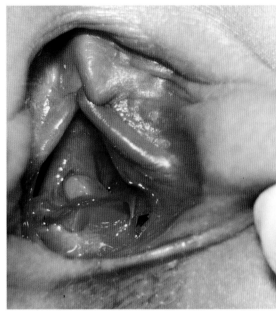

A 5-year-old with a history of straddle injury after an accident at school reported "blood in underwear." Note abrasion (arrow) with bleeding.

Peri-hymenal splinter. A 4-year-old with a wood splinter (arrow) from playground equipment. (See the two illustrations below.)

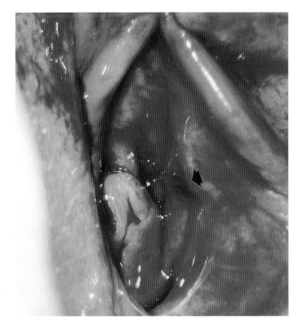

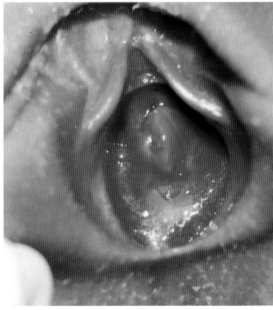

Peri-hymenal splinter removal. Left: The appearance of the hymen after splinter removal (arrow) using viscous xylocaine in clinic. **Right:** Healing 10 days later reveals a normal hymen with notches at 3-o'clock and 9-o'clock and ventral redundancy.

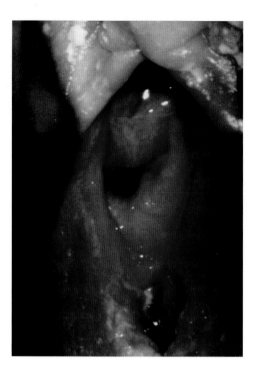

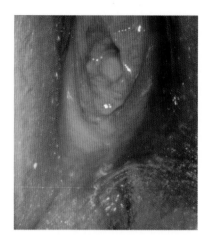

Accidental straddle injury. A 3½-year-old observed to sustain a straddle injury on the brick edge of swimming pool. Note acute laceration on posterior fourchette with normal hymen.

Accidental trauma—penetrating. Penetrating vaginal trauma in a 7-year-old with a history of jumping from dresser onto bedpost. The injury involved penetrating trauma to introitus, hymen, and vagina, requiring surgical repair. Marked scarring of the posterior fourchette and hymen from the 3-o'clock to the 9-o'clock position, extending into vagina. A remnant of normal hymen is apparent from the 12-o'clock to the 3-o'clock position. Photo taken 2 weeks after surgical repair.

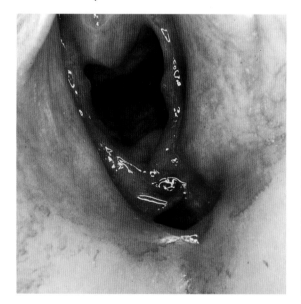

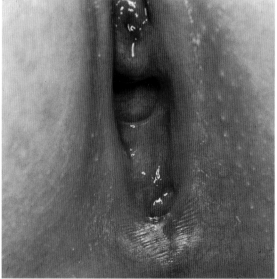

Penetrating injury of posterior fourchette and fossa through the base of hymen.
Left: Acute injury with damage to the fossa and posterior fourchette. **Right:** Post-healing, with persistence of post-traumatic fenestration at the base of the hymen at 6-o'clock.

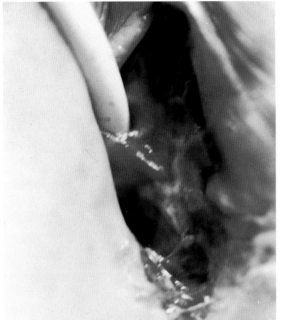
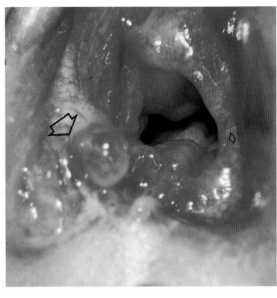
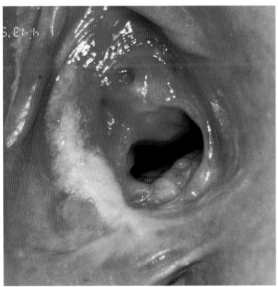
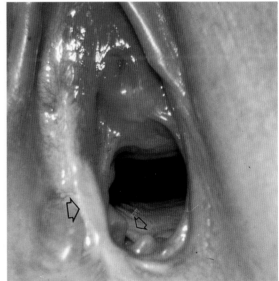

Healing series in a 7-year-old after accidental penetration of vagina.
Top left: Avulsion injury of right lateral perineum, posterior fourchette, fossa, and hymen from 6-o'clock to 10-o'clock. Catheter is in place prior to surgical repair.
Top right: Three months post-repair with formation of granulation tissue (large arrow). Note that the integrity of the hymen is preserved on the unaffected side (small arrow).
Lower panels: One year post-repair, granulation tissue is replaced by scar tissue (6-o'clock to 10-o'clock). Loss of hymen (small arrow) results in exposure of the intravaginal structures from 6-o'clock to 10-o'clock, which can be seen with the patient in both the supine (**left panel**) and prone (**right panel**) positions. Note the scar tissue (large arrow).

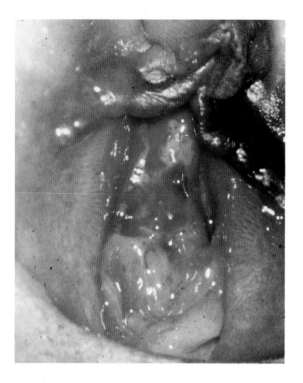

Straddle injury. A 4-year-old who slipped off a kitchen counter onto an open cabinet door, with injury to right labia minora and the peri-urethral mucous membranes. The hymen remains free of trauma and is crescentic with some redundancy and a vertical orientation of the opening.

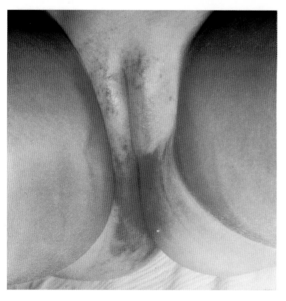

Genital hematoma. A 6-year-old rescued from the bottom of a spa. Genital hematoma involving the labia majora and inner thighs secondary to the suction of the water return in the family spa. (Courtesy of Dr. Lobe)

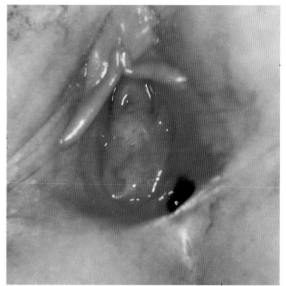

Pencil injury. A 3-year-old who reportedly "sat on a pencil," with a puncture wound at 5-o'clock. The injury resolved completely in two weeks.

FEMALE GENITAL MUTILATION

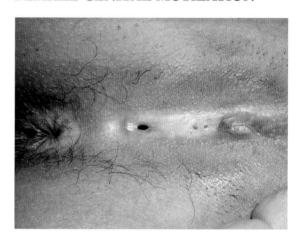

Genital mutilation. A 19-year-old pregnant Sudanese woman was seen for prenatal care. The appearance of the vulva is typical for female genital mutilation (FMG). The normal features of the vulva are absent. Note the small orifice in front of the vagina that permits intercourse and the two small openings in front of the urethra. (Courtesy of Sir John Dewhurst)

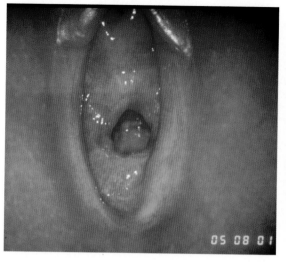

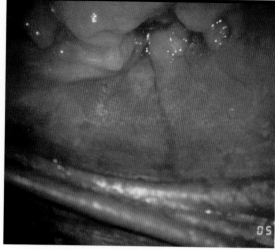

Acute trauma—digital penetration. Annular hymen in a 5-year-old with a history of attempted digital penetration. Note small cutaneous hemorrhages/abrasions of the hymen between the 2-o'clock and the 4-o'clock positions. (Jenny)

Acute trauma—attempted rape. Spoke-wheel abrasions of the vulva below the hymen in 14-year-old after attempted forceful vaginal penetration. (Jenny)

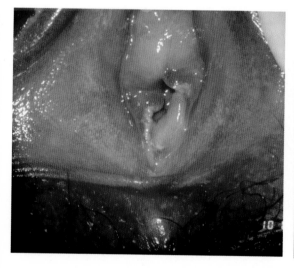

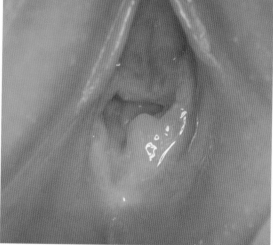

Acute trauma—sexual assault. Agglutinating hymenal lacerations 4 days after sexual assault. Normal-appearing hymen ventrally with discoloration of the torn hymenal surfaces at the 3-o'clock and 9-o'clock positions. (Jenny)

Healing trauma. Four days after witnessed multiple-assailant rape on a 9-year-old. Note the periurethral and intravaginal mucosal hemorrhages (arrow) and the healed hymenal tear and adjacent "mound" at the 6:30 position. (Stewart)

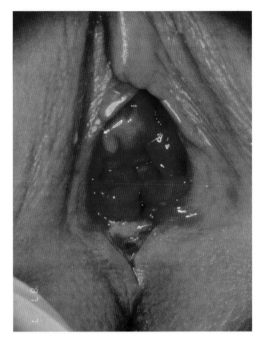

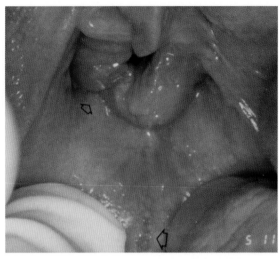

Acute mucosal abrasion and hymenal tear. Mucosal abrasions, superficial tear in posterior fourchette (large arrow), and tangential hymenal transection at the 7-o'clock position (small arrow), in a 14-year-old who had been raped 5 hours earlier. The tear is best demonstrated by spreading the hymen with a cotton-tipped applicator.

Acute trauma. A 1-year-old with disruption of hymenal and perineal tissues posteriorly. Mucosal hemorrhages of the hymen ventrally. (Pokorny)

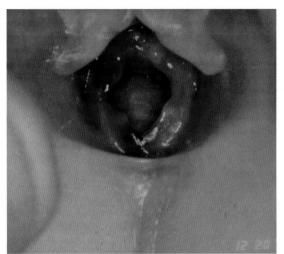

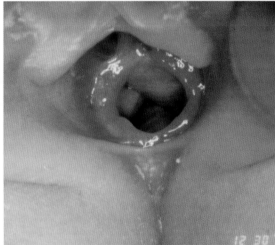

Acute trauma and healing. Left: Almost 3-year-old with submucosal hemorrhages at the 6-o'clock position and also from the 8-o'clock to the 10-o'clock position. Traumatic shallow transection at the 9-o'clock position. **Right:** Follow-up examination 10 days later. The hymen appears well healed without any clear indication of previous trauma. (Stewart)

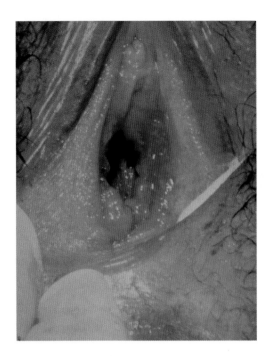 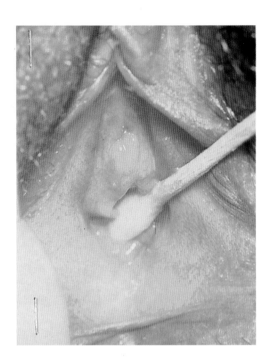

Acute trauma and healing. Left: Acute genital trauma in a 12-year-old requiring surgical repair of a large vaginal laceration. Photograph taken at the time of surgery within hours of rape. Trauma noted at base of hymen and laceration at the 1-o'clock and 2-o'clock positions with discoloration at the 2-o'clock and 10-o'clock positions. There is a blood-soaked gauze pad immediately inside the vagina. **Right:** One week following surgery, normal estrogenized appearing hymen ventrally. Acute trauma is healed and hymen now appears normal. (Pokorny)

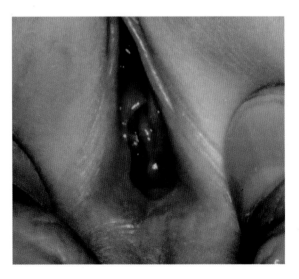 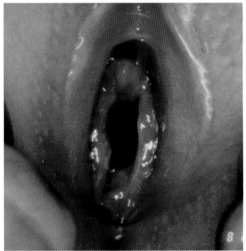

Acute trauma with healing. Left: A 3-year-old with a posterior tear of the hymen extending to the posterior fourchette at the 6-o'clock position. Abuse occurred 2 days prior to this examination. A 26-year-old male babysitter pled guilty to penile penetration. **Right:** Follow-up of vaginal/hymenal tear 2 months after assault. Note the well-healed transection at the 6-o'clock position. (Levitt)

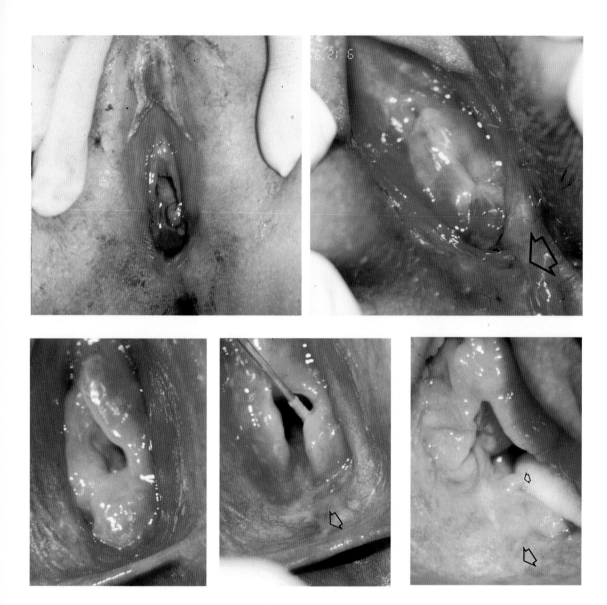

Acute sexual assault of a 9-year-old. A 9-year-old presented with a complaint of vaginal bleeding. **Top left:** Physical examination indicated penetrating trauma, and the child was taken to the operating room for examination under anesthesia and repair of posterior fourchette, fossa, and hymen. **Top right:** Examination one month later showed healing of the posterior fourchette (arrow). **Lower panels:** Four months after the assault (**left**) healing appears to be complete, and the hymen shows early effects of estrogen. Eight months after assault (**middle**) examination including use of a cotton-tipped applicator shows that transection of the hymen persists, and the posterior fourchette and fossa have completely healed. Note the avascular midline region, which corresponds to the original laceration (arrow). Three years after the assault, and after the onset of puberty (**right**) examination revealed persistence of the midline changes (large arrow), the transection of the hymen at 6-o'clock, and the regenerative effects of estrogen in the formation of redundant, fimbriated hymen with tag (small arrow).

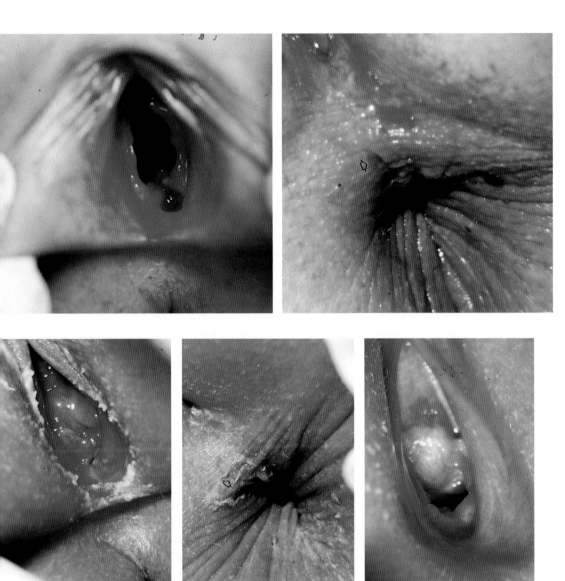

Longitudinal healing with hymenal repair in a victim of sexual assault. A 5-year-old was assaulted by a teenager in the school bathroom, causing acute transection of the hymen and laceration of the fossa navicularis and posterior fourchette (**upper left panel**) and anus (arrow, **upper right panel**) requiring surgical repair. Examination 6 days after surgical repair showed hymenal healing in the early stages (**lower left panel**) and complete healing of the anal tear (arrow, **lower center panel**). By 5 months post-surgery, the hymen was completely healed (**lower right panel**).

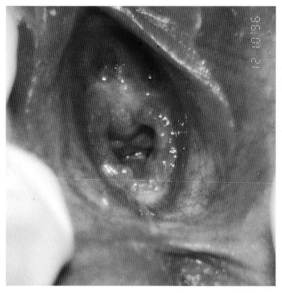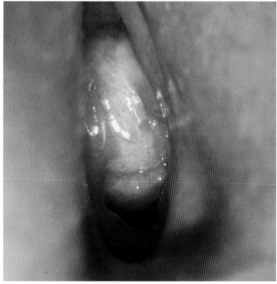

Follow-up examination of the 5-year-old victim of sexual assault. At 20 months after the assault, the hymen appears normal, except for slight persistence of an avascular, white area at the base (arrow) visualized with the patient lying supine (**left panel**) and prone (**right panel**). Note the smooth, sharp edge of the hymen.

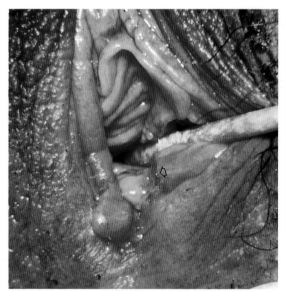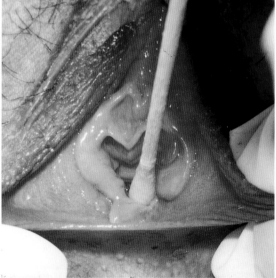

Sexual assault of an 11-year-old. An 11-year-old with a history of sexual assault by her stepfather. **Left:** Note acute laceration of the hymen (arrow) at 6-o'clock. **Right:** Two weeks later the healed transection is exposed with the use of a cotton-tipped applicator.

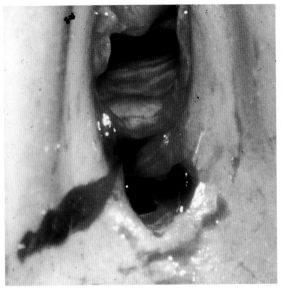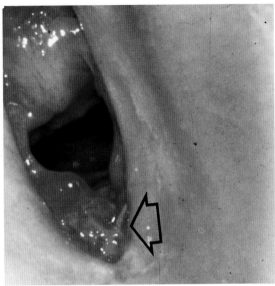

7-year-old assaulted by a stranger. **Left:** Two hours after a 7-year-old was found bleeding from the vagina, examination revealed a laceration extending from the posterior fourchette through the hymen, into the vagina. **Right:** After treatment with sitz baths and broad-spectrum antibiotics, examination 8 days later showed formation of midline granulation tissue (arrow).

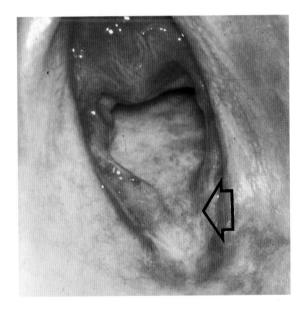

Follow-up of 7-year-old assaulted by a stranger. Examination at 6 months after the assault shows complete healing but persistence of the midline transection (arrow).

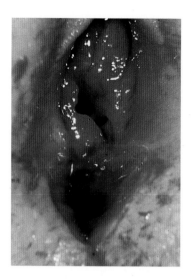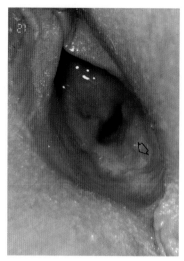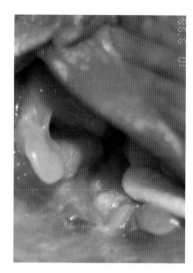

8-year-old assaulted by stranger. Acute injuries evaluated under anesthesia. **Left:** Repair of introital injuries was successful, but at 3 months the hymenal transection persists (arrow, **center panel**). **Right:** Two years later, at puberty, the hymen has become more redundant with response to estrogen, but the transection remains.

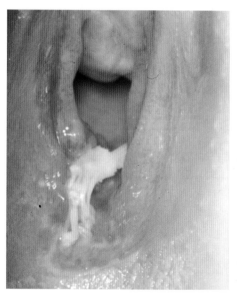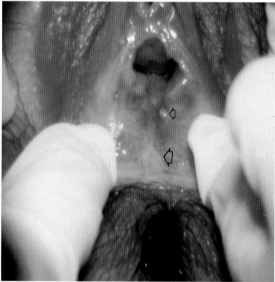

8-year-old lost to follow-up. An 8-year-old who presented to the local hospital with a history of being "found down" in a neighborhood park. She was taken to the operating room and a vaginal tear was "repaired" (no photographs taken; no police report filed). The child was discharged from the hospital without antibiotics and returned 5 days later with a serious abscess of the vaginal introitus, at which time the case was reported to Social Services. This child was then referred for examination after hospital discharge. **Left:** Note 6-o'clock transection with adherent white discharge. No history of sexual abuse was reported by the child, and the family was lost to follow-up. Five years later, the same child presented to the clinic after disclosing to school authorities that she had been sexually assaulted as a young child. **Right:** Examination revealed post-pubertal persistence of midline hymenal transection (small arrow) and avascular midline area of posterior fourchette (large arrow). Comparison of the two photographs suggests that the white perineal area is scar tissue.

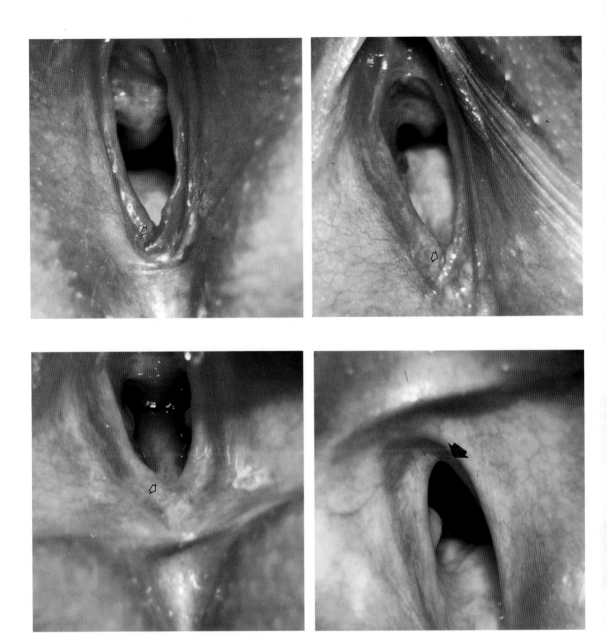

Tear of the vestibular hymenal mucosa and healing. A 9-year-old with a history of attempted penetration of vagina by a teenage stepbrother. The child came to the clinic with slight vaginal bleeding, and examination (**upper left**) revealed a mucosal tear of the hymen (arrow). One week later the area of the tear appears to be healing (upper right), and 6 weeks later examination with the patient in both supine (**lower left**) and prone (**lower right**) positions appeared normal. (arrows delineate precise area of acute injury)

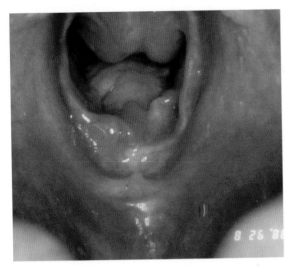

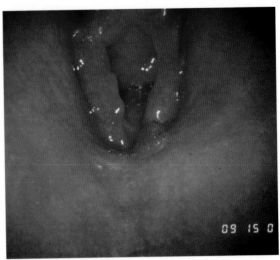

Healed trauma. Healed transection of the hymen at the 5-o'clock position in a 9-year-old. With the labial traction technique the hymenal opening is enlarged to 12 mm. Note scarring of the hymen at the 5-o'clock position, which extends across the fossa nevicularis and posterior fourchette at the midline. (Levitt)

Chronic changes of sexual abuse. A 3-year-old with annular hymen and healed transection at the 6-o'clock position. Condyloma acuminatum on posterior fourchette. (Jenny)

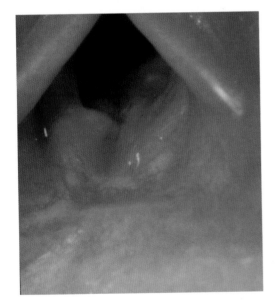

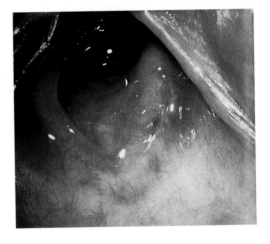

Chronic abuse. A 9-month-old with multiple fractures and sexual abuse. The hymenal dimensions were 5 mm transverse, 6–7 mm anterior-posterior. Note transection of the hymen at the 6-o'clock position. (From Emans SJ, Goldstein CP. *Pediatric and Adolescent Gynecology.* 3rd ed. Boston: Little, Brown, 1990. Reprinted by permission.)

Chronic penetration in a 6-year-old. Child referred with positive *N. gonorrhoeae* culture of the vagina and anal condyloma acuminatum. Normal-appearing hymen at the 1- to 5-o'clock position. Loss of hymen (attenuation) at the 6- to 11-o'clock position, with scarring and altered vascularity.

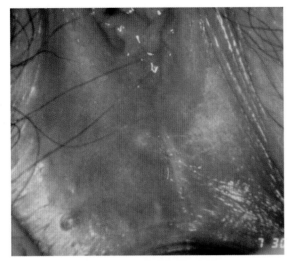

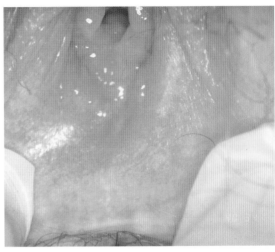

Healed trauma. A 14-year-old with healed trauma to the posterior fourchette and hymen. Well-healed scar of the posterior fourchette. Paramedian scar was palpable and can be differentiated from midline sparing. (Levitt)

Scarring of the posterior fourchette. Scarring of the hymen between the 6-o'clock and 8-o'clock positions, with loss of hymenal tissue (attenuation) and scar of the posterior fourchette midline with a change in surrounding vascularity. (Stewart)

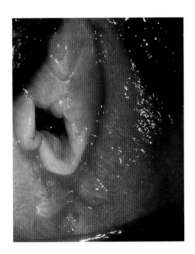

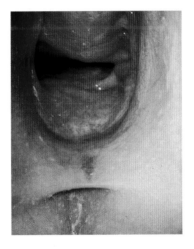

Adolescent victim of chronic abuse. A 13-year-old whose abuser confessed to chronic vaginal penetration since victim was age 5. Note transection of the hymen at the 7-o'clock position which extends to the base of the hymen. Normal estrogenized hymen ventrally. Skin tags in fossa navicularis.

Attenuation of the hymen. A 5-year-old with a history of chronic penetration by her stepfather. Note complete loss of hymen posteriorly with exposure of vaginal floor. The posterior fourchette is friable.

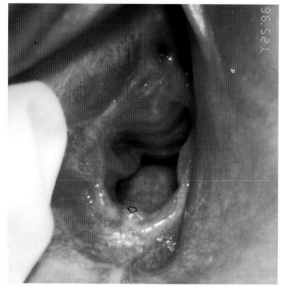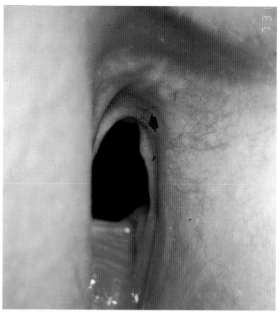

Delayed disclosure in an 8-year-old. This child reported a history of penile vaginal penetration by her mother's boyfriend, which had ended 6 months prior to this examination. **Left:** Supine with midline transection of hymen (small arrow). **Right:** Prone with double-layered appearance of hymen (large arrow).

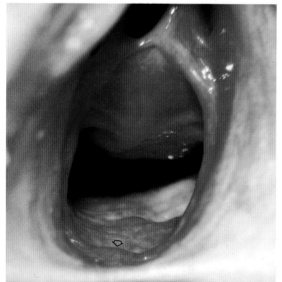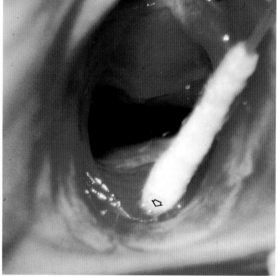

"Attenuation" in a 9-year-old. Diminished hymenal tissue in a 9-year-old with a history of repeated vaginal penetration. **Left:** A remnant (<1 mm) of hymen visible (small arrow) posteriorly. **Right:** Use of cotton-tipped applicator to illustrate remnant of hymenal tissue (arrow).

NORMAL ANI AND NONSPECIFIC CHANGES

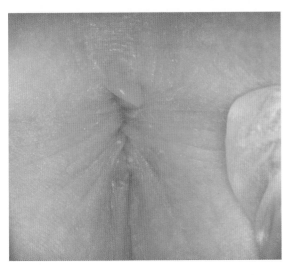

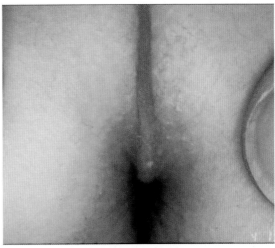

Normal anal fold. A 13-year-old with normal-appearing skin "fold" at the 12-o'clock position. (Stewart)

Median raphe. Prominent hyperpigmented median raphe in a 4-year-old boy. Raphe extends to anal verge as a skinfold at the 12-o'clock position. (Levitt)

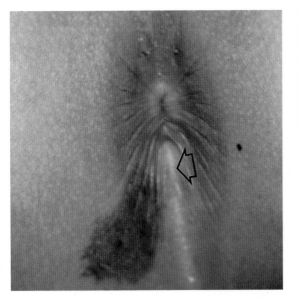

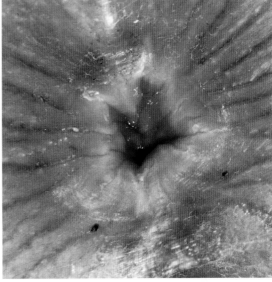

Pigmented nevus. A 9-year-old with a perineal pigmented nevus. Note hypo-pigmented median raphe and diastasis ani (arrow).

Pectinate line. A 10-year-old with pigmented anal folds, prominent pectinate line, and asymmetrical anal opening.

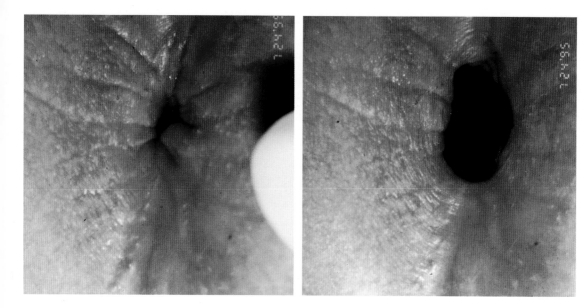

Reflex anal dilatation. Nonspecific reflex dilatation associated with gentle lateral traction. **Left:** Pre-traction. **Right:** With traction.

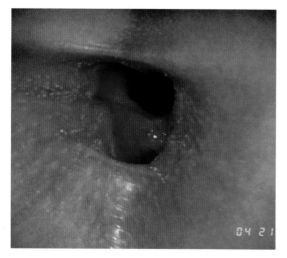

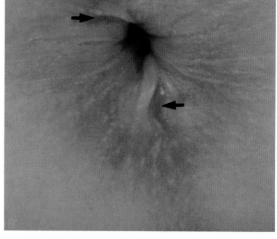

Anal dilatation caused by sedative medications. Child given demerol, phenergan, and thorazine prior to examination. Anal tone was normal after the sedative wore off. (Jenny)

Healing anal fissures. Healing anal fissures (arrow) in a 2½-year-old. (Pokorny)

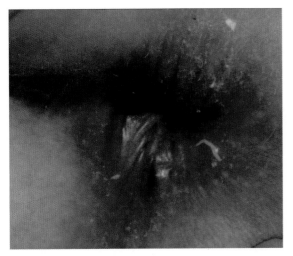

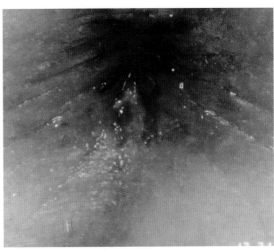

Pinworms. White, threadlike pinworm noted on anal examination in a young child. Note venous distension (arrow) in perianal tissues due to occlusion of venous return caused by spreading the anus open. (Levitt)

Perianal streptococcal cellulitis. A 2-year-old with perianal cellulitis and associated infected seborrheic dermatitis of the scalp. (Levitt)

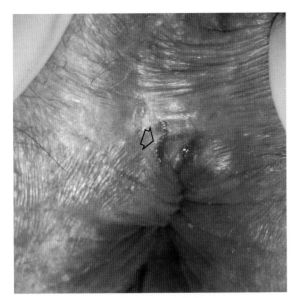

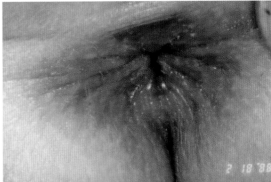

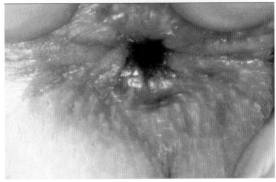

Anal fissures. A 12-year-old with midline anal fissures (arrow) and venous pooling. Anal fissures, in and of themselves, are a nonspecific finding; in this case, however, they are associated with a history of sodomy.

Venous lakes. Venous lakes in perianal tissue demonstrated in a 4-year-old. Lakes become more prominent with traction and disappear as traction is released. (Levitt)

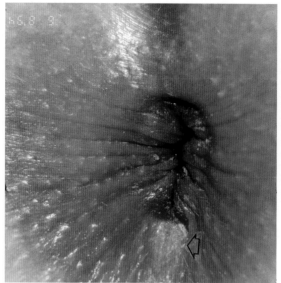

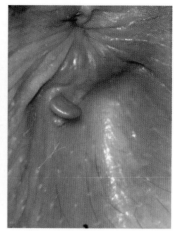

Venous lakes/congestion. A 4-year-old with prominent perianal venous lakes and diastasis ani (smooth area) at 6-o'clock.

Pigmented anal tag. An anal tag in a 3½-year-old with a history of anal laceration.

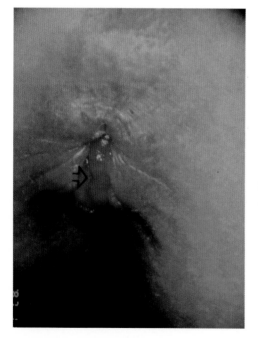

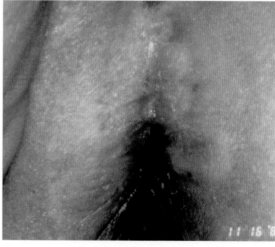

Perianal lichen sclerosus. An 18-month-old girl with perianal lichen sclerosus. Note the hypopigmentation and friability. (Levitt)

Rectal prolapse. A 3-year-old with rectal prolapse (arrow) found during examination for possible sexual abuse. Both rectal and vaginal cultures were positive for *Chlamydia trachomatis.* (Pokorny)

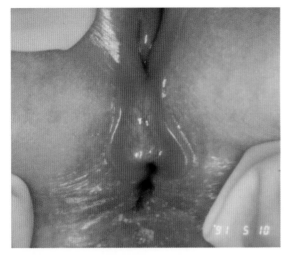

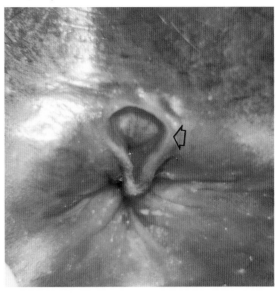

Failure of midline fusion. A 2-month-old with failure of midline fusion. Note how the midline congenital lesion extends from the posterior fourchette to the anus and is bounded by dermal ridges that are reddened. (Levitt)

A 5-year-old with congenital failed midline fusion of the anal verge. Note the typical rolled edges (arrow). This finding is easily differentiated from anal laceration by following for several weeks.

ANAL TRAUMA AND HEALING

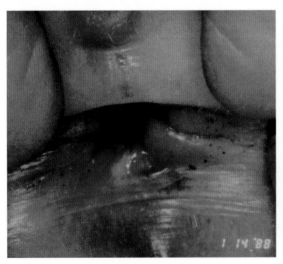

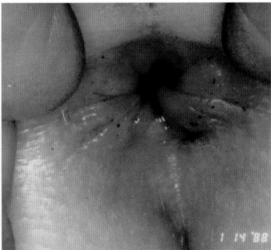

Acute anal trauma. Left: Perianal tear at the 6-o'clock position in a 3-year-old girl. **Right:** Tears more easily visualized with traction on the perianal skin. Note friability of the skin with traction. (Levitt)

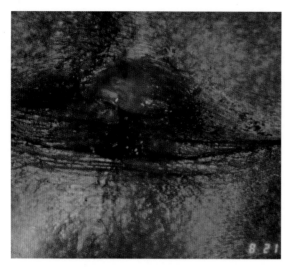

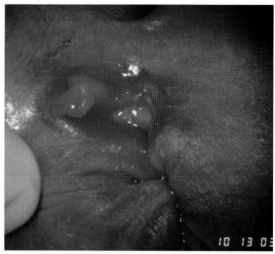

Acute anal laceration. Anal laceration at the 12-o'clock position in a 2-year-old boy. (Levitt)

Avulsed anal tag. Anal tag "avulsed" after acute assault. (Jenny)

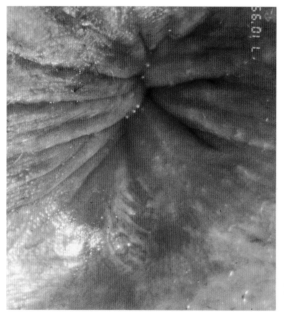

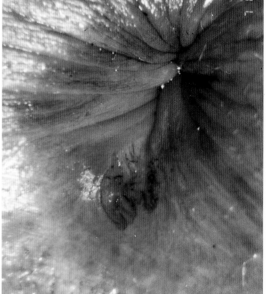

Anal laceration. A 5-year-old with a history of sexual abuse by a neighbor. **Left:** Acute anal laceration at 6-o'clock. **Right:** Use of toluidine dye to highlight laceration.

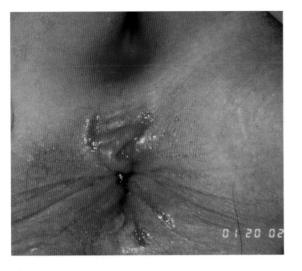

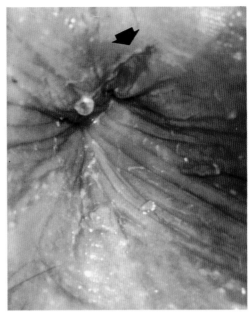

Stellate fissures. Fissures around the anus of small child after traumatic penetration. Note acute fissures at the 11-, 1-, 5-, and 6-o'clock positions. (Jenny)

Anal laceration. A 14-year-old girl abducted and assaulted by a stranger on her way to school. Note anal laceration at 12-o'clock position (arrow).

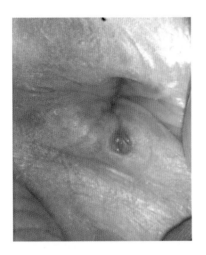 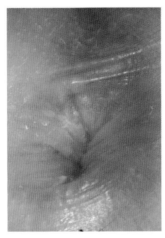

Anal laceration with healing. An 8-year-old with a history of painful sodomy by stepfather. **Left:** Acute laceration at the 11-o'clock position. **Right:** Two weeks later with healing of the laceration.

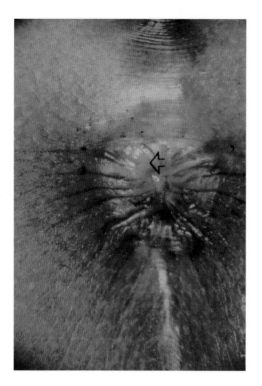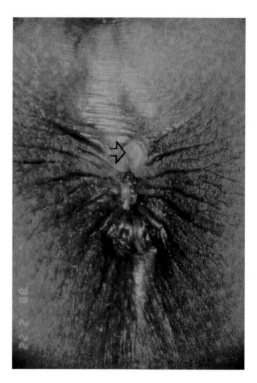

Acute trauma with healing. **Left:** An anal laceration at the 1-o'clock position in a 4-year-old girl initially evaluated for complaints of vulvovaginitis. Hymenal trauma was also noted. **Right:** At re-examination 3 years later a well-healed scar (arrow) with rolled margins is apparent. (Pokorny)

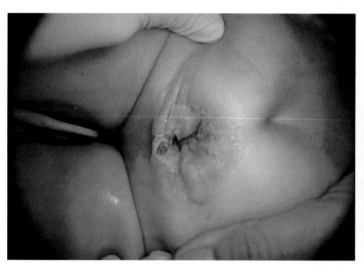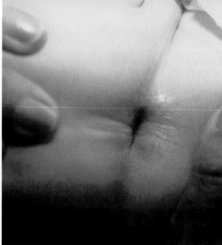

Acute trauma, with healing. **Left:** Severe anal burn (24 hours old), probably a curling iron injury to a 2-year-old male admitted in a coma with retinal hemorrhages and bilateral subdural hematomas. **Right:** Reexamination 2 months after acute injury. Note rapid healing with minimal scarring. (Stewart)

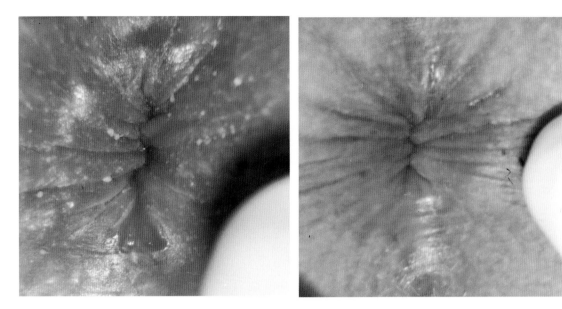

Anal laceration. An 8-year-old with a history of painful anal penetration evaluated one week after abuse (**left panel**) and then three months later (**right panel**).

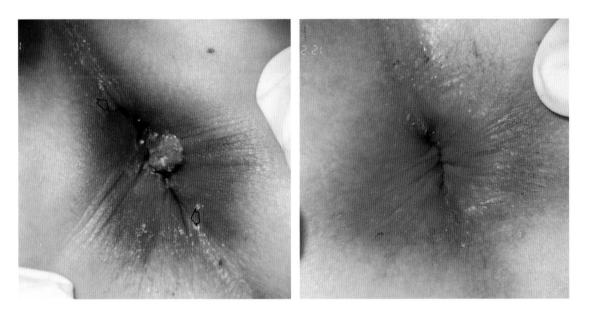

Anal trauma. A 14-month-old boy assaulted by the 15-year-old son of his babysitter. **Left:** The child was seen within hours of returning home from daycare with rectal bleeding. Note perianal hematoma, anal lacerations (arrows), and poor sphincter tone. **Right:** Ten days later the area appears completely normal.

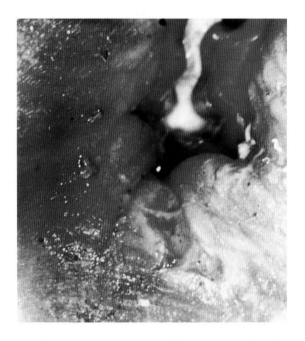
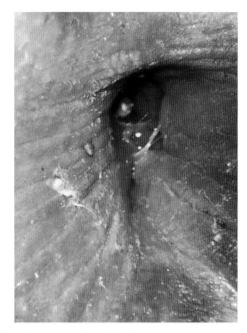

Anal trauma in a 2-year-old. Witnessed anal assault of 2-year-old girl by her 13-year-old brother. **Left:** Child presented with anal tear at 6-o'clock. **Right:** Two weeks later there was complete healing. Apparent persistent erythema can easily be confused with the pectinate line.

ADOLESCENTS

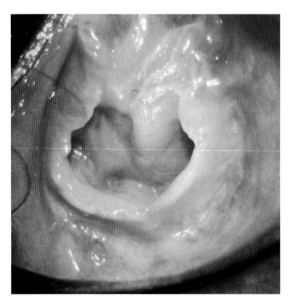
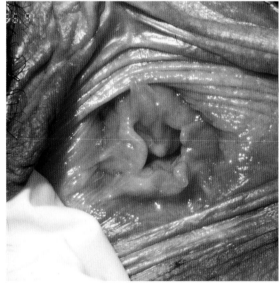

Normal estrogenized hymen. A 12-year-old with an estrogenized, sleeve-like, crescentic hymen.

Sexually active adolescent. A 17-year-old with a history of on-going sexual activity with numerous partners. Note redundant hymen, which appears normal with numerous partial clefts or notches, but without evidence of transections to the base of the hymen.

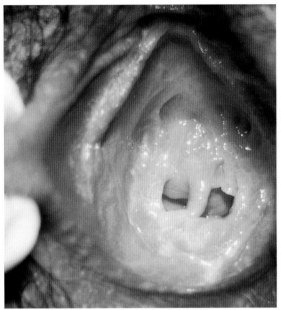 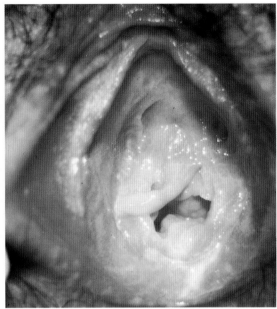

Hymenal tag. A 16-year-old with a hymenal tag, which mimics the appearance (**left panel**) of septate hymen, but the tag can be moved with a cotton-tipped applicator. Otherwise normal sleeve-like, hymen with multiple partial clefts and periurethral support bands at 10-o'clock and 2-o'clock.

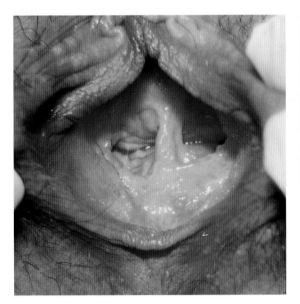 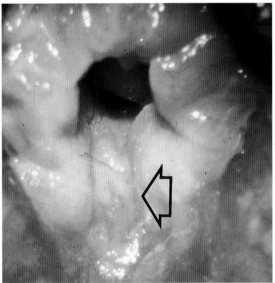

A 12-year-old with septate hymen.

Hymenal transection. A 15-year-old who described painful vaginal penetration at age 8 by her stepfather. Hymenal transection to the base of the hymen at 6-o'clock (arrow).

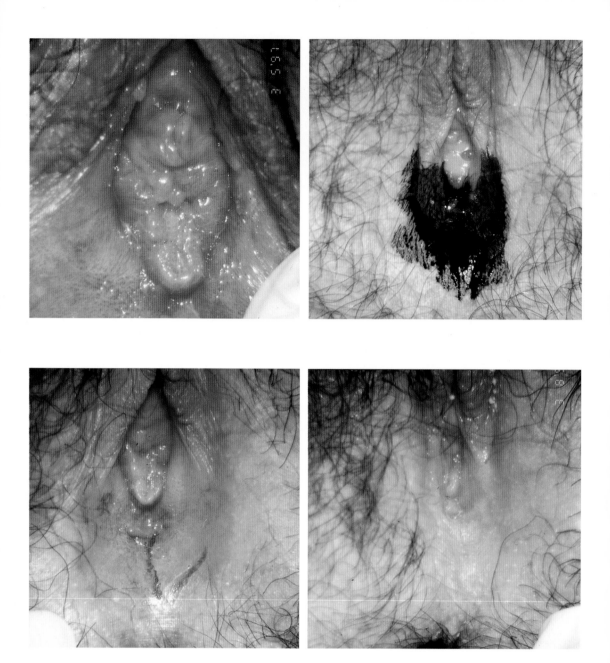

Introital trauma. A 16-year-old with a history of sexual assault by an acquaintance.
Top panels: Acute injuries of fossa and posterior fourchette; application of toluidine
dye (**right panel**) highlights acute lacerations. **Lower left panel:** hymen appears redundant, sleeve-like, and elastic.
Lower right panel: Lesions have healed three days after initial examination.

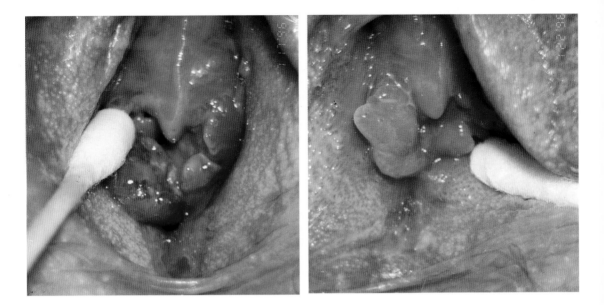

Hymenal trauma. A 14-year-old who was sexually assaulted by an acquaintance. **Left:** Hymenal bruising and abrasions, with transections at 3-o'clock and 5-o'clcok. Note additional abrasion of posterior fourchette below the 5-o'clock transection. **Right:** Complete healing at 5 days with persistence of the hymenal transections.

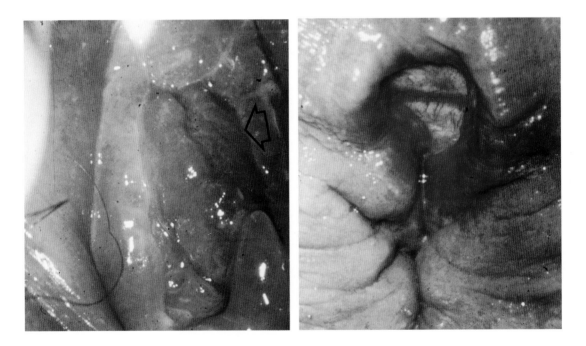

Pregnancy in a 10-year-old. An 80-pound 10-year-old who presented to the emergency department with a possible abdominal tumor. History of sexual abuse by father from age 8; ultrasound indicated a 16-week pregnancy. **Left:** The vaginal introitus. Note absence of hymen (arrow). **Right:** Acute anal trauma associated with a three-week history of daily sodomy.

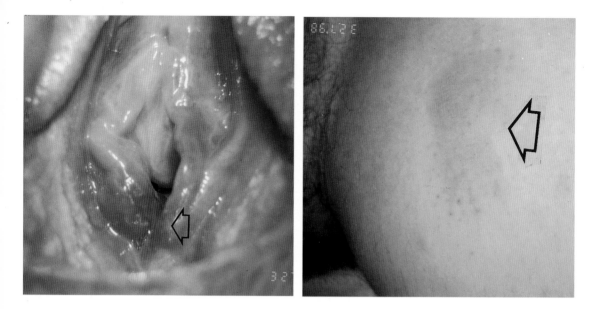

Sexual assault of a 14-year-old. Left: Acute hematoma, abrasions, and laceration (arrow) of hymen after assault by a stranger. **Right:** Hematoma of the inner thigh associated with the sexual assault.

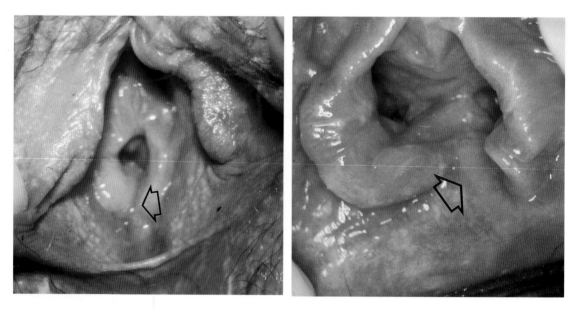

Follow-up examination of the 14-year-old sexual assault victim. After two weeks, there is complete healing and persistence of the hymenal transection at 6-o'clock.

Hymenal transection. A 16-year-old who described painful consensual first intercourse at age 14. Transection of hymen at 6-o'clock extends to the base (arrow).

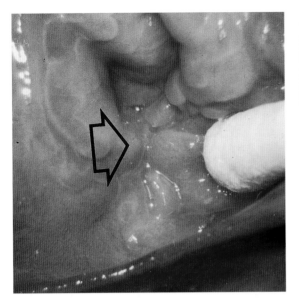

Hymenal transection. A 13-year-old incest survivor, 3 months post-abortion. Note transection of hymen (arrow) where redundant hymen is pulled aside by cotton-tipped applicator.

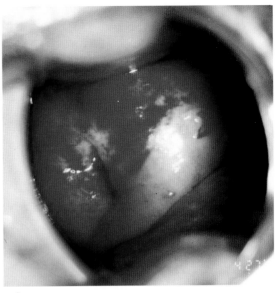

Abrasions of the cervix. Acute abrasions of cervix after sexual assault.

SEXUALLY TRANSMITTED DISEASES

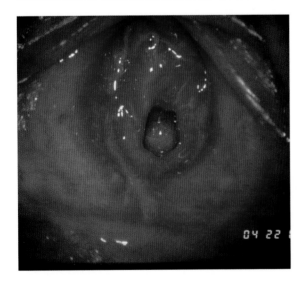

N. gonorrhoeae **vaginitis.** Profuse green vaginal discharge in a 5-year-old with a history of sexual abuse. Culture positive for *N. gonorrhoeae*. (Jenny)

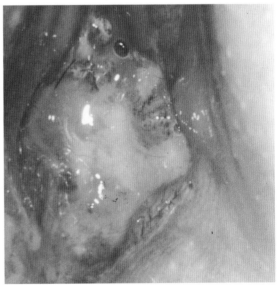

Gonorrhea in a 9-year-old.

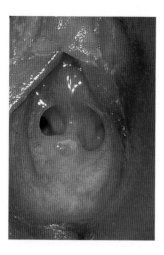

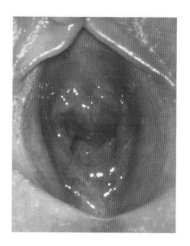

Septated hymen and vagina with positive *N. gonorrhoeae*. A 3-year-old referred with positive *N. gonorrhoeae* culture and septated hymen and vagina. Note smooth translucent hymenal edges with lacy, symmetrical vascularity and hymenal "dimple" in center of hymen.

Chlamydia trachomatis **vaginal infection.** Positive chlamydial culture in a child with normal hymenal configuration. The hymen is crescentic with a "figure 8" opening and longitudinal intravaginal ridges at the 3-o'clock and 9-o'clock positions.

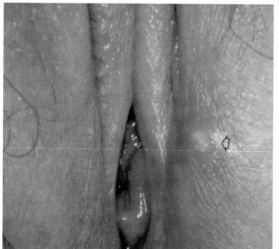

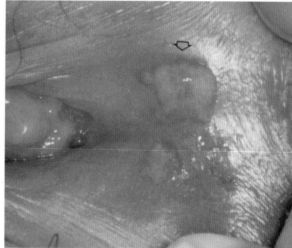

Herpes simplex type II. Left: Culture-proven herpes simplex type II. Note pustules (arrow). **Right:** Note ulcers (arrow). (Levitt)

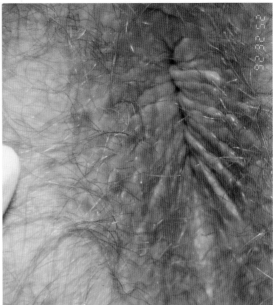

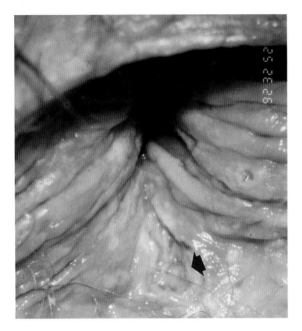

Herpes simplex, type II. Left: Acute anal laceration (arrow). **Right:** At follow-up 10 days later, examination showed healing of the anal laceration. Culture proved herpes simplex, type II.

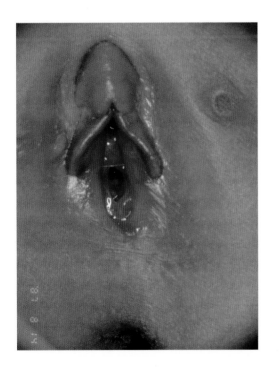

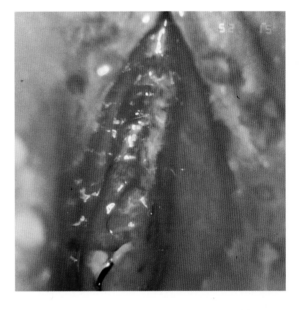

Herpes simplex type I. Culture-proven herpetic vulvar ulcers in a 3-year-old. (Pokorny)

Herpes simplex, type II. An 8-year-old complained of dysuria and bloody discharge. History from child that neighbor had sexually assaulted her two weeks earlier. Lesions cultured positive for herpes simplex, type II.

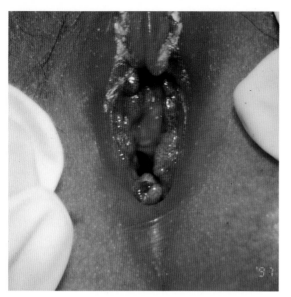

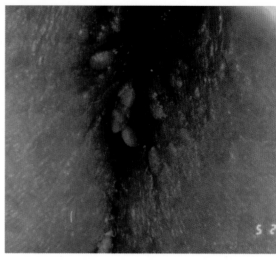

Condyloma acuminatum. A 3-year-old with a history of vaginal bleeding after being "kicked in her privates" at school. Note easy friability of condyloma at the 6-o'clock position (see Chapter 9).

Condyloma acuminatum. A 2-year-old with perianal condyloma acuminatum. (Levitt)

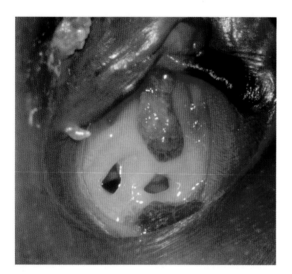

Condyloma acuminatum. Vaginal and anal lesions, including perihymenal lesions at the 6-o'clock position extending onto adjacent tissues via footlike projections. Septate hymen in a 2-year-old with history of maternal condyloma acuminatum at time of birth. The mother described the progression of lesions from the time the child was a few months of age.

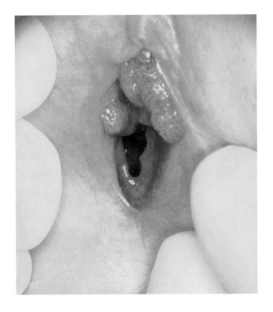

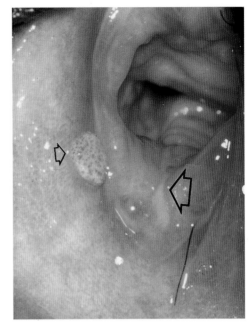

Condyloma acuminatum. Typical presentation of condyloma acuminatum in a 4-year-old. These lesions may become friable and can present as vaginal bleeding. (Pokorny)

Condyloma acuminatum. An 11-year-old with a history of delayed disclosure of ongoing sexual abuse by her stepfather. Note midline transection of the hymen (large arrow) with associated condyloma acuminatum (small arrow).

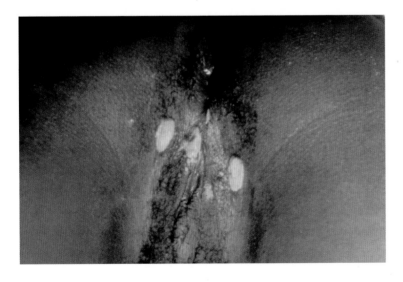

Condyloma latum (secondary syphilis). A 12-year-old with the typical lesions of secondary syphilis.

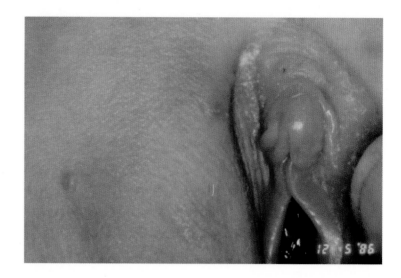

Molluscum contagiosum. Lesions of molluscum contagiosum in different stages on the labia of a 3-year-old. (Levitt)

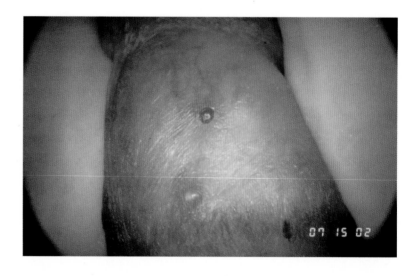

Molluscum contagiosum. Penile lesions in a young boy. Note central umbilication. (Jenny)

9

SEXUALLY
TRANSMITTED DISEASES

DAVID MURAM AND DEBORAH STEWART

The evaluation for sexually transmitted disease (STD) in the child or adolescent is a major focus of the medical examination for alleged sexual abuse. The presence of a potentially sexually transmitted organism can be an indication of prior sexual contact and thus has forensic as well as medical significance. Fortunately, the diagnosis of a sexually transmissible disease (STD) is a rare occurrence in childhood. Most survey studies estimate the incidence of STDs in sexually abused children to be 1%–5%. All STDs that have been reported in adults have also been reported in the pediatric population (Jenny, 1990). The histology and physiology of the genital tracts of prepubertal girls is markedly different from that of adults. (Table 9–1). Such differences affect the clinical presentation, the choice of appropriate diagnostic tests, and treatment options.

Table 9–1. Vaginal Physiology

Newborn	Child	Adolescent
Vaginal hypertrophy	Thin vaginal epithelium	Thick, mucus secreting
Glycogen (+)	Glycogen (−)	Glycogen (+)
Lactobacilli (+)	Lactobacilli (−)	Lactobacilli (+)
Cervical mucus	Thin labia	Cervical mucus
Hymen thick, elastic	Hymen thinner, more delicate	Hymen thick, elastic
Vaginal discharge white, bloody	No discharge	Leukorrhea
		Menses

GENERAL CONSIDERATIONS

This chapter is not intended to be a comprehensive text on sexually transmitted diseases. It focuses primarily on the manifestations of the various diseases in prepubertal children and the medico-legal aspects of STDs in children evaluated for possible sexual abuse. In addition, it lists some general recommendations regarding diagnosis and treatment.

Epidemiology

When the possibility or actual diagnosis of a STD is considered for any child, it is essential to consider all the possible sources of infection. Sexually transmitted organisms can infect children and adolescents through several routes.

- In utero transmission via the placenta and amniotic fluid, such as syphilis or human immunodeficiency virus (HIV).
- Perinatal acquisition via cervical secretions, such as *Neisseria gonorrhoeae*, *Chlamydia trachomatis*, human papillomavirus (HPV), or herpes simplex virus (HSV).
- Transmission through direct contact with infected secretions by one of the following:
  - sexual assault or molestation
  - consensual sexual contact in adolescents

    – nonsexual contact or autoinoculation

    – fomite transmission (extremely rare)

STD Screening

Table 9–2 lists the Centers for Disease Control recommendations for the screening for STDs during the evaluation of a child or adolescent patient suspected of having been sexually abused. The decision to evaluate a child for STDs must be made on an individual basis. It may be unnecessary to perform such evaluation in asymptomatic children whose history suggest a low risk for contracting a STD (CDC, 1998). STD screening is indicated for situ-

Table 9–2. Recommended Laboratory Procedures at Evaluation of Sexually Abused Children

Test	Girls	Boys
Initial Evaluation		
Inspection	Body	Body
	Oral cavity	Oral cavity
	Genitalia	Genitalia
	Anal & perianal	Anal & perianal
Cultures for *N. gonorrhoea*	Vaginal	Urethral*
	Anal	Anal
	Oral	Oral
Cultures for *C. trachomatis*	Vaginal	Urethral*
	Anal	Anal
Culture	Vaginal fluid	
Wet mount for *Trichomonas vaginalis*, amine test, clue cells, and other indicators of bacterial vaginosis (BV)		
Serum for serologic testing—syphilis, hepatitis, HIV		
Evaluation at 2-Week Follow-Up		
If indicated, obtain repeat cultures and wet mount evaluation in children who did not receive prophylactic therapy.		
Evaluation at 12-Week Follow-Up		
Obtain serologic tests for syphilis, HBV, and HIV.		

* Meatal specimen is sufficient when discharge is present.

ations in which there is an increased probability that the child has contracted an STD. These include the following:

- The child has signs or symptoms of an STD.
- The child has signs or symptoms of a genital infection that may have been transmitted through sexual contact.
- The known offender is known to harbor an STD.
- The known offender is at high risk of harboring an STD.
- There is a high prevalence of STD in the community.
- There is a history of penetration or ejaculation.
- Siblings or other household members are known to have STD or have signs or symptoms of STD.

The extent of the evaluation for STD may vary as well. A history of oral–genital, oral–anal, anal–genital, or genital–genital contact requires that relevant cultures be obtained. In very young children or in those unable to give a history, the examiner should consider culturing oral, genital, and anal sites. A reliable history of fondling over clothing in an asymptomatic older child or adolescent in conjunction with ongoing follow-up may not require testing. Indeed, GC cultures in asymptomatic children seen weeks after an assault are almost always negative (Muram et al, 1996; Ingram et al, 1992). The committee on Child Abuse and Neglect of American Academy of Pediatrics suggests certain criteria that should alert the examiner to screen for STD. Recent studies confirm that almost all girls with gonorrhea can be detected when these guidelines are followed (Hammershlag, 1998). However, there are insufficient data to determine the suitability of such recommendations for rectal and pharyngeal infections or genital infections in boys.

Histories must be evaluated carefully, and the examiner should be aware that infected genital secretions present on the hands of the perpetrator may spread STDs as well as genital contact. Any child or adolescent with ano-genital or oral symptoms should be evaluated regardless of the history. The physician should perform serologic testing for hepatitis B virus (HBV) in children who did not receive HBV vaccine as part of their vaccination. Since hepatitis B is a preventable disease, it is recommended that non-immunized children receive HBV vaccine if the history of serologic testing indicates that the child is susceptible. The first dose of the vaccine may be given immediately, the second dose 1–2 months later and the third dose 4–6 months later.

Serologic testing for HIV should be considered on an individual basis and requires repeat evaluations. There are insufficient data regarding the safety and efficacy of post-exposure prophylactic therapy for HIV in children.

If the child or adolescent is evaluated acutely after a single assault, then the CDC recommends that the tests listed in Table 9–2 be repeated within 2 weeks, except serologic tests for syphilis and HIV which should be repeated in 3 months and again in 6 months for HIV. A single examination may be sufficient if the last abusive episode occurred long before the medical evaluation. Some states now allow testing of the alleged perpetrator for the presence of communicable diseases such as syphilis and HIV infection. If the abuse has been ongoing, and if circumstances permit, the alleged offender may be evaluated in the above manner, and follow-up care for the child or adolescent can be appropriately modified.

Diagnostic Methods

Certain general principles apply to the diagnostic tools most useful in pediatric and adolescent populations. Because of the legal and psychological implications of a false-positive test, only the most specific and sensitive tests available should be used. Insensitive screening tests, such as direct fluorescent antibody (DFA) or enzyme immunoassay (EIA), should not be used in children or sexually assaulted young adolescents for the following reasons:

- The use of non-specific and non-sensitive tests in a low-prevalence population creates a much higher likelihood that a positive test will be a false positive and true positives will be missed. For example, if a test with a very high sensitivity and 95% specificity is used, and the prevalence of infection in the population is 5%, then the positive predictive value of the test would only be 50%.
- Most of the screening tests for STDs have been developed for and approved only for genital sites in the adult population. Existing organisms in the genital tract of children may interfere with these tests. For example, when non-culture tests for chlamydia are used for vaginal specimens, other organisms such as acinetobacter, *N. gonorrhoeae*, and *Gardnerella vaginalis* may interfere with the reading of the test causing false-positive results.
- The CDC recommends that all presumed isolates for *N. gonorrhoeae* should be confirmed by at least two tests that involve dif-

ferent principles. Furthermore, isolates should be preserved in case additional or repeat testing is needed. Similar considerations apply for the detection and confirmation of *C. trachomatis.*

- Sampling techniques must take into consideration the age and physical maturity of the patient. While mature adolescents can be sampled like adults, sampling from prepubertal children is different. Samples for *N. gonorrhoeae* and *C. trachomatis* should be collected from the vagina rather than the cervix. A meatal specimen of urethral discharge is an adequate substitute for an intra-urethral swab specimen in boys. Recovery of *C. trachomatis* from the urethra in boys is so low that the CDC does not recommend obtaining an intra-urethral swab for *C. trachomatis.* There are insufficient data to determine the sensitivity and specificity any of the PCR methods for the detection of *C. trachomatis* particles in a child's urine. Pharyngeal specimens for *C. trachomatis* are not recommended because the yield is low, perinatal acquired infections may persist into early childhood, and some laboratories cannot reliably distinguish *C. trachomatis* from *C. pneumoniae.*
- Biopsy of lesions, such as those suspected of being caused by HPV, may be useful in obtaining specimens for histopathologic evaluation and for subtyping using deoxyribonucleic acid (DNA) probe techniques. This is particularly important because of the potentially long incubation period of HPV in a child and the association of certain subtypes of HPV with genital cancers.

Medico-Legal Considerations

The presence of a sexually transmitted organism raises both medical and legal issues unique for children and adolescents.

Medical Considerations. The recommended prophylactic therapy against STDs for adolescents includes ceftriaxone (125 mg IM in a single dose) plus azithromycin (1 gm orally in a single dose) or doxycycline (100 mg orally twice a day for 7 days). As previously stated, the clinical manifestations in children are different than in adults. For example, *N. gonorrhoeae* and *C. trachomatis* rarely produce pelvic inflammatory disease or infectious arthritis in infected children. Therefore, prophylactic therapy is not indicated in asymptomatic children. There are no epidemiologic data available concerning age-related relative risks for sexual transmission following exposure. The only data available are from the adult literature. Long-term effects of STDs such as HPV remain unknown. Many clinicians are concerned about sequelae of childhood acquisition of STDs because of the much longer exposure to the organism.

It is unclear how often and in what circumstances bacterial vaginosis (BV) should be considered a sexually transmitted disease. Although BV may be an indicator of sexual activity, it is unclear whether BV is caused by an acquisition of sexually transmitted pathogens. Organisms associated with the clinical manifestations of BV, such as *G. vaginalis*, are also found in non-abused children or sexually inexperienced adolescents.

Treatment regimens for children may differ from those used for adults. This is particularly true for tetracycline treatment of *C. trachomatis* (contraindicated in children under 8 years of age) and podophyllin treatment for HPV infections because of the potential risk of neurotoxicity.

Legal Significance. The legal significance of the presence of a sexually transmitted organism in a child is often a critical piece of evidence. The clinician should consider the mode of transmission prior to reporting the patient to protective services. A careful maternal history must be taken to differentiate preexisting neonatal colonization from postnatal acquisition through direct contact. A medical examination of the mother, with appropriate diagnostic procedures, may be necessary. For infections with *C. trachomatis* and anogenital HPV, some data are available on the persistence of the perinatally acquired infection. Under federal evidence rules, medical examination and testing of the alleged perpetrator for STDs may be allowed following a court hearing.

The clinician interpreting STD evidence must have a solid knowledge base of the epidemiology, clinical manifestations, and treatment of the various STDs. This knowledge should include data on children, adolescents, and adults. Clinicians should avoid extrapolating adult data to children because the infectivity and clinical course may be quite different. Guidelines for reporting various STDs are listed in Table 9–3.

Lastly, when the only evidence of sexual abuse is the isolation of an organism or the detection of antibodies to a sexually transmissible agent, the findings should be confirmed and the implications considered carefully.

Table 9–3. Guidelines for Making the Decision to Report Sexual Abuse of Children

| Data Available | | Laboratory Findings | Response | |
History	Physical Examination		Level of Concern about Sexual Abuse	Report Decision
None	Normal	None	None	No report
Behavioral changes†	Normal	None	Variable depending upon behavior	Possible report*; follow closely (possible mental health referral)
None	Nonspecific findings	None	Low (worry)	Possible report*; follow closely
Nonspecific history by child or history by parent only	Nonspecific findings	None	Intermediate	Possible report*; follow closely
None	Specific findings‡	None	High	Report
Clear statement	Normal	None	High	Report
Clear statement	Specific findings	None	High	Report
None	Normal, nonspecific or specific findings	Positive culture for gonorrhea; positive serologic test for HIV; syphilis; presence of semen, sperm acid phosphatase	Very high	Report
Behavior changes	Nonspecific findings	Other sexually transmitted diseases	High	Report

* A report may or may not be indicated. The decision to report should be based on discussion with local or regional experts and/or child protective services agencies.

† Some behavioral changes are nonspecific, and other are more worrisome.

‡ Other reasons for findings ruled out.

Source: AAP Committee on Child Abuse and Neglect: Guidelines for the evaluation of sexual abuse of children. *Pediatrics.* 1999;103:186–191.

THE ORGANISMS

Neisseria gonorrhoeae

Biology. N. *gonorrhoeae* is a gram-negative intracellular diplococcus with absolute requirements for CO_2, an ambient temperature of 36°–38°C, and a pH of 7.2–7.6. Its predilection for infecting columnar or pseudostratified epithelium accounts for its presence in the endocervix of adolescents, and possibly the prepubertal vagina. The absence of endocervical glands on the ectocervix of the prepubertal child makes the cervix more resistant to infection, and ascending genital tract infection with N. *gonorrhoeae* is rare in children. Other sites of infection include the female and male urethra, conjunctivae, rectum, and pharynx. Secondary sites in adolescents and adults include gonococcal arthritis, sepsis, meningitis, endocarditis, myocarditis, and perihepatitis.

The overall incidence of gonococcal infection in the 0–9-year age group was reported at 6.5/100,000 (Pokorny, 1989). However, included in this group are neonates with gonococcal infection, most commonly ophthalmia neonatorum. Beyond the neonatal period, sexual contact is the almost exclusive cause of gonococcal infections in children (Sung and MacDonald, 1998). If gonorrhea is diagnosed in a child, all household contacts and close non-household associates should be cultured to identify asymptomatic carriers. Positive gonorrhea cultures have been found in 15% to 50% of household contacts of infected children (Alexander et al, 1984; Nair et al, 1986). In adults, transmission rates are dependent on the infected anatomic sites and the number of exposures (Hook and Handsfield, 1990) (Table 9–4).

Transmission rates in prepubertal children have not been established. Gonococcal infections are quite common in adolescents. Screening endocervical cultures were positive in 0.5%–13% of sex-

Table 9–4. Incidence of N. *gonorrhoeae* Transmission

Infected female to male (single exposure)	20%
Infected male to female (unknown number of exposures)	90%
Infected pharynx to other sites	Unknown
Fomites	Rare, if ever

ually active adolescents, with higher rates among those with a history of sexual abuse, those seen in inner city clinics, incarcerated teens, and those who engage in survival sex or risky sexual behaviors (Vermund et al, 1990; Roochuarg, 1991).

In purulent secretions, gonococci can remain viable from 2 hours to 3 days raising the possibility of fomite transmission (Srivastava, 1980; Ingram, 1989). However, there are no convincing data for any nonsexual mode of transmission, and there is only one documented case of an identified fomite transmission (Neinstein, 1984; Lipsitt et al, 1984). Branch and Paxton have shown that careful interviewing can detect the source of gonococcal infection in most children older than 1 year of age (1965).

The incubation period for *N. gonorrhoeae* is roughly one week, with symptoms generally appearing in 2–7 days. These children present with a vulvovaginitis accompanied by erythema, purulent vaginal discharge, and pruritus. Dysuria may result from the vulvitis or from urethritis. Untreated, this purulent vaginal discharge may be replaced by a serous discharge that can persist for several months (Nelson et al, 1976). Older studies of the natural history of untreated gonococcal vaginitis in girls have shown cases in which the discharge resolved without treatment leaving the children colonized (and, therefore, infectious) for up to 7 months. Some children then became culture negative without treatment. Populations of children studied in the preantibiotic era indicated a low incidence of peritonitis (Benson and Steer, 1937). Only a few cases of gonococcal salpingitis had been reported in prepubertal girls (Ingram, 1994; Kulhanjian and Hilton, 1991). Lastly, a very few children may have asymptomatic colonization with *N. gonorrhoeae* (DeJong, 1986).

In prepubertal boys, urethritis may be the only presenting symptom. Pharyngitis and proctitis have also been reported in children of both sexes. However, colonization of the pharynx and rectum is more common than symptomatic infection (Silber et al, 1983). Gonococcal conjunctivitis beyond the neonatal period has also been reported and generally presents with a febrile illness accompanied by a hyperpurulent conjunctivitis and periorbital cellulitis. This infection may result in visual impairment if not diagnosed promptly and treated appropriately.

Infection at more than one anatomic site is quite common. In one series, half the girls with positive vaginal cultures also had positive rectal cultures, and 15% had simultaneous positive vaginal and pharyngeal cultures. Only 3% had positive rectal cultures as the sole finding (Nelson et al, 1976). Other investigators reported similar observations (Ingram, 1994).

Diagnostic Methods. The use of indirect testing methods for *N. gonorrhoeae* is not recommended in children; both false-positive and false-negative tests have been reported with monoclonal antibody and direct flourescent antibody testing methods prior to adolescence (Whittington et al, 1988; Hammerschlag, 1989). DNA specific probes for gonorrhea and polymerase chain reaction (PCR) tests are quite useful in adolescents, with reported sensitivity and specificity rates of 97% and 99%, respectively. In addition, the DNA probes may be used as a reliable test of cure (Hanks et al, 1994). Ligase chain reaction tests were also found to be quite sensitive for the detection of *N. gonorrhoeae* (Liebling et al, 1994; Ching et al, 1995; Smith et al, 1995). However, there are no data regarding the utility of any of these methods in prepubertal children.

Culture via direct inoculation onto the Thayer-Martin plate or appropriate holding media is the only acceptable method of diagnosing *N. gonorrhoeae* in suspected sexual abuse. It is unwise to inoculate the specimen initially onto a nonselective medium because there are many *Neisseria* species in the normal oral flora. Presumptive positive isolates must be confirmed with two of the three current methods used to identify *N. gonorrhoeae*, carbohydrate degradation, enzyme substrate, or immunologic. It is also recommended that isolates obtained from children be stored at −70°C for additional confirmatory testing in case this is needed at a later date.

Treatment. The Centers for Disease Control and Prevention (CDC) recommends the use of ceftriaxone in children with gonococcal infections. Children weighing more than 45 kg are treated as adults. Children weighing less than 45 kg with uncomplicated infection (vulvovaginitis, urethritis, pharyngitis, or proctitis) may be treated with intramuscular ceftriaxone, 25–50 mg/kg, not to exceed 125 mg. Oral cefixime may be an alternative; however, efficacy data were gathered from adults, and until its efficacy is proven in prepubertal children, this regimen should be used only for children weighing >45 kg and in adolescents (Handsfield et al, 1991; Plourde et al, 1992). The treatment regimens are listed in Table 9–5.

Table 9-5. Treatment regimens for Gonorrhea

Treatment of Uncomplicated Infection	Treatment of Disseminated Infection
Children (<45 kg)	*Children (<45 kg)*
Ceftriaxone 125 mg IM in a single dose	Ceftriaxone 50 mg/kg IM or IV in a single dose daily for 7 days
Adolescents and Children (>45 kg)	*Adolescents and Children (>45 kg)*
One of the following:	**One of the following:**
Ceftriaxone 125 mg IM in a single dose	Ceftriaxone 1 g IM or IV every 8 hours
Cefixime 400 mg orally in a single dose	Cefotaxime 1 g IV every 8 hours
Ciprofloxacin 500 mg orally in a single dose	Ceftizoxime 1 g IV every 8 hours
Ofloxacin 400 mg orally in a single dose	**OR, for persons allergic to β lactam drugs:**
PLUS one of the following:	Ciprofloxacin 500 mg IV every 12 hours
Azithromycin 1 gm orally in a single dose	Ofloxacin 400 mg IV every 12 hours
Doxycycline 100 mg orally, twice daily for 7 days	Spectinomycin 2 g IM every 12 hours
	Continue treatment for 24–48 hours after improvement and then change to one of the following to complete a week of therapy:
	Cefixime 400 mg orally twice a day
	Ciprofloxacin 500 mg orally twice a day
	Ofloxacin 400 mg orally orally twice a day

Modified from Centers for Disease Control. Sexually transmitted diseases treatment guidelines. MMWR 1998;47(RR-1):1–116.

Spectinomycin 40 mg/kg may be used intramuscularly in children who cannot tolerate cephalosporins, but it is unreliable for the treatment of pharyngeal infections.

It is recommended that children over 8 years of age also receive azythromycin or doxycycline to cover concomitant infection with *C. trachomatis*. Children with complicated gonococcal infections, such as conjunctivitis, peritonitis, arthritis, or meningitis, should be given a more prolonged course of parenteral ceftriaxone (Table 9–5). Follow-up cultures should be obtained 10–14 days after treatment to ensure that the treatment has been effective. Prophylactic treatment for gonococcal infection in asymptomatic prepubertal children being evaluated for possible sexual abuse is not recommended.

Chlamydia trachomatis

Biology. C. trachomatis is an obligate intracellular parasite with 15 serotypes identified to date. The less common serotypes, L1, L2, and L3, are responsible for lymphogranuloma venereum; the serotypes D-K are responsible for inclusion conjunctivitis, pneumonia, vaginitis, non-gonococcal urethritis, cervicitis, and salpingitis. This obligate intracellular organism can be cultured only in a living cell host and not in artificial culture media. The primary modes of transmission of *C. trachomatis* all involve direct contact. Fomite transmission is extremely unlikely given the obligate intracellular nature of this parasite. Concomitant infection with *C. trachomatis* and *N. gonorrhoeae* is fairly common. In one study of prepubertal children with gonococcal infection, 27% were also positive for *C. trachomatis* (Rettig and Nelson, 1981). Transmission rates are dependent on the anatomic sites infected and number of exposures (Stamm and Holmes, 1990) (Table 9–6).

At birth, the neonate is inoculated by contact with infected secretions, and organisms then spread to the eyes, nasopharynx, vagina, and rectum. Vertical transmission at the time of cesarean

Table 9–6. Incidence of *C. trachomatis* Transmission

Infected female to male (unknown number of exposures)	30%
Infected male to female (unknown number of exposures)	90%

section performed after the rupture of membranes has also been reported. (Harrison and Alexander, 1984; Alexander, 1984; Frau and Alexander, 1985; Schachter et al, 1986). It appears that each site may be separately inoculated at birth, in addition to auto-inoculation from one site to another (Schachter et al, 1986).

Inclusion conjunctivitis is primarily a disease of the neonatal period. Beyond infancy, chlamydial infection in children is uncommon and generally presents as genital tract infection. Asymptomatic colonization of the genital tract may occur (Bell et al, 1987; Hammerschlag et al, 1978; Schachter, 1990). In Ingram's study (1986), 60% of children with positive vaginal cultures were asymptomatic. All of the children in this study with a positive oral or rectal culture were asymptomatic. However, as with gonococcal infection of the prepubertal genital tract, the "atrophic," unestrogenized vaginal epithelium may be directly infected with the organism, causing a true vaginitis. Children usually present with vaginitis, urethritis, and/or pyuria. Vulvar erythema, vaginal discharge, rectal pain, and vaginal bleeding are common complaints. *C. trachomatis* has also been reported as a cause of symptomatic urethritis in prepubertal boys (Rettig and Nelson, 1981).

There are no figures available for the incidence of chlamydial infection in children. However, a number of studies have suggested vertical transmission is common in infants delivered through an infected genital tract. The risk of inclusion conjunctivitis ranges from 18%–50%; chlamydial pneumonitis occurs in 10%–22% of exposed infants; and 60%–70% of exposed infants demonstrate serologic evidence of infection by 12 months of age (Harrison and Alexander, 1990; Alexander, 1984). *C. trachomatis* rectal or vaginal infection in sexually abused children is relatively infrequent, with prevalence of less than 5% (Schwarcz and Wittington, 1990). The infection is quite common in sexually active adolescents and young adults. The organism was isolated from endocervical cultures from 4%–17% of 16–24-year-old females enlisting in the U.S. Job Corps (CDC, 1997). In a recent study, prevalence was higher for non-Hispanic blacks (7%) than for Mexican-Americans (3%) and non-Hispanic whites (2%). Prevalence was higher for women than for men in non-Hispanic blacks (7% vs. 6%), Mexican-Americans (5% vs. 2%), and non-Hispanic whites (2% vs. 1%). In 15- to 19-year-old women, prevalence was 13% in non-Hispanic blacks, 11% in Mexican-Americans, and 5% in non-Hispanic whites (Mertz et al,

1998). In girls who have reported sexual abuse, the overall incidence of chlamydial infection is generally reported to be between 2%–6% (Cupoli and Sewell, 1988; Keskey et al, 1987). However, the incidence varies greatly in different areas and different clinics. In one series of preadolescent sexually abused girls, 43% of cultures were positive (Keskey et al, 1987), while in another series the prevalence was 13%. (Muram, 1989). However, in a subsequent large study, the prevalence of *C. trachomatis* was only 1.2%. (Ingram et al, 1992).

As with gonococcal infection, multi-site infection with *C. trachomatis* has been reported. In Ingram's population of suspected sexual abuse victims, 8% of children had positive vaginal cultures. He also found 2.4% positive rectal and 0.8% positive pharyngeal cultures in this group (Ingram et al, 1986). An earlier study by the same author noted a 3% incidence of positive pharyngeal and concomitant vaginal and rectal cultures in a population of abused children (Ingram et al, 1984). A significant number of child and adolescent patients had multiple culture sites that were positive for chlamydial genital infection. As with gonococcal infection, many of these positive cultures were obtained from anatomic sites that the children had not mentioned in their initial disclosures of abuse (Keskey et al, 1987).

In the neonatal period, infection with *C. trachomatis* most commonly presents with the development of inclusion conjunctivitis at 5–7 days–of–age. Initially, a mucoid discharge is present that may become purulent within a few days. Without treatment, colonization of the conjunctiva may persist for up to 2 years and may produce chronic sequelae. Perinatal exposure to *C. trachomatis* may also result in pneumonitis presenting at 3 to 11 weeks of age with a history of prolonged cough and congestion (Harrison and Alexander, 1990).

Perinatal exposure may also result in colonization of the vagina and rectum (Schachter et al, 1979). Longitudinal studies of asymptomatic infants exposed to *C. trachomatis* at birth have shown carriage of the organism up to 55 weeks in the rectum and 53 weeks in the vagina (Bell et al, 1992). Because by the age of 1–3 years the majority of children have been treated with antibiotics to which the organism is sensitive, the issue of persistence often become less likely, and the potential for sexual transmission as the source of infection becomes much greater.

Cell culture using a monolayer of suspectible cells, such as

McCoy cells, is regarded as the optimal method of diagnosis. Because this organism is intracellular, it is important to obtain epithelial cells for the culture rather than culturing any discharge that is present. In prepubertal children, a careful vaginal or urethral culture is necessary. The use of an adequate growth and/or transport media, such as minimal essential media (MEM), is also important. Urethral swabs of calcium alginate are often useful in obtaining samples from children because of their small diameter, but they must be batch tested to ensure there is no toxicity to the growth of *C. trachomatis* (Mahony and Chernesky, 1985). Alternatively, the clinician may use male urethral and nasopharyngeal polyester swabs. When positive culture results are obtained, freezing of the organism at $-70°$ C may be indicated. This is especially important if forensic confirmation is needed later.

Antigen detection testing has become increasingly popular in response to the expense and limited availability of cell cultures for *C. trachomatis*. These testing methods employ one of the following: a direct flourescent monoclonal antibody (for example, Microtrak), an enzyme linked immunoassay (ELISA; for example, Chlamydiazyme), DNA probes (such as Pace 2, Gen-Probe), PCR (such as Amplicor), ligase chain reaction (LCR), or transcription mediated amplification (Gen Probe Amplified). These tests are most useful in adolescents and other high-risk populations with high sensitivity and specificity rates (Clarke et al, 1993; Schachter et al, 1994). However, sensitivity and specificity data were generated in high-prevalence populations such as adult STD clinics. Because of the legal ramifications associated with the diagnosis of chlamydial infection in children, the CDC recommends using appropriate cultures in prepubertal children. The low prevalence of *C. trachomatis* infection in sexually abused children and the need to test anatomic sites other than the cervix and urethra contribute to unacceptable sensitivity and specificity rates. Up to 50% false-positive and false-negative rates have been reported with the use of some antigen detection methods in children (Hammerschlag et al, 1988; Hammerschlag, 1997). Serologic testing for the presence of antibodies to *C. trachomatis* has not been clinically useful in children because seroconversion is common during the childhood years.

Finally, the CDC guidelines suggest that when cultures for *C. trachomatis* are unavailable one may use DNA amplification tests (CDC, 1998). Preliminary data comparing cultures and PCR performed on vaginal washings in prepubertal girls show sensitivity and specificty rates of 100% and 89.7%, respectively (Embree et al, 1996).

Azithromycin 1g orally in a single dose or doxycycline (100 mg twice daily for 7 days) is recommended for children 8 years of age or older. Children who are younger than 8 years but who weigh 45 kg or more may be treated with azithromycin 1g orally in a single dose. Erythromycin (50 mg/kg/day for 10 to 14 days) is the treatment of choice for genital chlamydial infections in children who weigh less than 45 kg. The effectiveness of erythromycin therapy in children is approximately 80%, and a second course of therapy may be required. Adolescents may be treated with a single dose (1g) of azithromycin or alternatively with doxycycline (100 mg twice daily for 7 days).

Prophylactic treatment for *C. trachomatis* in prepubertal children is not indicated. The low prevalence and minimal risk for upper genital tract disease allow the practitioner to await culture results prior to instituting treatment. Because of the relatively high association of infection with *N. gonorrhoeae* and *C. trachomatis* in children, coverage for *C. trachomatis* should be included in treatment for children with gonococcal infection if chlamydial cultures are not available. Follow-up cultures should be obtained to ensure eradication of the organism.

Herpes Simplex Virus

Genital herpes is caused by an infection with the double stranded DNA herpes simplex virus (HSV). The virus has two subtypes, HSV-1 and HSV-2. Although it once was thought that HSV-1 occurred only in oral lesions, and HSV-2 in genital lesions, it is well documented that infection with a particular HSV type is not site specific. Each HSV type generates its own specific antibody response, with antibody against one HSV type not providing immunity to the other type (Corey, 1990). The virus can survive in host cells in a latent state for long periods of time. Reactivation of these latent infections can occur by factors that are not well understood. HSV is readily inactivated at room temperature and by drying.

Herpes simplex virus is transmitted by close contact with an individual who is shedding the virus with the virus entering mucosal surfaces through an epithelial break (Corey, 1990). Infectivity may be as high as 50%. Transmission by sexual contact is the most common source of childhood genital herpes (Hibbard, 1985; Gushurst, 1985; Kaplan et al, 1985; Nahmias et al, 1968; Gardner and Jones, 1984). Autoinnoculation from nongenital lesions has been documented as a source of some genital herpes during childhood (Miller et al, 1987). The possibility of nonsexual transmission through close contact has been implicated in the high incidence of antibodies to HSV 2 among children in certain geographic areas. However, the casual transmission of genital herpes to a child through nonsexual contact has not been proven. Similarly, fomite transmission has not been documented (Douglas and Corey, 1983).

Congenital HSV infection from transplacental passage may occur, although it is uncommon. Vertical transmission of the virus during vaginal delivery has been described well as the cause of potentially devastating neonatal herpes infection. Perinatal transmission is an uncommon cause of childhood genital herpes, but if the genitalia are the site of neonatal cutaneous infection, the possibility for recurrent genital lesions exists (Taieb et al, 1987).

During childhood, herpes simplex virus infection most commonly presents as gingivostomatitis. This may appear as a mild gingivitis or as a more severe infection with painful vesicular lesions of the lips and oral cavity that later ulcerate. A pharyngitis may also develop. Multifocal disease is quite common in children with primary HSV infection (Sweet and Gibbs, 1990).

Genital herpes lesions, caused by both HSV-1 and -2, have been reported in children. The clinical presentation of primary genital herpes is very similar to that described in adults. After an incubation period of 2–20 days, The initial outbreak of lesions is often accompanied by pruritis and swelling, followed by the development of papules and vesicles that subsequently ulcerate in 1–3 days. Grouped vesicles, if present, are pathognomonic; lesions may be found on the vulvae, vagina, cervix, or rectum; and inguinal adenopathy is common (Sweet and Gibbs, 1990).

These vesicles later ulcerate and often are accompanied by systemic symptoms such as inguinal adenopathy, fever, malaise, nausea, and headache. Urinary retention may develop. Lesions due to HSV-1 and -2 may be clinically indistinguishable, but HSV-2 is four times more likely to cause recurrent genital herpes. Secondary lesions are generally less severe with less viral shedding and no systemic symptoms. Symptoms of primary infections usually resolve within 10–21 days. Symptoms of recurrent genital disease are milder and more localized to the genital region. External genital lesions may be unilateral. Prodromal symptoms may vary from mild tingling to severe sacral neuralgia occurring as early as five days prior to the outbreak. Symptoms of recurrent disease may last from 1 to 14 days. In non-primary first infections, symptoms are milder than in primary, but greater than in recurrent, episodes.

HSV-1 and HSV-2 may cause perianal infections. These infections are often associated with acute onset of pain, bloody/mucoid discharge, tenesmus, constipation, fever, malaise, myalgia, and urinary retention. External lesions may be visible on only 50% of those infected. Anoscopy or sigmoidoscopy may reveal friability of the lower 10 cm of the rectum and occasionally demonstrate discrete ulcerations. The differential diagnosis includes herpes zoster, syphilis, chancroid, trauma, Behçet's disease, and other less common disorders (Christian et al, 1997).

The diagnosis of genital herpes in a child is made by viral culture of suspicious lesions. It is recommended that positive herpes cultures in children be subjected to confirmatory testing. False negative cultures may occur if specimens are obtained from lesions with decreased viral shedding, such as recurrent lesions or those that are ulcerated or crusted. Antigen detection testing has not been evaluated in children and is not recommended for the reasons discussed previously.

A recent study illustrates the advantage of rapid PCR diagnosis of herpes simplex virus and varicella zoster virus in vesicle fluids. The investigators tested vesicular fluid from 132 patients using PCR technique. The PCR did not differentiate between HSV-1 and HSV-2, but the sensitivity and specificity were 100%. The sensitivities of virus isolation and electron microscopy for detection of herpes simplex virus were 56% and 80%, respectively (Beards et al, 1998).

Serologic diagnosis is most useful in detecting prior infection or showing that the current infection is primary. It may be a helpful adjunct to culture or immunologic diagnosis. It may be particularly useful when lesions are cultured in the ulcerative stages. Paired sera must be obtained if there are indications of active or recent infection. The absence of antibodies on two occasions, two to three weeks apart, excludes the diagnosis. A rise in IgM antibodies followed by a rise in IgG antibodies is indicative of a recent infection.

The antibody testing performed by many commercial laboratories has cross-reactivity between HSV-1 and HSV-2. Thus, a fourfold increased in the titer is difficult to interpret because it may represent a significant new infection or a new infection with another type.

There are no treatment guidelines for children with genital herpes infection. Acyclovir (400 mg orally three times a day for 7 to 10 days, or 200 mg five times a day for 7 to 10 days), famcyclovir (250 mg orally three times a day for 7 to 10 days) and valacyclovir (1 g orally twice daily for 7 to 10 days) have been demonstrated to be effective in adults for the treatment of primary herpes. Regimens for suppressive treatment of secondary lesions require lower doses of these drugs (acyclovir; 400 mg orally twice daily, famcyclovir; 250 mg orally twice daily, valacyclovir; 500 mg or 1 g daily) (CDC, 1998). Since the therapeutic safety of acyclovir during childhood has been demonstrated, many clinicians treat children with primary genital herpes with acyclovir, 30–60 mg/kg/day for 10 days. Others prefer to use only symptomatic treatment of the genital lesions with local care, sitz-baths, and drying agents. Superimposed bacterial infection is uncommon but when present may require antibiotic therapy (Kesson, 1998).

Bacterial Vaginosis

Biology. Bacterial vaginosis is a syndrome associated with an overgrowth of multiple organisms including *Gardnerella vaginalis, Mycoplasma hominis, Mobiluncus sp., Bacteroides sp.,* and gram-negative organisms. In conjunction with polymicrobial overgrowth is a relative lack of hydrogen-producing lactobacilli, and a resultant alkaline vaginal pH. The presence or absence of any of these individual organisms (such as *G. vaginalis*) neither confirms nor negates the diagnosis of bacterial vaginosis.

Epidemiology. Bacterial vaginosis (BV) is relatively common in adolescents and adult women and is likely a marker of sexual activity (Chambers et al, 1987; Hillier and Holmes, 1990). It is found in increased frequency with other STDs and is thought to be a precedent for some forms of pelvic inflammatory disease. *G. vaginalis* and the syndrome of BV may be present in sexually inexperienced adolescents as well. Some studies concluded that *G. vaginalis* was found significantly more often in sexually abused children than in asymptomatic, non-abused controls (Chambers et al, 1987; Hillier and Holmes, 1990; Bartley et al, 1987; Hammerschlag, 1985). However, Ingram and colleagues reported that the prevalence of *G. vaginalis* was similar among abused girls and controls (Ingram et al, 1992). Other modes of transmission may occur, but there is very little data regarding vertical, casual, or fomite transmission. It is unclear how often and in what circumstances BV should be considered a sexually transmitted disease.

Clinical Syndromes. In bacterial vaginosis, an odorous, non-viscous, homogeneous vaginal discharge may be present in prepubertal and adolescent girls. Although *G. vaginalis* is present in most patients with BV, this organism may be present in asymptomatic girls. Abdominal pain, pruritus, or dysuria are not associated with a clinical diagnosis of BV. Some investigators believe that the presence of BV may predispose the pubertal female to an increased risk of both obstetric infections, such as chorioamnionitis, and gynecological infections, such as pelvic inflammatory disease (Eschenbach et al, 1988). No clinical counterpart of BV has been described in males.

In pubertal females, the diagnosis of BV is made by the presence of three of the following criteria: (1) homogeneous discharge, (2) development of a fishy odor when 10% KOH is added to vaginal secretions (positive whiff test), (3) presence of >20% of epithelial cells as clue cells (small coccobacillary organisms coating granulated epithelial cells), (4) a vaginal pH higher than 4.5. The sensitivity of the clue cell is approximately 70%–90%, with approximately 95% specificity. The gram stain adds sensitivity and characteristically shows a decrease in lactobacilli and an abundance of gram-variable coccobacilli consistent with *G. vaginalis* or *Bacteroides spp.* The sensitivity and specificity of these diagnostic methods are not well documented for prepubertal children. Because the prepubertal pH is physiologically high, pH cannot be used as criterion. The CDC guidelines for the evaluation of children and adolescent victims of sexual abuse do not currently recommend obtaining cultures for *G. vaginalis*.

Treatment of asymptomatic individuals is controversial. Adolescents with bacterial vaginosis may be treated with metronidazole (500 mg orally twice a day for 7 days), clindamycin cream 2% (one full applicator intravaginally at bedtime for 7 days), or metronidazole gel, 0.75% (one full applicator intravaginally once or twice daily for 5 days). Alternative regimens consist of metronidazole (2 g orally in a single dose) or clindamycin (300 mg orally twice daily for 7 days). Partner treatment can be considered in recurrent symptomatic cases, but is controversial.

Human Papillomavirus

Over 60 biotypes of HPV have been described. The majority of these biotypes infect cutaneous sites, but over 14 biotypes that infect mucosal sites have been described. Two of these mucosal biotypes, HPV–13 and HPV–32, infect the oral cavity exclusively, but the genital tract acts as a reservoir for the others. Each genital subtype has a different set of lesion morphology, predilection for extragenital site infection, and oncogenic potential. The organism infects epithelial cells, which undergo transformation and proliferation. Transmission occurs via direct contact with infected skin or mucous membranes and has been described during gestation and delivery and with direct contact, including sexual abuse. Nongenital sites may be infected by genital warts. The most common non-genital site is the anus. Anal warts can be found in association with genital warts or may occur without genital infection. Transmission of HPV through oral–genital contact has been described and can include lesions on the lips, tongue, or palate. Multiple studies have demonstrated the role of sexual transmission of anogenital warts. Recent studies done by teams skilled in child and adolescent sexual assault suggest that the vast majority of children older than 12–18 months with anogenital HPV have acquired their infection as a result of direct sexual contact (Boyd, 1990; Herman-Giddens et al, 1998; Jenison et al, 1990). The most common types of anogenital HPV infections are subtypes 6 and 11, followed by 16 and 18, and, rarely, 31 (Jones et al, 1993; Craighill et al, 1993).

Perinatal transmission of HPV infections from infected mothers to their infants has been well documented. Although the predominant method of infection occurs through direct contact with infected lesions in the birth canal, a single case of congenital anal condyloma has been reported, suggesting in utero transmission of HPV (Tang, 1978). As the incubation period for HPV infection averages 2–3 months in adults, but has been described up to 20 months, a young infant with anogenital warts may have acquired them through vertical transmission from the mother. Perinatally transmitted lesions of HPV infection may not become obvious to caretakers or clinicians until many months after their initial clinical expression. Also, HPV lesions may spontaneously resolve and then subsequently recur, making the timing of the initial exposure more difficult to ascertain.

Non-sexual transmission of HPV infections to the anogenital area has been postulated. Theoretically, it is possible to acquire certain subtypes of HPV through non-sexual direct contact such as diapering, sexual play, and co-bathing. There is little, if any, direct evidence that hand and common warts (commonly types 1–4) can be spread to the anogenital area through autoinoculation, direct contact, or fomites. There is no increased incidence of anogenital warts in a child or family with common warts.

Genital warts possibly resulting from casual contact have been described in children and adolescents whose close household contacts have HPV infection (Pacheco et al, 1991). In this study, the investigators excluded sexual abuse by detailed histories, concluding that casual daily contact may permit transmission of HPV. However, few of the children disclosed abuse or admitted to some kind of sexual contact without penetration. Therefore, before sexual abuse can be excluded as the source of the genital warts, a thorough, careful social and medical evaluation is necessary.

Anogenital warts may be found in association with other STDs in children. In one small study of 11 girls aged 1.5–11 years with anogenital HPV infections, 65% had coexisting vaginal infections with organisms associated with sexual activity (Herman-Giddens et al, 1988).

Children and adolescents with anogenital HPV infections can present with genital bleeding, pain, genital discharge, or asymptomatic lesions discovered on a routine physical examination. HPV anogenital lesions have different morphologies, including exophytic, papular, "microwarts," or flat. The term *condyloma acuminata* refers to a specific morphology of genital HPV lesions (exophytic, "pointy," soft, fleshy lesions) and should not be used as a synonym for anogenital HPV infections. These lesions are most often associated with HPV subtypes 6 and 11 in adults. Papular lesions are usually found in the anogenital area, the penile shaft, and the labia majora and perineum. Recently, "microwarts" have been described as flat warts of the vulva that manifest as fissuring and can be seen only with the application of acetic acid and colposcopy. Flat warts may be seen on the cervix or the penile shaft only after application of acetic acid and the use of colposcopy. In pubertal females, genital lesions first appear at the posterior fourchette and adjacent labia, later appearing on the adjacent genital sites; 20% extend to the perineum and anus, but rarely can be found on adjacent thigh or trunk. On males, lesions usually appear first at the frenum, coronal sulcus, and meatus. Anal condylomata may spread to the anal canal, and endoscopy is desirable for complete evaluation. Lesions should be differentiated from other genital growths, such as verruca vulgaris (biopsy), condylomata lata (serologic test for syphilis), and molluscum contagiosum (clinical appearance), as well as other anatomical variants, such as vulvar epithelial papillae on small vulvar sebaceous glands in the estrogenized female. In men, grouped yellow sebaceous glands on the prepuce may be mistaken for HPV infection.

In children, the HPV genital lesions may appear much different than those seen in adults. On the unestrogenized mucosa they may appear friable, soft, unkeratinized, exophytic lesions. HPV infections with certain subtypes, particularly 16, 18, and 31, have been found to be associated with certain genital epithelial neoplasms, including cervical, vulvar, penile, and anal (Davis et al, 1989).

HPV has not yet been grown in tissue culture, so diagnostic methods are limited to more indirect methods, such as light microscopy, DNA probes, and radioactive probes. Traditionally, the diagnosis in sexually active adolescents and adults has been through visual inspection, often aided by colposcopy, with biopsy reserved for unclear cases or those not responding to therapy. Because the diagnosis in children and nonsexually active adolescents is often highly suspicious for prior sexual contact, obtaining tissue for confirmation and subtyping should be strongly considered. Biopsy specimens of exophytic or papular lesions or scrapings of flat lesions should be sent for light microscopy and DNA subtyping.

Vaginal washing may be used to identify viral particles from infected children (Gutman et al, 1992). Amplification of small quantities of viral DNA can be achieved by PCR techniques (Gutman et al, 1994; Pakarian et al, 1994). In adolescents, cytology has been the method most commonly used to detect HPV in cervical scrapings (Pap smear). However, there are a significant number of false negatives with this technique. Histopathologic methods include hematoxylin and eosin staining of biopsy specimens looking for the characteristic koilocytosis. Histopathologic detection of HPV via identification of koilocytosis is a fairly sensitive and specific technique for HPV in expert hands, but in forensically sensitive cases this method should be combined with a DNA identification method that can identify subtypes, such as Southern blot, in situ hybridization, Vira-Pap, Vira-Type, and PCR. The Southern blot is an extremely time-consuming and costly method requiring biopsy material. It is the gold standard by which all other methods are compared.

In situ hybridization is useful for examining paraffin-embedded biopsy specimens, although exfoliated cell scrapings have been used. It lacks some sensitivity when compared to the Southern blot. The Vira-Pap identifies the presence of HPV DNA using a radioactive-labeled nucleic acid probe. This is a commercial kit designed for use like the Pap smear. The Vira-Type identifies the specific genital subtype of HPV DNA. The PCR amplification method is useful when only small quantities of DNA material are available. False positives are possible if contamination occurs. It should be noted that all DNA hybridization tests can have false-negative results for many reasons. If a false-negative result is suspected, reanalysis should be attempted with a new clinical sample.

The goal of therapy should be symptomatic treatment, aimed at the eradication of lesions and of associated symptoms. There are no data to suggest that any therapy alters the long-term consequences of HPV infections. HPV has been demonstrated in normal tissue adjacent to laser-excised lesions and frequently recurs even when the original lesions are treated. Patient preference, physician experience, and available resources guide the selection of a treatment modality.

In general, treatment modalities are divided into two major groups, patient-applied and provider-applied. Patient-applied therapy consists of the application of podofilox 0.5 percent solution or gel to the visible lesions. The patient applies the medication to the lesions twice daily for 3 days, followed by 4 days of no therapy. This 7-day cycle should be repeated for no more than four cycles. Another regimen consists of imiquimod 5% cream. The patient applies the medication at bed time, three times a week for as long as 16 weeks.

Various provider-applied therapies include of the following:

- Topical application of tricholoroacetic acid (TCA) or bi-choloroacetic acid (BCA), 80%–90%. These agents may be used for external genital/perianal, vaginal, and anal warts. Lesions may be treated as frequently as 3 times per week. Discomfort from treatment of lesions can be modified by the use of wet towels, topical gels, and hand-held fans. Although effective, TCA treatment can be painful and may not be optimal in the very young patient or in the patient with extensive lesions.
- Cryotherapy with liquid nitrogen has been used for anogenital warts in children and adolescents. The cryoprobe may be used for external exophytic or cervical warts. Freezing should be continued until an iceball 1–2 mm larger than the diameter of the wart is noted. Topical/local anesthetic should be used because cryotherapy is painful. Cryotherapy should probably not be used for infants and children with extensive lesions.
- Podophyllin in tincture of benzoin has been used for the treatment of external genital or perianal warts. A 10%–25% solution is usually applied. Because podophyllin is potentially neurotoxic, the CDC recommends that no more than 0.5 cc should be applied per treatment session, and that an area no larger than 10 cm^2 of keratinized skin or 2 cm^2 of vaginal mucosa should be treated per session. It should be washed off in 1 to 4 hours and repeated weekly. Some experts caution against vaginal application of podophyllin because of concern about systemic absorption. Podophyllin is contraindicated during pregnancy and is not recommended for treatment of lesions in highly vascularized tissue such as cervical, anal, and oral warts. Use in small children should be judicious; many centers do not use podophyllin for children. Podophyllin is a resin with a high degree of variability of concentration. If poor results are obtained, a new bottle should be used. It may also be used in conjunction with other therapies, for example, immediately following cryotherapy or TCA treatment.
- Surgical removal, either by electrosurgery, sharp excision, or laser ablation, may be necessary in patients with extensive lesions, in patients who failed topical therapy, or in young patients who require general anesthesia for the removal of warts. Some centers prefer to use a carbon dioxide laser in the superpulse mode for all prepubertal children, noting that this technique minimizes the amount of eschar and adjacent tissue damage leading to a shorter healing time (Davis et al, 1989).

- Some centers employ interferon, either as therapy for patients who failed other therapies, or in combination with other treatment modalities. Systemic interferon is not effective. It must be injected, subcutaneously, IM, or directly into the lesions. Because of the inconvenient routes of administration, interferon is not recommended for routine use.
- Vaginoscopy and/or anoscopy in anogenitally infected children may be necessary for recalcitrant cases.

All adults and adolescent women with anogenital warts should have at least a yearly Pap smear. Some clinicians recommend follow up every 6 months. Recommendations have not been established for the frequency and duration of follow-up of HPV-infected children. However, many experts believe that essentially all HPV-infected children should be examined on an annual basis, particularly those infected with genital subtypes associated with genital cancers (Pakarian et al, 1994).

Syphilis

Infection with *Trichomonas pallidum* increased dramatically in the late 1980s, but syphilis rates have declined since then (CDC, 1991). Perinatal transmission of syphilis occurs most often by hematogenous transplacental passage of the organism, rather than by direct exposure at the time of birth. Congenital and acquired syphilis usually can be distinguished by examining results of maternal serology and cord blood/neonatal serology obtained at the time of birth. However, there is a latent period between infection and conversion to positive serology. If the infant is delivered during this "window" of time, congenital syphilis may result despite negative perinatal serologies. This possibility should be considered when a child under one year of age presents with possible acquired syphilis (Zenker et al, 1991; Dorfman et al, 1990; Mobley et al, 1998).

Primary syphilis has a very similar presentation in the pediatric and adult population, generally appearing as a painless genital chancre at an average of 21 days after exposure. Primary lesions may also present in the oral cavity and perianal area. Perianal chancres have been confused with simple perianal fissures. The differential diagnosis of these lesions may include condyloma acuminata, trauma, and ulcerative lesions such as those due to *Herpes simplex* (Ginsburg,

1983). At this stage, serologies are frequently negative. Non-treponemal testing, such as RPR and VDRL, generally takes 4–8 weeks to convert after initial exposure; these tests may be positive during the first week after the chancre is present. Treponemal serologies of MHA-TP and flourescent treponemal antibody absorption tests may also be negative during the incubation period and early primary syphilis. For that reason, the clinician faced with a possible syphilitic chancre in a child should obtain a darkfield examination.

Secondary syphilis has also been reported during childhood. Secondary syphilis often presents as a skin rash within one to several months after exposure (Sung and MacDonald, 1998). The differential diagnosis of such a rash would include pityriasis rosea, psoriasis, and tinea versicola, as well as viral illnesses and drug reactions. Again, a relatively high index of suspicion is needed to accurately diagnose the infrequent condition of secondary syphilis in the pediatric population (Lim et al, 1995).

In the absence of perinatal transmission, syphilis is nearly always sexually transmitted. Accidental transmission in laboratory accidents and during surgery on infected individuals has been described. Transmission during transfusion of blood, by contact with syphilitic lesions on the breast of a nursing mother, and by "nonsexual" kissing have all been described; however, these forms of transmission are very rare (Neinstein et al, 1984).

Except in rare situations, syphilis in a child beyond the neonatal period is acquired through sexual contact. Fortunately, this is one of the least common STDs noted among sexually abused children. White's series (1983) reported six cases of positive serologies among the 108 children screened; this represents one of the highest syphilis rates noted in the literature. Much lower prevalence rates of positive syphilis serologies in sexually abused children have been reported; one positive serology was reported out of 532 children evaluated by DeJong (1986). Cupoli (1988) found only one in 1,059 serologies to be positive, and the Center for Child Protection in San Diego found only two positive serologies in over 6,000 children screened (Horowitz and Chadwick, 1990). This clearly indicates that syphilis is one of the least common STDs transmitted to children during sexual abuse, yet most protocols require serologic testing for syphilis, a requirement most examiners fail to fulfill (Bays and Chadwick, 1991).

Treatment of syphilis depends on the stage of the disease. Post-assault prophylaxis against gonorrhoeae and chlamydia should eradicate incubating syphilis, but at least one case has been reported in which ceftriaxone given post-rape did not apparently eradicate incubating syphilis (Siqueira et al, 1991).

Trichomonas vaginalis

The *T. vaginalis* organism is a flagellated protozoan with an affinity for alkaline urogenital environments. In adults and adolescents it is almost exclusively sexually transmitted. The neonatal infection risk is low (0%–5%). It may persist 3–6 weeks in the neonatal vagina, owing to maternal estrogenization, and cause vaginitis. It can be maintained in the urinary tract after disappearance from the vagina. It is found only rarely in the vagina of prepubertal girls.

T. vaginalis has not been shown to colonize the mouth or the GI tract. A related species, *T. tenax*, is associated with oral gingivitis, while *T. hominis* can reside in the large bowel. Thus these three species are particularly site specific. The survival of *Trichomonas* has been described on wet cloths used for genital wiping, although there are no documented cases of transmission through fomites (Lossick, 1989). Beyond the newborn period, the presence of *Trichomonas* in the vagina is highly suggestive of sexual contact.

Asymptomatic infections do occur, but vaginitis is the most common clinical manifestation of infection in adolescents and adults. Concurrent infection with *G. vaginalis* and *Candida albicans* is common.

For diagnosis, in pubertal females the wet mount is 50% sensitive. The Pap smear has an equivalent or lower sensitivity to the wet mount but may have false positives. Cultures done in trichosel broth medium are 95% sensitive. Monoclonal antibody and ELISA techniques appear promising, but both suffer from the same problems seen with chlamydia infection when used in the sexually abused population. There are no data on the efficacy of diagnostic methods in prepubertal children.

Trichomonas may be treated with a single doze of metronidazole 2 g or 500 mg twice daily for 7 days in adolescents. In children, use a single oral dose of 40 mg/kg (maximum 2g) or 7 days of 15 mg/kg/day given in two divided doses (maximum 1 g per day).

Molluscum contagiosum

Molluscum contagiosum is a DNA-containing poxvirus that replicates in the cytoplasm, producing cytoplasmic inclusions and hyperplasia of infected cells. Transmission is through direct contact with the infected skin and has been reported to occur among wrestlers, patients of surgeons with hand lesions, and children sharing baths, and by contact with infected towels and examination equipment. The incubation period ranges from 1 week to 6 months.

The lesions are classically described as fleshy umbilicated papules that are usually asymptomatic, but may on occasion cause pruritus, tenderness, or pain. Duration of infection is approximately 2 months per papule and 3 years per infection. There are two forms. In children, lesions are found most commonly on the face, trunk, or limbs and are caused by person-to-person or fomite contact. Genital lesions in children may be the result of sexual abuse. In adults, the most common method of transmission is sexual, and the infection is commonly found with other STDs.

Diagnosis is made by the characteristic gross appearance of the lesions. If necessary, a biopsy will show a characteristic molluscum body on hematoxylin and eosin stain. Virus may be directly visualized by electron microscopy. A fluorescent antibody test is available.

Treatment of the lesions often is not necessary, but if desired they may be treated by curettage, electrodessication, or laser (Jones and Muram, 1993). Physical or chemical irritants such as cryotherapy, silver nitrate, podophyllin, or phenol may be applied, but modalities should not produce scarring.

OTHER SEXUALLY TRANSMITTED DISEASES

Hepatitis B

Universal immunization of children and adolescents has been recommended by a number of professional organizations. In the nonimmune patient, hepatitis B surface antigen testing should be obtained if epidemiological evidence warrants it or if the patient or parent requests it. Testing should be done if it is known that the assailant has had multiple sexual partners, participates in IV drug abuse or has a partner who does so, or engages in homosexual intercourse. Some states have laws allowing for assailant testing. The child should be tested and given the first dose of hepatitis B vaccine and instructions to complete the series of immunizations.

Human Immunodeficiency Virus

HIV infection among the young sexually abused population has been reported, but is uncommon. Nonetheless, cases have been described of transmission of the virus to children through sexual molestation (Gutman et al, 1991). Of great concern is the high frequency of high-risk sexual acts, such as sodomy, in child sexual abuse. Because of this, and because of the serious nature of the infection and recent clinical improvements in HIV testing and treatment, many experts are now recommending HIV screening for all alleged sexual abuse victims, particularly in high-prevalence geographic areas. Screening should be done at the time of entry into the program. Consideration should be given to testing at 3, 6, and possibly 12 month later. Most states require informed consent by the patient and/or parents prior to testing. In all cases of child abuse involving contact, the issue of AIDS should be addressed with the child victim and/or his or her family. Some states allow for assailant testing. In neonates and infants, a positive HIV serology can occur from passive transmission of maternal antibody. Thus, serial maternal and infant testing must be done. Some centers now provide post-assault HIV drug therapy. However, the efficacy of such prophylactic therapy is unknown. The physician also should consider the known toxicity and risks of these antiretroviral drugs and the strict requirements for compliance and monitoring.

Genital Mycoplasmas

In adults, colonization with either *Mycoplasma hominis* or *Ureaplasma urealyticum* is highly correlated with sexual experience. In one study of abused children, both organisms were isolated more frequently in the abused population than in the controls (Hammerschlag, 1987). However, these organisms have been found in children without a history of sexual contact. Colonization was not associated with symptoms, although an exudative vaginitis in a 10-year-old child has been reported in association with *M. hominis* (Waites et al, 1983). Neonatal transmission does occur, and may persist at least 12 months. More prevalence studies are needed. At present, it is difficult to interpret the isolation of this organism from the vagina or rectum as a marker for sexual contact.

REFERENCES

Alexander, ER. Maternal and infant sexually transmitted diseases. *Urol Clin North Am.* 1984;11:131–139.

Alexander, WJ, H Griddith, JG Housch, and JR Holmes. Infections in sexual contacts and associates of children with gonorrhea. *Sex Transm Dis.* 1984; sSII:156–158.

Bartley, DL, L Morgan, and ME Rimsza. *Gardnerella vaginalis* in prepubertal girls. *Am J Dis Child.* 1987;141:1014–1017.

Bays, J, and D Chadwick. The serologic test for syphilis in sexually abused children. *Adolesc Pediatr Gynecol.* 1991;4:148–151.

Beards, G, C Graham, and D Pillay. Investigation of vesicular rashes for HSV and VZV by PCR. *J Med Virol.* 1998;54(3):155–7.

Bell, TA, WE Stamm, CC Kuo, SP Wang, KK Holmes, and JT Grayston. Delayed appearance of *Chlamydia trachomatis* infections acquired at birth. *Pediatr Infect Dis J.* 1987;6:928–931.

Bell, TA, WE Stamm, SP Wang, CC Kuo, and KK Holmes. Chronic *Chlamydia trachomatis* infections in infants. *JAMA* 1992;267;400–402.

Benson, RA, and A, Steer. Vaginitis in children. *Am J Obstet Gynecol.* 1937;53:806.

Boyd, AS. *Condylomata acuminata* in the pediatric population. *Am J Dis Child.* 1990;144:817.

Branch, G, and P Paxton. A study of gonococcal infections among infants and children. *Public Health Rep.* 1965;80:347–352.

Centers for Disease Control. Primary, secondary syphilis—U.S., 1981–1990. *JAMA.* 1991;265(22):2940.

CDC. *Chlamydia trachomatis* genital infections—US 1995. *MMWR.* 1997;46:193.

Centers for Disease Control. Sexually transmitted diseases treatment guidelines. *MMWR.* 1998;47(RR-1):1–116.

Chambers, CV, MA Shafer, H Adger, M Ohm-Smith, SG Millstein, CE Irwin, J Schachter, and R Sweet. Microflora of the urethra in adolescent boys: relationships to sexual activity and nongonococcal urethritis. *J Pediatr.* 1987; 110:314–321.

Ching, S, H Lee, EW Hook 3rd., MR Jacobs, and J Zenilman. Ligase chain reaction for detection of *Neisseria gonorrhoeae* in urogenital swabs. *J Clin Microbiol.* 1995;33(12):3111–4.

Christian, CW, ML Singer, JE Crawford, and D Durbin. Perianal herpes zoster presenting as suspected child abuse. *Pediatrics.* 1997;99(4):608–10.

Clarke, LM, MF Sierra, BJ Daidone, N Lopez, JM Covino, and WM McCormack. Comparison of the Syva MicroTrak enzyme immunoassay and Gen-Probe PACE 2 with cell culture for diagnosis of cervical *Chlamydia trachomatis* infection in a high-prevalence female population. *J Clin Microbiol.* 1993;31(4): 968–71.

Corey, L Genital herpes. In: Holmes, KK, PA Mardh, and PF Sparling, (Eds.) *Sexually Transmitted Diseases.* 2nd ed. New York: McGraw-Hill, 1990:391–413.

Craighill, M, B O'Connell, C McLachlin, H Kozakewich, and C Crum. HPV PCR analysis of prepubertal genital lesions. *Adolesc Pediatr Gynecol.* 1993;6:183.

Cupoli, JM, and PM Sewell. One thousand fifty-nine children with a chief complaint of sexual abuse. *Child Abuse Neglect*. 1988;12:151–162.

Davis, AJ, and SJ Emans. Human papilloma virus infection the pediatric and adolescent patient. *J Pediatr*. 1989;115:1–9.

DeJong, AR. Sexually transmitted diseases in sexually abused children. *Sex Transm Dis*. 1986;13:123–126.

Dorfman, DH, and JH Glaser. Congenital syphilis presenting in infants after the newborn period. *N Engl J Med*. 1990;323:1299–1302.

Douglas, JM, and L Corey. Fomites and herpes simplex viruses: A case of nonvenereal transmission? *JAMA*. 1983;250:3093.

Embree, JE, D Lindsay, T Williams, RW Peeling, S Wood, and M Morris. Acceptability and usefulness of vaginal washes in premenarcheal girls as a diagnostic procedure for sexually transmitted diseases. The Child Protection Centre at the Winnipeg Children's Hospital. *Pediatr Infect Dis J*. 1996;15(8):662–7.

Eschenbach, DA, S Hillier, C Critchlow, C Stevens, T DeRouen, and KK Holmes. Diagnosis and clinical manifestation of bacterial vaginosis. *Am J Obstet Gynecol*. 1988;158:819–828.

Frau, LM, and ER Alexander. Public health implicatons of sexually transmitted diseases in pediatric practice. *Pediatr Infect Dis. J*. 1985;4:453–467.

Gardner, M, and J Jones. Genital herpes acquired by sexual abuse of children. *J Pediatr*. 1984;104:243–244.

Ginsburg, CM. Acquired syphilis in prepubertal children. *Pediatr Infect Dis*. 1983; 2:232–234.

Gushurst, CA. The problem of genital herpes in prepubertal children. *Am J Dis Child*. 1985;139:542–545.

Gutman, LT, KK St Claire, C Weedy, ME Herman-Giddens, BA Lane, JG Niemeyer, and RE McKinney Jr. Human immunodeficiency virus transmission by child sexual abuse. *Am J Dis Child*. 1991;145:137–141.

Gutman, LT, K St. Claire, ME Herman-Giddens, WW Johnston, and WC Phelps. Evaluation of sexually abused and nonabused young girls for intravaginal human papillomavirus infection. *Am J Dis Child*. 1992;146(6):694–9.

Gutman, LT, KK St. Claire, VD Everett, DL Ingram, J Soper, WW Johnston, GG Mulvaney, and WC Phelps. Cervical-vaginal and intraanal human papillomavirus infection of young girls with external genital warts. *J Infect Dis*. 1994;170(2):339–44.

Hammerschlag, M. Pitfalls in the diagnosis of sexually transmitted diseases in children. *ASPAC News*. 1989;1989:4–5.

Hammerschlag, MR. Diagnosis of chlamydial infection in the pediatric population. *Immunol Invest*. 1997;26(1-2):151–6.

Hammershlag, MR. The transmissibility of sexually transmitted diseases in sexually abused children. *Child Abuse Neglect*. 1998;22:623–633.

Hammerschlag, MR, S Alpert, I Rosner, P Thurston, D Semine, D McComb, and WM McCormack. Microbiology of the vagina in children: normal and potentially pathogenic organisms. *Pediatrics* 1978;62: 57–62.

Hammerschlag, MR, B Doraiswamy, and P Cox. Colonization of sexually abused children with genital mycoplasmas. *Sex Transm Dis*. 1987;14:23–25.

Hammerschlag, MR, M Cummings, B Doraiswamy, P Cox, and WM McCormack. Nonspecific vaginitis following sexual abuse in children. *Pediatrics*. 1985;75: 1028–1031.

Hammerschlag, MR, PJ Rettig, and ME Shields. False positive results with the use of chlamydial antigen detection tests in the evaluation of suspected sexual abuse in children. *Pediatr Infect Dis J*. 1988;7:11–14.

Hanks, JW, CT Scott, CE Butler, and DW Wells. Evaluation of a DNA probe assay (Gen-Probe PACE 2) as the test of cure for *Neisseria gonorrhoeae* genital infections. *J Pediatr.* 1994;125(1):161–2.

Handsfield, HH, WM McCormack, EW Hook 3d., JM Douglas Jr., JM Covino, MS Verdon, CA Reichart, and JM Ehret. A comparison of single-dose cefixime with ceftriaxone as treatment for uncomplicated gonorrhea. The Gonorrhea Treatment Study Group. *N Engl J Med.* 1991;325(19):1337–41.

Harrison, HR, and ER Alexander. Chlamydial infections in infants and children. *Sexually Transmitted Diseases.* 2nd ed. New York: McGraw-Hill, 1990: 811–820.

Herman-Giddens, ME, LT Gutman, and NL Berson. Association of coexisting vaginal infections and multiple abusers in female children with genital warts. *Sex Transm Dis.* 1988;15:63–67.

Hibbard, RA. Herpetic vulvovaginitis and child abuse. *Am J Dis Child.* 1985; 139:542.

Hillier, A, and KK Holmes. Bacterial Vaginosis. In: Holmes, KK, PA Mardh, PF Sparling. (Eds.) *Sexually Transmitted Diseases.* 2nd ed. New York: McGraw-Hill, 1990.

Hook, EW, and HH Handsfield. Gonococcal infections in the adult. In: KK Holmes, PA Mardh, and PF Sparling (Eds.) *Sexually Transmitted Diseases.* 2nd ed. New York: McGraw-Hill, 1990.

Horowitz, S, and DL Chadwick. Syphilis as a sole indicator of sexual abuse: Two cases with no intervention. *Child Abuse Neglect.* 1990;14:129–132.

Ingram, DL. The gonococcus and the toilet seat revisited (letter). *Pediatr Infect Dis.* 1989;8:191.

Ingram, DL. Neisseria gonorrhea in children. *Pediatr Annals.* 1994;23(7):341–5.

Ingram, DL, DK Runyan, AD Collins, ST White, MF Durfee, AW Pearson, and AR Occhiuti. Vaginal *Chlamydia trachomatis* infection in children with sexual contact. *Pediatr Infect Dis J.* 1984;3:97–99.

Ingram, DL, ST White, AR Occhiuti, and PR Lyna. Childhood vaginal infections: association of *Chlamydia trachomatis* with sexual contact. *Pediatr Infect Dis J.* 1986;5:226–229.

Ingram, DL, D Everett, PR Lyna, ST White, and LA Rockwell. Epidemiology of adult sexually transmitted diseases in children being evaluated for sexual abuse. *Pediatr Infect Dis J.* 1992;11:945–950.

Jenison, SA, XP Yu, JM Valentine, LA Koutsky, AE Christiansen, AM Beckmann, and DA Galloway. Evidence of prevalent genital-type human papillomavirus infections in adults and children. *J Infect Dis.* 1990;162:60.

Jenny, C. Child sexual abuse and STD. *Sexually Transmitted Diseases.* 2nd ed. New York: McGraw-Hill, 1990: 895–900.

Jones, CE, and D Muram. Use of CO_2 laser in treatment of *Molluscum contagiosum:* A report of four cases. *Adolesc Pediatr Gynecol.* 1993;6:154–156.

Jones, CE, D Muram, BR Hostetler, and O Lasater. The use of HPV DNA-typing in the management of ano-genital condyloma in prepubertal girls. *Adolesc Pediatr Gynecol.* 1993;6:184.

Kaplan, KM, GR Fleisher, JE Paradise, and HN Freidman. Social relevance of genital herpes simplex in children. *Am J Dis Child.* 1984;138:872–874.

Keskey, TS, M Suarez, N Gleicher, J Friberg, and HB Levy. *Chlamydia trachomatis* infection in sexually abused children. *Mt. Sinai J Med.* 1987;54:129–134.

Kesson, AM. Use of acyclovir in herpes simplex virus infections. *J Pediatr Child Health.* 1998;34(1):9–13.

Kulhanjian, JA, and NS Hilton. Gonococcal salpingitis in a premenarchal female following sexual assault. *Clin Pediatr.* 1991;30(1):53–5.

Liebling, MR, DG Arkfeld, GA Michelini, MJ Nishio, BJ Eng, T Jin, and JS Louie. Identification of *Neisseria gonorrhoeae* in synovial fluid using the polymerase chain reaction. *Arthritis Rheum.* 1994;37(5):702–9.

Lim, HK, WL Smith, Y Sato, and J Choi. Congenital syphilis mimicking child abuse. *Pediatr Radiol.* 1995;25(7):560–1.

Lipsitt, HJ, and AJ Parmet. Nonsexual transmission of gonorrhea to a child (letter). *N Engl J Med.* 1984;311:470.

Lossick, JS. Epidemiology of urogenital trichomoniasis. In: Honigbertg, BM. (Ed.) *Trichomonas Parasitic in Humans.* New York: Springer–Verlag, 1989.

Mahony, JB, and MA Chernesky. Effect of swab type and storage temperature on the isolation of *Chlamydia trachomatis* from clinical specimens. *J Clin Microbiol.* 1985; 22: 865–867.

Mertz, KJ, GM McQuillan, WC Levine, DH Candal, JC Bullard, RE Johnson, ME St. Louis, and CM Black. A pilot study of the prevalence of chlamydial infection in a national household survey. *Sexually Transmitted Diseases.* 1998; 25(5):225–8.

Miller, RG, WL Whittington, RM Coleman, and SM Nigida. Acquisition of concomitant oral and genital infection with herpes simplex virus type 2. *Sex Transm Dis.* 1987;14:41–43.

Mobley, JA, RE McKeown, KL Jackson, F Sy, JS Parham, and ER Brenner. Risk factors for congenital syphilis in infants of women with syphilis in South Carolina. *Am J Public Health.* 1998;88(4):597–602.

Muram, D. Child sexual abuse—Genital findings in prepubertal girls. I. The unaided medical examination. *Am J Obstet Gynecol.* 1989;160:328–333.

Muram, D, PM Speck, and M Dockter. Child sexual abuse examination: Is there a need for routine screening for *N. gonorrhoeae?* *Adolesc Pediatr Gynecol.* 1996; 9:79–80.

Nahmias, AJ, WR Dowdle, ZM Naib, WE Josey, and CF Luce. Genital infection with herpesvirus hominis types 1 and 2 in children. *Pediatrics.* 1968; 42:659–666.

Nair, PM, E Glazer-Semmel, C Gould, and E Ruff. *Neisseria gonorrhoeae* in asymptotomotic prepubertal household contacts of children with gonococcal infection. *Clin Pediatr.* 1986;25:160–163.

Neinstein, LS, J Goldering, and S Carpenter. Nonsexual transmission of sexually transmitted diseases: An infrequent occurrence. *Pediatrics.* 1984;74:67–75.

Nelson, JD, E Mohs, AS Dajani, and SA Plotkin. Gonorrhea in preschool and school-aged children: Report of the prepubertal gonorrhea cooperative study group. *JAMA.* 1976;236:1359–1364.

Pacheco, BP, DP Guillermo, JMM Ribas, S Vighi, and NG Rueda. Vulvar infection caused by human papilloma virus in children and adolescents without sexual contact. *Adolesc Pediatr Gynecol.* 1991;4:136–142.

Pakarian, F, J Kaye, J Cason, B Kell, R Jewers, NW Derias, KS Raju, and JM Best. Cancer associated human papillomaviruses: perinatal transmission and persistence. *British Journal of Obstet Gynecol.* 1994;101(6):514–7.

Plourde, PJ, M Tyndall, E Agoki, J Ombette, LA Slaney, LJ D'Costa, JO Ndinya-Achola, and FA Plummer. Single-dose cefixime versus single-dose ceftriaxone in the treatment of antimicrobial-resistant *Neisseria gonorrhoeae* infection. *J Infect Dis.* 1992;166(4):919–22.

Pokorny, SF. Child abuse and infections. *Obstet Gynecol Clin North Am.* 1989; 16:408–413.

Rettig, PJ, and JD Nelson. Genital tract infection with *Chlamydia trachomatis* in prepubertal children. *J Pediatr* 1981;99:206–210.

Roochvarg, LB, and JC Lovchik. Screening for pharyngeal gonorrhea in adolescents. A reexamination. *J Adolesc Health*. 1991;12(3):269–72.

Schachter, J. Biology of *Chlamydia trachomatis*. *Sexually Transmitted Diseases*. 2nd ed. New York: McGraw-Hill, 1990: 167–180.

Schachter, J, M Grossman, and J Holt. Infection with *Chlamydia trachomatis*: Involvement of multiple anatomic sites in neonates. *J Infect Dis*. 1979;139: 232.

Schachter, J, M Grossman, and RL Sweet. Prospective study of perinatal transmission of *C. trachomatis*. *JAMA*. 1986; 255:3374–3377.

Schachter, J, WE Stamm, TC Quinn, WW Andrews, JD Burczak, and HH Lee. Ligase chain reaction to detect *Chlamydia trachomatis* infection of the cervix. *J Clin Microbiol*. 1994;32(10):2540–3.

Schwarcz, SK, and WL Whittington. Sexual assault and sexually transmitted diseases: Detection and management in adults and children. *Rev Infect Dis*. 1990;12:S682–S689.

Silber, TJ, and G Controni. Clinical spectrum of pharyngeal gonorrhea in children and adolescents. *J Adoles Health Care*. 1983;4:51–54.

Siqueira, LM, SH Barnett, E Kass, and M Gertner. Incubating syphilis in an adolescent female rape victim. *J Adolesc Health Care*. 1991;12:459–461.

Smith, KR, S Ching, H Lee, Y Ohhashi, HY Hu, HC Fisher 3rd., and EW Hook 3rd. Evaluation of ligase chain reaction for use with urine for identification of *Neisseria gonorrhoeae* in females attending a sexually transmitted disease clinic. *J Clin Microbiol*. 1995;33(2):455–7.

Srivastava, AC. Survival of gonococci in urethral secretions with reference to the nonsexual transmission of gonococcal infection. *J Med Microbiol*. 1980;13: 593–596.

Stamm, WE, and KK Holmes. *Chlamydia trachomatis* infections of the adult. In: Holmes, KK, PA Mardh, and PF Sparling. (Eds.) *Sexually Transmitted Diseases*. 2nd ed. New York: McGraw-Hill, 1990.

Sung, L, and NE MacDonald. Gonorrhea: A pediatric perspective. *Pediatr Rev*. 1998;19(1):13–16.

Sung, L, and NE MacDonald. Syphilis: A pediatric perspective. *Pediatr Rev*. 1998;19(1):17–22.

Sweet, RL, and RS Gibbs. Perinatal infections. *Infectious Diseases of the Female Genital Tract*. 2nd. Baltimore: Williams and Wilkins, 1990: 290–319.

Taieb, A, S Body, I Astar, P duPasquier, and J Maleville. Clinical epidemology of symptomatic primary herpetic infection in children. *Acta Paediatr Scand*. 1987;76:128–132.

Tang, CK. Congenital *Condyloma acuminata*. *Am J Obstet Gynecol*. 1978;131: 912–913.

Vermund, SH, T Alexander-Rodriguez, S Macleod, KF Kelley, and T Alexander-Rodriguez. History of sexual abuse in incarcerated adolescents with gonorrhea or syphilis. *J Adolesc Health Care*. 1990;11(5):449–52.

Vlaspolder, F, JA Mutsaers, F Blog, and A Notowicz. Value of a DNA probe assay (Gen-Probe) compared with that of culture for diagnosis of gonococcal infection. *J Clin Microbiol*. 1993;31(1):107–10.

Waites, KB, MG Brown, S Stagno, J Schlachter, S Greenberg, GP Hemstreet, and GH Cassell. Association of genital mycoplasmas with exudative vaginitis in a 10 year old: A case of misdiagnosis. *Pediatrics*. 1983;71:250–252.

White, ST, FA Loda, DL Ingram, and A Pearson. Sexually transmitted diseases in sexually abused children. *Pediatrics*. 1983;72:16–21.

Whittington, WL, RJ Rice, JW Biddle, and JS Knapp. Incorrect identification of Neisseria gonorrhoeae from infants and children. *Pediatr Infect Dis J*. 1988; 7:3–10.

Zenker, PN, and SM Berman. Congenital syphilis: Trends and recommendations for evaluation and management. *Pediatr Infect Dis J*. 1991;10:516–522.

10

TESTIFYING AS AN EXPERT WITNESS

KENNETH R. FREEMAN

Few experiences are as stressful as testifying in court. This is true not just for experts, but for all witnesses. Their recollections may be cloudy, and the way they are allowed to relate information is different from everday experience. Usually they are not permitted to narrate their answers, cannot explain ambiguous answers, and are frequently interrupted by objections from the lawyers and comments from the judge.

The expert witness has the additional burden of being scientifically correct while at the same time communicating effectively to

Kenneth R. Freeman is a judge on the Los Angeles Superior Court. He is a past Department of Justice Visiting Fellow and a former deputy district attorney. Portions of this article were prepared under NIJ Grant #86-IJ-CX-0082. Points of view or opinions expressed in this chapter are those of the author and do not necessarily reflect the official position or policies of the U.S. Department of Justice or of the Los Angeles Superior Court.

the judge and jury. Because an expert must depend upon lawyers to ask questions that will permit an opinion to be accurately expressed, being effective may sometimes seem to be an impossible task, outside the control of the expert. Although cases and lawyers vary, there is much that can be done to ensure smooth presentation of testimony.

It is the aim of this chapter to present practical suggestions that accomplish this purpose and restore a measure of control to the expert. The chapter contains a summary of applicable law regarding expert testimony.[*] Where appropriate, examples of actual instructions given by judges to juries are cited.[†]

THE ROLE OF AN EXPERT WITNESS

An expert witness is one who possesses special knowledge or skill on a subject that is beyond common experience (this definition is codified as California Evidence Code §720). It is the task of an expert witness to help the judge or jury understand specific evidence or to determine a fact in issue. This is done by providing qualified, appropriate, unbiased, and neutral opinion, that is scientifically sound, regarding evidence or a fact in issue (Table 10–1).

> A person is qualified to testify as an expert if [the witness] has special knowledge, skill, experience, training, or education sufficient to qualify [the witness] as an expert on the subject to which [the witness'] testimony relates.

---

[*] Throughout the chapter, California Law is cited as an example of state laws regarding expert testimony. All references to the Evidence Code refer to the California Evidence Code. Although the information presented in this chapter is consistent with California Law, the concepts and principles stated are generally true throughout the United States.

[†] All references to jury instructions are taken from *California Jury Instructions, Criminal*, 6th ed., Committee on Standard Jury Instructions, Criminal, Superior Court (CALJIC), West Publications, St. Paul, Minn., 1996. These are actual instructions that are given to jurors before deliberation. Although these instructions are based upon criminal trials, the same principles apply to civil cases. It is worthwhile for the expert to consider these jury instructions when testifying. Individual instructions are cited, where applicable, throughout the chapter. Each instruction is numbered as indicated.

Table 10–1. Qualities of an Effective Expert

Ideal qualities to communicate to the jury
  Unbiased
  Neutral
  Knowledgeable about field
  Scientifically sound opinions
  Willing to explain opinions

A witness who has special knowledge, skill, experience, training, or education in a particular subject has testified to certain opinions. Any such witness is referred to as an *expert witness*. In determining what weight to give to any opinion expressed by an expert witness, you should consider the qualifications and believability of the witness, the facts or materials upon which each opinion is based, and the reasons for each opinion.

An opinion is only as good as the facts and reasons on which it is based. If you find that any fact has not been proved, or has been disproved, you must consider that in determining the value of the opinion. Likewise, you must consider the strengths and weaknesses of the reasons on which it is based.

You are not bound by an opinion. Give each opinion the weight you find it deserves. You may disregard any opinion if you find it to be unreasonable (CALJIC 2.80)

Helping the Judge and Jury

Although an expert is usually engaged by one side or another, the expert works for the court as opposed to working for either side. An expert could be sought and hired by the court. As a practical matter, an expert is usually sought and hired by one side or the other.

Although an expert may be hired by either side, the expert is sometimes paid by or appointed by the court. Being appointed by the court is not the same as being hired by the court. It usually occurs in criminal cases where the side requesting appointment persuades the court to pay for an essential expert. Occasionally, some experts, who are hired by one side, attempt to create the false impression that they are hired by the court. This is not a recommended procedure because opposing counsel may bring out the true facts on cross-examination and damage the expert's credibility.

Specific Evidence

The expert must render an opinion about specific evidence that is before the court. Evidence is before the court when it has been offered either before or concurrent with the opinion about that evidence. Expert opinion must always be given either (1) in response to a hypothetical question or (2) based upon in-court or out-of-court observation of real evidence.

> If a witness is testifying as an expert, [the witness'] testimony in the form of an opinion is limited to such an opinion as is:
> . . .
> (b) Based on matter (including [the witness'] special knowledge, skill, experience, training, and education) perceived by or personally known to the witness or made known to [the witness] at or before the hearing, whether or not admissible, that is of a type that reasonably may be relied upon by an expert in forming an opinion upon the subject to which his [or her] testimony relates, unless an expert is precluded by law from using such matter as a basis for his [or her] opinion. (Evidence Code §801)

If in response to a hypothetical question, the question must contain a summary of the evidence and based upon facts that have been already presented to the jury.

> In examining an expert witness, counsel may ask a hypothetical question. This is a question in which the witness is asked to assume the truth of a set of facts, and to give an opinion based on that assumption.
> In permitting such a question, the court does not rule, and does not necessarily find that all the assumed facts have been proved. It only determines that those assumed facts are within the possible range of the evidence. It is for you to decide from all the evidence whether or not the facts assumed in a hypothetical question have been proved. If you should decide that any assumption in a question has not been proved, you are to determine the effect of that failure of proof on the value and weight of the expert opinion based on the assumed facts. (CALJIC 2.82)

If pertinent facts are left out, or if facts are included that have not been presented to the jury, then the question is objectionable and should not be permitted by the court.

Real evidence is evidence that consists of objects, writings, recordings, or photographs as opposed to testimonial evidence.

Real evidence is usually before the court as an exhibit, but does not have to be.

Qualified and Appropriate Opinion

As Table 10–2 indicates, before an opinion may be admitted into evidence, certain requirements must be met. An opinion is appropriate if the area to which it is testified is properly subject to expert opinion. An area is properly subject to expert opinion if it is sufficiently beyond common experience that expert opinion would help the judge or jury understand the evidence or decide a fact in issue.

> The court may, and upon objection shall, exclude testimony in the form of an opinion that is based in whole or in significant part on matter that is not a proper basis for such an opinion. In such case, the witness may, if there remains a proper basis for his [or her] opinion, then state his [or her] opinion after excluding from consideration the matter determined to be improper. (Evidence Code §803)

The qualification of a witness to testify as an expert must relate to the particular subject about which he or she is asked to express an opinion.

A witness may establish qualification as an expert by testifying to his or her special knowledge, skill, experience, training, or education. This is referred to as establishing a foundation that the witness is qualified. The qualification of a witness to testify as an expert must relate to the particular subject about which the witness is asked to express an opinion.

Unbiased and Neutral Testimony

To be considered credible, an expert must appear intelligent, unbiased, and neutral. To be effective, the expert must overcome the

Table 10–2. Foundational Requirements before Expert
Opinion Is Admitted

Expert is qualified.
Opinion is scientifically valid.
There is a factual basis for opinion.

skeptic's view that an expert will offer a biased opinion that favors the party who hired the expert witness.

Scientific Opinion

An expert may offer an opinion based upon his or her scientific background or may testify regarding the results of a scientific method, procedure, or instrument. The expert must give the facts upon which his or her opinion is based. This is known as the factual foundation for the expert's opinion.

If the expert testifies about the results of a scientific test or procedure, the expert must demonstrate that the method or procedure is based upon approved scientific principles, generally accepted within the scientific community.

As stated in *Fry v. United States** (D.C. Cir. 1923) 293 F.1013, 1014:

> Just when a scientific principle or discovery crosses the line between the experimental and demonstrable stages is difficult to define. Somewhere in this twilight zone the evidential force of the principle must be recognized, and while courts will go a long way in admitting expert testimony deduced from a well–recognized scientific principle or discovery, the thing from which the deduction is made must be sufficiently established to have gained general acceptance in the particular field in which it belongs.

If the expert testifies about the results of a scientific instrument, the expert must, besides the above, show that the device was working properly at the time it was used and that the instrument was operated correctly to obtain the result. This is known as establishing a scientific foundation for the instrument, test, or procedure.

Fact in Issue

The expert must testify regarding a fact in issue and may not offer an opinion on an ultimate issue to be determined by the judge or jury. By way of example, an expert may not properly offer the opinion that the defendant is guilty or not guilty.

---

*Note that for federal trials, the United States Supreme Court has held that the *Fry* case was superseded by the Federal Rules of Evidence and that expert testimony could be admitted if the District Court deemed it both relevant and reliable. See *Daubert v. Merrell Dow Pharmaceuticals, Inc.*, 509 U.S. 579.

DIFFERENCES BETWEEN LAY AND EXPERT TESTIMONY

A lay witness may offer a relevant opinion about items within ordinary knowledge.

> If a witness is not testifying as an expert, [the witness'] testimony in the form of an opinion is limited to such an opinion as is permitted by law, including but not limited to an opinion that is: (a) Rationally based on the perception of the witness; and (b) Helpful to a clear understanding of his [or her] testimony. (Evidence Code §800)

A lay witness must limit testimony to items about which he or she has personal knowledge. Personal knowledge is knowledge obtained by actual observation obtained while witnessing an event. This is sometimes referred to as percipient knowledge or that the witness is a percipient witness.

A lay witness may offer an opinion about matters of everyday experience such as age or demeanor of a person, distance, and so forth.

> In determining the weight to be given to an opinion expressed by any witness who did not testify as an expert witness, you should consider [the witness'] credibility, the extent of [the witness'] opportunity to perceive the matters upon which [the witness'] opinion is based and the reasons, if any, given for it. You are not required to accept such an opinion but should give it the weight, if any, to which you find it entitled. (CALJIC 2.81)

A lay witness can be compelled to testify about matters personally observed. An expert cannot be compelled to testify about his or her opinion unless the expert is also a percipient witness regarding the same subject matter.

PREPARATION FOR EXPERT TESTIMONY

It may appear to some experts that whether or not a case will flow smoothly is based upon the random chance that an examining attorney will understand how to present testimony correctly. It would be frustrating to testify while trying to overcome what appears to be the examining attorney's lack of insight and skill and general ignorance. Success in presenting expert testimony need not be random. It is possible to prepare for and to minimize most of the common problems experienced during testimony.

Successful presentation depends upon proper communication. The two most common pitfalls are (1) the expert and lawyer are on different wave-lengths and are at cross-purposes and (2) the expert and lawyer are on the same wavelength but fighting each other.

The first problem is the more serious, because it is a case of total break-down of communication between expert and lawyer. The expert doesn't understand and doesn't know what the attorney is trying to prove. The expert answers each question by itself, not knowing where the question is leading. Because of this, the expert answers each question literally. The lawyer is not happy with the answer, but doesn't know how to rephrase the question to get answers he or she wants the jury to hear. Because of this, both expert and lawyer appear confused, frustrated, and sometimes angry.

The second situation is where both lawyer and expert know what the lawyer is trying to prove, but the lawyer keeps asking questions that don't accomplish the task. The expert becomes frustrated because the lawyer doesn't ask the appropriate and "obvious" question. The expert tries to guide the lawyer with "leading" answers, but the lawyer doesn't seem to take the hint.

Preparation should be a joint effort of attorney and expert. Both must meet beforehand, well before testimony. If the examining attorney does not want to meet in advance, the expert must explain the purpose and importance of this meeting. A meeting far before trial is an important part of thorough preparation. It permits the expert and the attorney to discuss the case in a relaxed and non-pressured environment. It gives the attorney a chance to discuss what will happen and what can be expected. This relieves the anxiety caused by the unknown. Early meetings allow planning of testimony and permit forewarning of other problem areas in time to take action. Like everything else, preparation is the secret to effective expert testimony. Because an expert must rely on an attorney to ask the right questions during direct examination, preparation must be a joint effort of both attorney and expert. If the attorney refuses to meet in advance for this preparation, the expert should consider declining the assignment.

When meeting with the examining attorney, it is important that the following areas be covered.

1. Establish the purpose of the expert at trial. What is it that the attorney is trying to prove? What are the key issues that can be resolved with expert opinion? What are the problem areas? What kind of opposing expert opinion can be expected? What is the best way to present the opinion?

2. Discuss how the testimony will be presented. The attorney and the expert should discuss what questions will permit the expert to narrate background and expertise. The expert can help the attorney by developing a set of questions and answers that will ensure that the appropriate opinion is elicited at trial. These questions may then be practiced to see if the expert's answers flow properly. Surprises can be avoided by agreeing that no questions will be asked on direct examination at trial that were not asked at the practice session.

3. Discuss possible cross-examination areas. The expert should mentally examine the opinion for weak points or flaws. It is helpful to imagine how another qualified expert might differ. The lawyer can be alerted to these areas with discussion about why the contrary position is incorrect or misguided.

4. Learn what testimony to expect and establish communication. If necessary, the expert should explain the vocabulary of the field of expertise to the lawyer and ask about any puzzling legal jargon. Questions should be asked to learn how the lawyer thinks. Find out what is expected from the testimony. Problem areas should be discussed and solutions planned. If there has never been a meeting with the lawyer, the lawyer's knowledge of what the expert will say is based upon the written reports or other prior testimony. If a meeting occurs and the basis of an opinion discussed, it will usually be found that there is some misunderstanding between reports and probable expert testimony. By going over the opinion and its basis, both lawyer and expert will learn what areas need to be clarified. More importantly, both will gain insight into ways to ask and answer questions that are easiest for the judge and jury to understand.

   The expert and lawyer may find it is helpful to rehearse the exact questions that the lawyer is planning to ask when in court. This helps pinpoint possible misunderstandings, makes communication in court smoother, and can reduce stress. The known is always less stressful than the unknown.

5. Identify and alleviate problem areas. Another benefit of going

over the questions to be asked in court is that both lawyer and expert learn problem areas that will be encountered on direct and cross-examination. Understanding these problems in advance and guarding against them can avoid much stress. Although some problems will be unique to a particular case, some problems continually recur. It might be helpful to discuss these common problems and look at possible solutions.

THE DAY OF TRIAL

Guidelines to Follow While Waiting to Testify

There are many dilemmas that an expert witness faces while waiting to testify. The expert should avoid sitting or standing around before trial. If possible, the expert should arrive exactly when it is necessary to testify and not sooner. Because witnesses are usually excluded from the courtroom, experts often find themselves waiting in the hall in front of the courtroom doors or sitting on a hallway bench. This is a position of vulnerability because the expert usually does not know anyone, but everyone is aware of who the expert is. It would be best if there were no waiting period and the expert could arrive, walk into the courtroom, testify, and leave, but this rarely happens. What follows are tips to minimize problems that could occur.

It should be borne in mind by the expert that the qualities listed in Table 10–1 need to be communicated at all times and not just when the expert is on the witness stand.

Should the expert talk to the opposing attorney? If the expert refuses to talk to the opposing attorney, the expert will probably be accused of bias. If the expert talks to the attorney, anything said can and will be used in court. If the expert would rather not talk to opposing counsel, the expert should keep busy (make phone calls, write memos, read unrelated reports, etc.).

If the expert talks to opposing counsel, the expert should be polite and open. If the expert has literature that relates to testimony, it should be shown to the lawyer if requested (but nothing should be volunteered). Attempts to befriend an attorney may cause problems. It is unwise to try to convince the lawyer his or her side is "wrong." Lawyers are paid to believe in their client's cause. It is also unwise to say something that is "off the record." Nothing is off the record to a lawyer who wants to win a case.

Last-minute material from opposing counsel should not be read. Immediately before testifying, it is generally unwise for an expert to take material from an opposing attorney and read it. If an expert takes something from the lawyer and reads it, the expert may be cross-examined on that material and it may be received into evidence, even if it is totally without merit. The rule is that an expert cannot be cross-examined on anything that was not used to form an opinion.

TESTIFYING AT TRIAL

When answering questions, an expert must be aware of demeanor. It's helpful to be aware of the instruction which the court charges the jury regarding evaluation of any witness' testimony, including expert testimony.

> Every person who testifies under oath is a witness. You are the sole judges of the believability of a witness and the weight to be given the testimony of each witness.
> In determining the believability of a witness you may consider anything that has a tendency in reason to prove or disprove the truthfulness of the testimony of the witness, including but not limited to any of the following:
> The extent of the opportunity or the ability of the witness to see or hear or otherwise become aware of any matter about which the witness has testified;
> The ability of the witness to remember or to communicate any matter about which the witness has testified;
> The character and quality of that testimony;
> The demeanor and manner of the witness while testifying;
> The existence or nonexistence of a bias, interest or other motive;
> Evidence of the existence or nonexistence of any fact testified to by the witness;
> The attitude of the witness toward this action or toward the giving of testimony. . . . (CALJIC 2.20)

The expert should listen carefully to all questions and look at the person asking the question when answering. Some experts feel it is important to look at the jury when testifying. This should be done with caution. A good rule of thumb is that the expert should look only at the jury when the question asks for something to be explained to the jury.

The expert should remain calm and in control. If the expert becomes angry during cross-examination, the jury's confidence in the expert's opinion may be affected. A neutral expert is calm and in control. Charts, diagrams, and "chalk talks" are effective because they create the image that the expert is the teacher and everyone else is the student. Overhead slides or other lights–out material may distract jurors because of viewing problems.

Badgering can be avoided by telling the lawyer that the answer needs to be explained and that, accordingly, a yes or no answer would be meaningless. A court should permit an expert to explain his or her answer.

> A witness testifying in the form of an opinion may state on direct examination the reasons for his opinion and the matter (including, in the case of an expert, his special knowledge, skill, experience, training, and education) upon which it is based, unless he is precluded by law from using such reasons or matter as a basis for his opinion. The court in its discretion may require that a witness before testifying in the form of an opinion be first examined concerning the matter upon which his opinion is based. (Evidence Code §802)

SURVIVING CROSS-EXAMINATION

Opposing counsel wants the expert to appear biased, dishonest, stupid, and ignorant.

> In resolving any conflict that may exist in the testimony of expert witnesses, you should weigh the opinion of one expert against that of another. In doing this, you should consider the relative qualifications and credibility of the expert witnesses, as well as the reasons for each opinion and the facts and other matters upon which it was based. (CALJIC 2.83)

He or she wants the expert to appear to be a literature reviewer only with no real knowledge. The lawyer will try to show that the expert has insufficient background or expertise. Opposing counsel may try to maneuver the expert into being inconsistent or make the expert appear foolishly consistent. This may be done by using the expert's scientific training to analyze material a certain way and by confusing scientific principles with legal principles.

For example, the word "possible" has a different meaning in the courtroom than in the outside world. In the courtroom, "possible" means reasonable scientific probability, whereas in the scientific world "possible" means anything that is conceivable.

The Form of a Question Is Important

The expert should be careful about the form of the question. Some questions cannot be answered in the form they are asked. What follows are tips for answering various improperly formed questions.

Answer Compound Questions with a Statement.

Q: Was it your opinion doctor that the child was sexually and physically abused?
A: My opinion was the child was sexually abused.

Answer Assumptive Questions with a Statement.

Q: Did you inform the police that the nurse failed to take a history?
A: The nurse did take a history.

Answer Leading Questions with a Statement.

Q: That wasn't exactly the truth, was it?
A: It was exactly the truth.

Hypothetical Questions Must Always Fit the Facts. For this example, the hypothetical case being tried involves a physically abused child with multiple bruises of varying ages and types and a spiral fracture of the right elbow. One of the injuries contained in the example is a circular bruise to the right shoulder.

Q: Doctor, you testified that it was your opinion that the child in this case was a battered child, didn't you?
A: Yes.
Q: Doctor, I'd like to ask you questions about each injury separately. With respect to the first injury, the bruise on the right shoulder.

Q: Isn't it true that it would be possible to get the injury in an accidental manner?

A: Do you mean in the context of this case, or in another manner?

Q: Let's say in the context of this case.

A: In the context of this case, it is my opinion that the bruise was intentionally inflicted.

Q: But is it possible that it was accidentally caused?

A: Using reasonable scientific probability, it is not.

Q: What about taken by itself, not in the context of this particular case—would your opinion change?

DA: Objection, your honor, no foundation. The hypothetical is not based upon facts of this case.

Court: Sustained.

Handling Prior Statements

A common occurrence is the situation where the expert is faced with what appears to be his or her own inconsistent prior statement, either in a written report or in previous testimony. Experts often give preliminary opinions or speculate, only to find out later that, based upon a more complete analysis, the opinion or speculation changes. When the opposing counsel discovers this change, there is an effort to use the change to force an expert into admitting fallibility or, worse, lying. This technique attempts to confuse the expert based upon the scientist's belief that truth is absolute. Consider the following example:

Q: Doctor, you stated in your report that the temperature of the solution was 90 degrees centigrade, didn't you?

A: Yes.

Q: But the temperature was really 91.7 degrees, wasn't it?

A: Yes.

Q: So, your statement in the report is not exactly the truth, is it?

A: Yes, it was the truth.

Q: If the temperature was in reality 91.7 degrees, how could your statement that it was 90 degrees be the truth, doctor?

A: Because at the time that I stated it was 90 degrees, I believed it to be 90 degrees.

The concept of truth has one meaning in science and another meaning in the courtroom. In science, truth is absolute. If something is false, it cannot be true. In the courtroom, truth is the absence of deceit. In the courtroom, a person lies when that person has the intent to deceive. If a person believes a statement is true, then he or she is telling the truth. In this example, the expert demonstrates an awareness of courtroom standards for evaluating truth and thus avoided the trap set by the questioning attorney.

CONCLUSION

This chapter has presented tips and techniques on how to testify as an expert witness. While it is true that the expert is dependent upon the lawyer conducting the examination to effectively ask questions that elicit opinion, there is much the expert can do to ensure smooth presentation of testimony. Of primary importance is preparation for the testimony by meeting with the examining attorney in advance of the court appearance. This allows both the expert and the lawyer to learn how to communicate with each other. It also presents the opportunity for the expert to educate the lawyer about the basis for the opinion and the possible strengths of the opposing opinion.

The expert can also maximize presentation by understanding what cross-examination techniques may be used by opposing counsel to confuse and confound. Examples have been presented to demonstrate these techniques and suggestions made to neutralize them.

The role of an expert is an important one. Proper preparation and understanding permit the expert to convert what may be a frustrating experience to a rewarding and challenging opportunity.

Glossary

Abrasion: an area of the body surface denuded of skin or mucous membrane caused by an abnormal process.

Abscess: a localized collection of pus in a cavity formed by the disintegration of tissue.

Adnexa: a term that collectively describes the ovaries, uterine tubes, and ligaments of the uterus.

Anal canal: the terminal portion of the large bowel extending from the rectum to the anus.

Anterior commissure: the junction of the labia majora anteriorly, at the lower border of the symphysis pubis.

Anus: the distal orifice of the gastrointestinal tract.

CDC: Centers for Disease Control and Prevention.

Cervical os: an opening in the cervix leading into the uterine cavity.

Clitoral hood: a covering fold of skin over the clitoris. Also called clitoral prepuce.

Clitoris: a small, elongated, erectile body, situated between the labia just beneath the mons pubis; homologous with the male penis.

Contusion: a superficial injury produced by impact without laceration (a bruise).

Ecchymosis: an extravasation of blood under the skin.

Epididymis: an elongated cord-like structure which attaches the spermatic cord to the posterior border of the testis.

Fossa navicularis: a hollow or depressed area in the vestibule anterior to the posterior commissure and inferior to the vagina.

Hymen: a membranous fold which partially occludes the external orifice of the vagina.

Labia majora: an elongated fold running downward and backward from the mons pubis in the female, one on either side of the vestibule.

Labia minora: a small fold of skin located on each side of the vestibule and medial to the labia majora.

Laceration: a wound made by tearing. Occasionally used to describe a wound caused by sharp objects.

Midline raphe: a ridge along the midline of the perineum, from the posterior commissure to the anus. In the male, it is continuous with the raphe scroti.

Mons pubis: a rounded fleshy prominence over the symphysis pubis. In adulthood this area is covered by pubic hair.

Penis: the male genital organ consisting of a root, body, and a glans. The root is attached to the pubic bones. The body consists of two parallel cylinders of erectile tissue, the corpora cavernosa, and beneath them, a third cylindrical structure, the corpus spongiosum, through which the urethra passes. The glans is a thickening at the tip of the penis and is covered by a prepuce (foreskin) and is demarcated from the body of the penis by a ridge, the corona. The penis is homologous with the clitoris.

Perineum: the area between the anus and the posterior commissure.

Petechia: a very small, round, non-raised purplish-red spot caused by intradermal or submucosal hemorrhage.

Posterior commissure: the apparent junction of the labia majora posteriorly. Also called the posterior fourchette.

Prostate: a gland which surrounds the neck of the bladder and urethra. It is made up partly of glandular elements, the ducts from which empty into the prostatic portion of the urethra, and produces the majority of seminal fluid.

Rectum: the distal portion of the large intestine beginning at the third sacral vertebra as a continuation of the sigmoid colon and ending in the anal canal.

Scrotum: a skin pouch which contains the testes. A midline ridge, the raphe scroti, is continuous with the midline raphe of the perineum.

Seminal vesicles: a pair of sacculated pouches attached to the posterior part of the urinary bladder, the duct of each joins the ipsilateral vas deferens to form the ejaculatory duct.

Synechia: adhesion of parts or tissues, e.g., hymen to vestibule.

Testes: the male gonads.

Transection: a cross-section. In this text it denotes a perpendicular cut through the hymenal tissue.

Urethra: a canal conveying urine from the bladder to the exterior of the body.

Urethral meatus: the opening of the urethra into the vestibule in the female, or into the glans in the male.

Uterine cervix: the lower and narrow end of the uterus that opens into the vagina.

Uterus: a pear-shaped organ in which the embryo grows and develops.

Vagina: a canal extending from the vestibule to the uterine cervix.

Vaginal fornix: a recess formed between the vaginal wall and the vaginal part of the cervix.

Vas deferens: an excretory duct of the testis which unites with the excretory duct of the seminal vesicle to form the ejaculatory duct.

Vestibule: a space or cavity at the entrance to a canal. In the female genitalia, the vestibule denotes the space between the labia minora into which the urethra and the vagina open.

Vulva: the female external genitalia, including the labia majora, labia minora, mons pubis, clitoris, perineum, and vestibule of the vagina.

ANNOTATED BIBLIOGRAPHY
1992–1998

Adams, J. Sexual abuse and adolescents. *Pediatric Annals.* 1997 May; 26(5): 299–304.

Adams, JA, and S Knudson. Genital findings in adolescent girls referred for suspected sexual abuse. *Archives of Pediatrics and Adolescent Medicine.* 1996 Aug; 150(8): 850–7.

A study of 204 adolescent girls with a history of probable or definite sexual abuse revealed that normal or nonspecific results of genital examinations were commonly found, unless the abuse was very recent. Further studies are needed to document the healing of genital injuries in victims of acute assault and the frequency of hymenal findings in nonabused, nonsexually active adolescent females.

Adams, JA, K Harper, S Knudson, and J Revilla. Examination findings in legally confirmed child sexual abuse: It's normal to be normal. *Pediatrics.* 1994 Sep; vol. 9493:310–7.

A review of 236 cases of sexual abuse with perpetrator convictions. Genital findings were normal in 28 percent, nonspecific in 49 percent, suspicious in 9 percent and abnormal in 14 percent. Abnormal anal findings were found in only 1 percent. Conclusion is that abnormal genital findings are not common in sexually abused girls.

Adams, JA, and R Wells. Normal versus abnormal genital findings in children: How well do examiners agree? *Child Abuse Neglect.* 1993 Sep-Oct; 17 (5):663–75.

Colposcopic photographs of the anogenital area of 15 patients were shown to 170 medical examiners. The agreement between the participants and the experts on the abnormal cases (mean 81 percent) was significantly higher than on the normal cases (mean 71 percent, p < .001) and on genital findings (78 percent) than on anal findings (63 percent). Higher experience level (more cases seen per month) was associated with significantly higher agreement between the participants and the experts on five of eight normal cases and two of four abnormal cases. Use of a colposcope was also associated with higher overall agreement with experts (74 percent vs. 44 percent < .0001)

American Medical Association. Diagnostic and treatment guidelines concerning child abuse and neglect. Chicago: AMA, 1985.

Pamphlet for physicians giving the diagnostic and treatment guidelines for child sexual abuse. Includes introductory information, physical signs (including a hymenal diameter of greater than 4 mm), and behavioral indicators.

Bays, J, and D Chadwick. Medical diagnosis of the sexually abused child. *Child Abuse Neglect.* 1993 Jan-Feb; 17 (1):91–110 Review Article 90 REFS.

Bays, J, and C Jenny. Genital and anal conditions confused with child sexual abuse trauma. *Am J Dis Child.* 1990;144:1319–1322.

Case review article using seven children to illustrate how dermatologic, traumatic, infectious and congenital disorders may be confused with sexual abuse. Excellent illustrations.

Bays, J, and LV Lewman. Toluidine blue in the detection at autopsy of perineal and anal lacerations in victims of sexual abuse. *Arch Path Lab Med.* 1992 June; 116:620–1.

Brief description of the use of dye at autopsy to aid in the detection of genital and anal injuries due to child sexual abuse. Cites four case examples.

Berenson, AB, AH Heger, and S Andrews. Appearance of the hymen in newborns. *Pediatrics.* 1991;87:458–465.

An article designed to answer the question raised in all "normal studies": Are these truly normal, non-abused girls or have they not disclosed their abuse? This study evaluated female newborns before they left the nursery, and documents the presence of clefts, bumps, tags, and ridges which may later be confused with post-traumatic changes.

Berenson, AB, AH Heger, JM Hayes, RK Bailey, and SJ Emans. Appearance of the hymen in prepubertal girls. *Pediatrics.* 1992;89:387–394.

A review of 211 girls selected for non-abuse. The article describes the types of hymens, presence of bumps, tags, vestibular bands (periurethral), longitudinal intravaginal ridges, and notches. Hymenal diameters were also studied. Important to note that attenuation and scarring/disruption was found in only one girl, who was lost to follow-up.

Berkowitz, CD. Sexual abuse of children and adolescents. *Adv Pediatr.* 1987;34: 275–312.

Chapter with overview on sexual abuse including information on definitions, incidence, medical assessment and management, the medical history, and behavioral assessment. Detailed information on the physical examination including techniques, information on the normal anatomy, hymenal diameter, and abnormal findings consistent with trauma. Includes examination of the male victim and information regarding anal trauma. The section on laboratory evaluation includes the forensic examination and the evaluation and treatment of sexually transmitted diseases. The psychological interview is also included with recommended therapy. Legal obligations and involvement with the court are briefly discussed. Extensive bibliography.

Berkowitz, CD. Pediatric Abuse: New patterns of injury. *Emerg Med Clin North Am.* 1995 May; 13(2):321–41.

A review article with 110 references covering the spectrum of abusive symptomatology. Aim of article is to heighten the awareness of emergency department physicians to the range of clinical signs and symptoms in the diagnosis and treatment of abused children. Article reviews both physical and sexual abuse.

Berkowitz, CD, SL Elvik, and M Logan. A simulated "acquired" imperforate hymen following the genital trauma of sexual abuse. *Clin Pediatr.* 1987;26:307–309.

Case report of a five-year-old originally evaluated for acute vaginal bleeding. This child showed scarring and tearing of the vaginal introitus. Follow-up evaluation showed progressive healing with replacement of the hymen with a thick scar.

Black, CM. Current Methods of Laboratory Diagnosis of *Chlamydia trachomatis* infections. *Clin Micro Rev.* 1997 Jan; 10(1):160–184.

This article discusses the different patient populations of *Chlamydia trachomatis* infection, including victims of sexual assault and abuse. Information regarding specimen collection and transport for both culture and nonculture testing. Even though

DNA amplification techniques are being performed more frequently and are an evolving "gold standard," in cases of suspected sexual abuse or assault, only culture tests should be used. It is also the recommended method for detection of *C. trachomatis* in the urethra of asymptomatic boys, the anorectum of patients of all ages, the nasopharynx of infants, and the vagina of prepubertal girls because of the lack of sufficient evaluation of the performance of nonculture tests, including nucleic acid amplification tests, on these specimens. Specimens must be transported in *C. trachomatis*-specific medium, and depending on the acuity of the exposure, a follow-up culture should occur two weeks later.

Blythe, MJ, and DP Orr. Childhood sexual abuse: guidelines for evaluation. *Indiana Med.* 1985;78:11–18.

Review article covering basic introductory information on sexual abuse including definitions and behavioral and medical indicators. Details of genital and anal findings include disruption of hymenal integrity, changes in vaginal opening, anal tears and changes in tone. Recommends medical and psychological follow-up.

Bond, GR, MD Dowd, I Landsman, and M Rimsza. Unintentional perineal injury in prepubescent girls: A multicenter, prospective report of 56 girls. *Pediatrics.* 1995 May; 95(5):628–31.

Prospective study to determine the pattern of perineal injuries and frequency of hymeneal involvement resulting from unintentional trauma in prepubescent girls. 56 cases presenting to emergency departments were evaluated. Most injuries were minor with the majority of injuries anterior or lateral to the hymen. 34 percent were posterior to the hymen, with thigh injuries in older children engaged in bicycle riding or outdoor play. Only one patient had hymeneal involvement and this was a two year old who fell, abducting her legs with a pinpoint abraded area on the hymeneal surface at 3 o'clock. Conclusions were that hymeneal damage is extremely rare in accidental perineal injuries.

Bond, GR, et al. Unintentional perineal injury in prepubescent girls: A multicenter prospective report of 56 girls. *Pediatrics.* 1995; (95):628–631.

All accidents were observed or occurred during risky activities. No photographs were taken. Injuries were documented with drawings. Results: Most injuries were minor, involved the labia minora, and were anterior and lateral to the hymen. 34 percent involved injury posterior to the hymen. In only one case was the hymen involved. Conclusion was that without penetration the hymen is rarely involved.

Botash, A. Examination for sexual abuse in prepubertal children: An update. *Pediatric Annals.* Year?; 26(5):312–320.

A review article which discusses the complete sexual abuse evaluation, and informs the physician how to make appropriate referrals to centers of excellence.

Britton, H, and K Hansen. Sexual abuse. *Clinical Obstetrics and Gynecology.* 1997 Mar; 40(1):226–40.

This article provides an excellent overview of the evaluation of sexual abuse, discussing definitions, recognition of signs and symptoms, history-taking, the medical examination, sexually transmitted diseases, the use of the forensic rape kit, legal implications, long-term consequences, and follow-up. Photographs accompany the article.

Budayr, M, RN Ankney, and RA Moore. *Condyloma Acuminata* in infants and children—A survey of colon and rectal surgeons. *Diseases of the Colon and Rectum.* 1996 Oct; 39(10):1112–1115.

Cannon, AF, GP Davidson, and DM Moore. Anal size in children: the influence of age, constipation, rectal examination and defecation. *Med J Aust.* 1990;153: 380–383.

Review of 54 children who were free from any anorectal diseases who were evaluated for anal size 30 seconds after exposure of the anus for examination. The results showed that the antero-posterior diameter was less or equal to 10.0 mm and the transverse diameter was less or equal to 2.0 mm. Age, sex, digital-rectal examination, time since defecation, or position had no effect on the results. The authors recommend a standardized examination approach to all children with a set time at which measurements will be taken. They recommend that the inspection time be 30 seconds in a cooperating conscious child.

Cantwell, H. Vaginal inspection as it relates to child sexual abuse in girls under 13. *Child Abuse Neglect.* 1983;7:171–176.

A review of 247 cases in which vaginal inspection and measurements of the horizontal hymenal diameter were done. With horizontal diameters greater than 4 mm there was a confirming history of past sexual abuse in 75% of these girls.

Cantwell, H. Update on vaginal inspection as it relates to child sexual abuse in girls under thirteen. *Child Abuse Neglect.* 1987;11:545–546.

A follow-up study to the initial 1983 study in which a review of histories with additional disclosures of abuse suggested that an enlarged hymenal diameter was correlated with an abuse history in 80%. Repeat examinations on some of the victims included in the original study showed that the hymenal diameter may become smaller with time and further abuse.

Clayden, G. Anal appearances and child sexual abuse. *Lancet.* 1987;March:620–621.

A letter to the editor in response to Hobbs and Wynne's articles on anal findings in child sexual abuse states that "apart from recent violent abuse . . . the appearance of the anus . . . is unlikely to provide reliable evidence to confirm or exclude penetration."

Claytor, RN, KL Barth, and CI Shubin. Evaluating child sexual abuse: observations regarding ano-genital injury. *Clin Pediatr.* 1989;28:419–422.

A retrospective review of 944 children who had been examined by one pediatrician. 64% of the females and 34% of males had positive findings. Study also tried to correlate hymenal opening size with abuse. (Note: these statistics are exactly the reverse of what most investigators have described.)

Cowell, C. The gynecology examination of infants, children and young adolescents. *Pediatr Clin North Am.* 1981;28:247.

Chapter with useful chart on the anatomy and physiology of the reproductive tract. Includes information on the changes of the external and internal anatomy with maturation.

Darmstadt, GL. Perianal lymphangioma circumscriptum mistaken for genital warts. *Pediatrics.* 1996 Sep; 98(3:1):461–3.

De Jong, AR, and M Rose. Frequency and significance of physical evidence in legally proven cases of child sexual abuse. *Pediatrics.* 1989;84:1022–1026.

This is a study to determine the frequency and significance of physical evidence of genital or anal injury, sexually transmitted diseases, and seminal fluid in legally proven child sexual abuse felony cases. A total of 45 cases were reviewed retrospectively. No significant difference in rate of felony conviction was found in cases with or without physical evidence. Of cases resulting in felony convictions, physical evidence was present in only 23%. The authors conclude that the essential element in the prosecution of cases is the quality of the history obtained and the ability of the child to testify effectively.

Derksen, DJ. Children with *Condylomata accuminata.* *J Fam Prac.* 1992 Apr; 34:419–23.

Review of seven children (2 to 12 years old) who had genital HPV infections. Each child was interviewed and examined with colposcopy. A shave biopsy of the genital lesions was sent for pathology and HPV typing. Results: six of seven children had Perianal warts. The seventh had labial lesions. Five of the children had been sexually abused, as determined by history, physical examination, or an investigation by CPS.

Viral typing showed that five had HPV type 6 or 11, one had HPV type 16 or 18. Conclusions: Genital types of HPV (6, 11, 16, 18) should alert the family physician to proceed with careful assessment for sexual abuse. HPV can be the result of sexual abuse and HPV typing is a useful too in diagnosis.

Dowd, MD, et al. The interpretation of urogenital findings in children with straddle injuries. *Journal of Pediatric Surgery.* 1994; (29)1:7–10.

Retrospective study of 100 emergency room patients evaluated for "accidental" straddle injuries. Cases were not documented photographically. Results showed that most injuries were minor lacerations and abrasion of the genitalia. 11 percent had injury of the PF and hymeneal and vaginal injuries were caused by penetrating mechanisms. Five patients were felt to have been sexually abused based on historical information and physical findings. In boys the majority had scrotal and penile lacerations, ecchymosis and swelling.

Dubowitz, H, M Black, and D Harrington. The diagnosis of child sexual abuse. *AJDC.* 1992 June; (146):688–693.

Purpose of the article was to assess how 132 children were evaluated in an interdisciplinary team for possible sexual abuse. The social worker interviewed the parents, a psychologist interviewed the children. Parents completed a *Child Behavior Check List* and the child's reaction to the medical examination was noted. Results: The history from the child and abnormal physical findings were significantly associated with the team's diagnosis of sexual abuse, whereas the presence of sexualized behavior, somatic problems, and the child's response to the examination did not make an additional contribution. Article reviews the characteristics of the abuse as well as the physical findings divided into normal and abnormal findings. The examination was performed without colposcopy or magnification, no photographs were taken, and the maximum transverse diameter of the hymeneal opening was measured relative to the known width of the examiners index finger. Examiners documented vaginal opening >4 mm, acute trauma, scarring, adhesions, increased friability, discharge, hymeneal asymmetry, discontinuity, rounding, bumps, and clefts. The authors concluded that there was significant correlation of hymeneal opening size, adhesions, asymmetry, and rounding with the likelihood of abuse, however all these findings were present in both the group judged to be abused and the non-abused group. Scarring and hymeneal discontinuity were only found in the abused group.

(Note: difficult to review findings as well as accuracy of the hymeneal opening sizes without photographs taken with magnification.)

Emans, SJ. Vulvovaginitis in the child and adolescent. *Pediatr Rev.* 1986;8:12–19.

Review article covering the etiology, evaluation, and management of vulvovaginitis. A thorough evaluation will include a history, general physical examination, and careful genital examination and cultures. Specific information on the adolescent patient is also included. Provides detailed information on specific organisms and treatment with charts listing normal flora and treatment of vaginal discharge. Findings noted to be specific for sexual abuse were lacerations of hymen, attenuation, dilation of hymen, adhesions from hymen to vagina.

Emans, SJ, et al. Hymenal findings in adolescent women: Impact of tampon use and consensual sexual activity. *J Peds*. 1994; 125(1):153–160.

Prospective study of 300 post menarcheal females comparing hymenal anatomy between girls who were: 1) tampon users 2) non-sexually active and 3) sexually active. Other factors were assessed including prior gynecological examination and factors related to the ease of examination. Important to professionals diagnosing sexual abuse in children and adolescents was the finding that girls who were sexually active were significantly more likely than tampon users to have "complete clefts" in the posterior 180 degrees.

Emans, SJ, MR Laufer, and DP Goldstein. *Pediatric and Adolescent Gynecology*. 4th ed. Philadelphia: Lippincott Raven, 1990.

General pediatric gynecology text, with sections devoted to developmental and normal genital anatomy. Also covers genital trauma and sexual abuse.

Emans, SJ, ER Woods, NT Flagg, and A Freeman. Genital findings in sexually abused, symptomatic and asymptomatic girls. *Pediatrics*. 1987;79:778–785.

A review of 20 different genital findings in three groups of girls: (1) sexually abused girls (n = 119), (2) normal girls with no genital complaints (n = 127), and (3) girls with other genital complaints (n = 59). Comparisons of findings and hymenal diameter measurements were made for each group. Magnification with colposcope or otoscope is discussed. There were marked differences between groups 1 and 2, but group 3 had significant similarities with group 1. Some of the girls in group 3, especially those with scars, may have been sexual abuse victims. Vulvar inflammation may lead to some findings similar to group 1 findings.

Ellerstein, NS, and JW Canavan. Sexual abuse of boys. *Am J Dis Child*. 1980;134: 255–257.

Retrospective review of 145 cases of sexually abused children in which 11% were male. Physical findings are documented with only 50% of the boys having any positive findings. A comparison is made between the male and female patients as to characteristics of the abuse and abuser, where it occurred, and presence of physical findings.

Enos, WF, TB Conrath, and JC Byers. Forensic evaluation of the sexually abused child. *Pediatrics*. 1986;78:385–398.

Results of a 16-year forensic study of 162 cases. Includes examination protocol, the taking of laboratory specimens, and evidence collections. Also includes anatomical chart and illustrations of female abuse trauma. One hundred and thirty-two victims were female; 30 were male. Sexual abuse criteria included (1) positive tests for ejaculation, (2) patterns of wounds including condition of hymen and/or anal sphincter, (3) foreign body materials, (4) eyewitness accounts, and (5) history from victim. Based on these criteria 41.7% of females and 40.0% of males had a positive evaluation. Describes the examination of the hymen and normal anatomy. Accidental trauma does not cause hymenal damage. Significance of enlarged hymenal diameter also discussed. The younger the child, the less likely there will be a positive test for sperm.

Feldman, K. Inflicted penile incision injuries (letter). *Child Abuse and Neglect*. 1997 Mar; 21(3):253–4.

Finkel, KC. Sexual abuse of children: an update. *Can Med Assoc J*. 1987;136: 245–252.

General overview of child sexual abuse with background information on the psycho-social issues, pedophilia, and the role of the physician. Excellent review of medical and behavioral indicators with long list of references and charts. Focuses considerable attention on the difficult aspects of sexual abuse.

Finkel, MA. Anogenital trauma in sexually abused children. *Pediatrics*. 1989;84: 317–322.

Review of seven cases of children who experienced acute genital and/or anal trauma. The author describes the process of healing involving either (1) regeneration or (2) repair. Superficial wounds occurring in the genital area go through a process of regeneration which may be complete in a matter of 2–3 days. Five of the seven children had healing without residua. When more serious injuries occur, healing involves a process of repair with the formation of granulation tissue and scarring. The author concludes that trauma can heal with little or no residua and that the history continues to be the most important part of evaluating a child for possible sexual abuse, noting that the absence of medical findings should not rule out that abuse has occurred.

Frith, K. Rape, divorce and nullity. *Br J Hosp Med*. 1970;4:762–767.

A forensic guide to the evaluation of the rape victim. Primary focus is on the adult victim. Emphasizes need for careful history. Describes normal hymenal anatomy as a "thin piece of skin" and notes that hymens may be very elastic and therefore it may be difficult to determine if penetration has occurred. Well-illustrated documentation of the rupture of intact hymens with fingers and objects simulating penile penetration in virginal adult women under anesthesia. Tears occurred posteriorly with simulated penile penetration, and laterally or postero-laterally with finger rupture.

Frith, K. Sexual offences, divorce and nullity. In: *Gradworhl's Legal Machine*. 3rd ed. Bristol, VK.: Wright, 1976.

Follow-up article to above with emphasis on the forensic examination of different-age victims. Describes examination of rape victims and the various configurations of hymens. The hymen may be lax or have evidence of old scars. Anal examination should document (1) smoothness of the mucosa, (2) thickening of the mucosa, (3) fissures or tears with fresh or old scars, (4) funnel appearance, and (5) hemorrhoids or tags. Includes extensive information on the forensic evaluation.

Gabby, T, et al. Sexual abuse of children; the detection of semen on skin. *AJDC*. 1992 June; 146:700–703.

Long-standing protocols have required the evaluation of all children with history of possible sexual abuse within the previous 72 hours. Part of this evaluation was the use of the Wood's lamp, a UV light that cased semen to fluoresce. In this study, four forensic laboratory techniques were compared to determine their sensitivity over time. Technique: Semen was placed on the skin of volunteers. Samples of the dried semen were assessed during a 28 hour period with 1) Wood's Lamp 2) Microscopy 3) Acid phosphatase assay and 4) two assays for prostatic protein p 30. Results: the usefulness of the Wood's lamp diminished drmatically by 28 hours but fluorescence of urine persisted up to 80 hours. Overtime, the p 30 enzyme-linked immunosorbent assay was more sensitive than all other assays. Conclusions: Wood's lamp is not a sensitive screening tool and the p30 assay by enzyme-linked immunosorbent techniques is the most sensitive assay for the presence of semen.

Gardner, JJ. Descriptive study of genital variations in health, non-abused premenarchal girls. *J Peds*. 1992 Feb; 120:251–7.

Evaluation under anesthesia of 19 premenarchal girls who were asymptomatic and
selected for non-abusive histories. The study demonstrated wide anatomic variations.
Certain anatomical variations were noted. These variations included "increased vascularity (44 percent), midline avascular areas (27 percent), ragged posterior
fourchette (10 percent), peri-hymeneal tethers (14 percent), bumps (11 percent), and
asymmetry of the hymeneal tissue (9 percent). The author recommends caution
when interpreting small anatomical variations.

Gellert, GA, et al. Situational and sociodemographic characteristics of children infected with human immunodeficiency virus from pediatric sexual abuse. *Pediatrics*. 1993 Jan; 91:39–44.

Results of a survey sent to 2,147 professionals in health and social services. In cases
where HIV infection was reported, further questionnaires were sent to assess the de-
mographics, living situations, alternative risks, basis for diagnosis, profiles of the perpetrators, and types of abuse. Results: of 5622 HIV tests, 28 children were infected
with HIV and lacked alternative transmission routes. 64 percent of victims were female, and 71 percent were black. Mean age was nine years. Infection with other
STD's occurred in 33 percent. Basis for HIV testing included: 1) finding suggestion
of disease, 2) HIV positive or high risk perpetrators, 3) Presence of another STD.
Perpetrators were child's parent in 42 percent of cases and another family member in
25 percent.

Gibbons, M, and ED Vincent. Childhood sexual abuse. *Am Fam Phys*. 1994 Jan;
49(1):125–36. Review Article: 43 REFS.

Goff, CW, KR Burke, C Rickenback, and DP Buebendorf. Vaginal opening measurement in prepubertal girls. *Am J Dis Child*. 1989;143:1366–1368.

A review of 273 prepubertal girls who were preselected for non-abuse. Vaginal opening diameter tended to enlarge with age and to be larger in the supine frog-leg position. An opening greater than 4 mm was rare.

Gutman, LT, ME Herman-Giddens, and RE McKinney. Pediatric acquired immunodeficiency syndrome; Barriers to recognizing the role of child sexual
abuse. *AJDC*. 1993 July; 147(7):775–80. Review Article: 68 REFS.

Gutman, LT, et al. Evaluation of sexually abused and nonabused young girls for intravaginal human papillomavirus infection. *AJDC*. 1992 June; 146:694–9.

Parallel studies to evaluate prevalence of HPV infections in these two groups. Vaginal wash samples from index and control patients were assayed for HPV-1, -2, -4,
-6, -11 and -16. PAP smears were examined from index patients. Results: 33 percent
of index patients were positive for HPV-6, -11, -16 compared with none of the control patients. This study supports sexual contact as a major route in the transmission
of anal-genital HPV disease in children. Evaluation of the intravaginal specimens was
necessary to identify infection with HPV, since these results did not correlate with
the present or absence of external anal-genital warts.

Handley, J, W Dinsmore, et al. Anogenital warts in prepubertal children; Sexual
abuse or not? *Int J STD AIDS*. 1993 Sep/Oct; 4(5):271–9.

Findings suggest (a) the majority of children with AG warts do not acquire these sexually. (b) vertical transmission is an important means by which young children acquire AG warts, (c) household members of children with AG warts should be routinely screened for NG and AG warts, CIN lesions (mothers only) and other AG

infections or STDs (adults only), (d) HPV typing of AG warts in children may help to clarify their mode of transmission, (e) spontaneous resolution of AG warts in children does occur, (f) scissor excisions combine with electrocautery is a safe and efficacious treatment for AG warts in children.

Hanson, RM, Sexually transmitted diseases and the sexually abuse child. *Curr Opin Ped.* 1993 Feb; 5(1):41–49. Review Article: 74 REFS.

Heger, A. *Response: Child sexual abuse, a medical view.* Los Angeles, United Way, Inc., 1985.

Training manual to accompany video aimed at teaching physicians in training to recognize and diagnose sexual abuse. Includes protocols, bibliography of medical articles, and prevention materials. Color plates illustrate both normal and abnormal genital and anal anatomy.

Heger, A, M Durfee, and B Woodling. Medical evaluation chapter, *Sexual Abuse of Young Children.* By Kee MacFarlane and Jill Waterman et. al. (New York: The Guilford Press, 1986).

Introductory chapter on the medical evaluation of the sexually abused child in textbook with extensive information on the preschool-aged sexual abuse victim.

Heger, A, and SJ Emans. Introital diameter as the criterion for sexual abuse. *Pediatrics.* 1990;85:222–223.

A commentary questioning the reliability of using measurements of the hymenal opening as a sensitive and/or specific sign of sexual abuse. Questions the use of measuring antero-posterior diameters, since hymen morphology varies, and recommends conservative, scientific approach to the diagnosis of sexual abuse.

Herjanic, B. Sexual abuse of children. *JAMA.* 1978;239:331–333.

Description of general management of the child sexual abuse victim, including developing a high index of suspicion on the part of the practitioner. Describes techniques for taking a history from the victim without having parents present. Also recommends that a social history should be taken from the responsible adults. Recommends tape-recording all initial interviews.

Herman-Giddens, ME. Vaginal foreign bodies and child sexual abuse. *Archives of Pediatrics and Adolescent medicine.* 1994 Feb; 148(2):195–200.

Retrospective review of 12 cases involving girls under the age of ten who present with vaginal foreign bodies. Two of the girls had STDs, and eight met diagnostic criteria for confirmed sexual abuse, three for suspected abuse, and in one case the abuse status was unknown. The author concludes that girls presented with VFBs need to be evaluated for possible abuse.

Herman-Giddens, ME, and TE Frothingham. Prepubertal female genitalia: examination for evidence of sexual abuse. *Pediatrics.* 1987;80:203–208.

A review of 375 cases discussing the techniques for evaluating sexual abuse victims and the types of injuries, both vaginal and anal, that occur with abuse. Uses two case reports to illustrate evaluation process. Recommends good history and careful examination noting hymenal opening, evidence of recent trauma, scars, bruising, discharge, bleeding, lacerations, notches, etc. An anal exam often yields no findings, but one may find gaping anus, skin tags (not at the 12-o'clock position), fissures, scars, hyperpigmentation, and thickening of skin. Reviews normal hymenal variants.

Herman-Giddens, ME, and NL Berson. Harmful genital care practices in children: a type of child abuse. *JAMA.* 1989;261:577–579.

A review of 17 cases in which harmful genital care practices produced physical and psychological harm. These practices were primarily unusual and ritualistic handling and inspection of the child's genitals.

Hibbard, RA, and GL Hartman. Components of child and parent interviews in cases of alleged sexual abuse. *Child Abuse Negl.* 1993 Jul/Aug; 17(4):495–500.

This study demonstrates some professional bias in interviewing children and parents and suggests that having a single interview or interviewer may not always by optimal for a thorough evaluation. Increased communication and teamwork among professionals and cross-training among disciplines should facilitate both the recognition of the appropriateness of some multiple interviews, as well as provide efforts to consolidate interviews when possible.

Hobbs, CM, and JM Wynne. The sexually abused battered child. *Arch Dis Child.* 1990;65:423–427.

A review of 130 children who were identified as being victims of both sexual and physical abuse/neglect. Mean age for girls (n = 77) was 5.7 years and for boys (n = 53) was 6.8 years. The patterns of injury that suggested sexual abuse included bruises, scratches, and burns on the lower trunk and genital area. Four deaths were reported.

Hobbs, CJ, and JM Wynne. Child abuse: buggery in childhood—a common syndrome of child abuse. *Lancet.* 1986;2:792–796.

A review of 35 cases, ages 14 months to 8 years, with a history and physical signs of sodomy. Twenty-seven had history of abuse from child or perpetrator. Anal findings include fissures, dilatation, loss of sphincter, shortening and eversion of the anal canal, external venous congestion, and generalized reddening and thickening of the perianal tissues. Associated vaginal signs were found in 14 girls, but penile penetration was uncommon. Excellent illustrations.

Hobbs, CJ, and JM Wynne. Sexual abuse of English boys and girls: the importance of anal examination. *Child Abuse Neglect.* 1989;13:195–210.

A review of 608 cases of suspected child sexual abuse of which 337 were confirmed or probable cases. A wide variety of abuses were included: 30% gave a history of digital or penile penetration of the anus and 42% had positive anal findings. Sixty percent of those children under the age of 5 had positive anal findings. Anal findings included erythema, swelling, laxity, shortening or eversions, RAD, fissures, venous congestion, skin changes, twitching, funneling, hematoma and bruising, and infection. The authors noted a general absence of these findings in a group of children who were not abused. Recommends thorough anal examination of all children suspected to have been sexually abused, but does not recommend invasive procedures or digital examination. Note: Most case evaluations were done acutely, and follow-up examination showed virtually complete healing, with very few showing permanent scarring.

Huffman, J, CJ Dewhurst, and VJ Copraro. *The Gynecology of Childhood and Adolescence.* 3rd ed. Philadelphia: W.B. Saunders, 1981.

Pediatric and adolescent gynecology text with information on normal genital development, normal genitalia and hymenal configurations, congenital anomalies, and changes caused by trauma. Includes information on changes that occur with hormonal changes and maturation.

Hymel, KP, and C Jenny. Child sexual abuse. *Pediatrics in Review*. 1996 Jul; 17(7):236–49. Review article discussing the medical evaluation of suspected child sexual abuse in pediatric primary care.

Horowitz, DA. Physical examination of sexually abused children and adolescents. *Pediatr Rev*. 1987;9:25–29.

Intended as a detailed description of the vaginal examination of the prepubertal child and adolescent. Includes information on approach to the child, issues of privacy and control, different positions, and obtaining specimens. Minimal information on physical findings other than a hymenal opening larger than 4 mm may suggest penetration.

Ingram, DL, et al. Ureaplasma urealyticum and large colony mycoplasma colonization in female children and its relationship to sexual contact, age, and race. *Child Abuse Negl*. 1992 Mar/Apr; 16(2):265–75.

Prospective study of 452 female children age 1 to 12 years in which cultures were taken and correlated to introital diameter, age, and race. Although there were correlations between an increased hymeneal diameter and history of sexual abuse, and the presence of these organisms was higher in black girls, there was no significant correlation that would indicate that colonization with UU and LCM was useful marker for sexual contact.

Jenny, C, MLD Kuhns, and F Arakawa. Hymen in newborn female infants. *Pediatrics*. 1987;80:399–400.

A review of 1,131 female infant examinations in which all were found to have hymens.

Jones, JG. Sexual abuse of children. *Am J Dis Child*. 1982;136:142–146.

Introduction to the sexual abuse of children with information on definition, incidence, types of abuse, pedophilia, and rape. Describes behavioral indicators and interview techniques. Recommends the use of a forensic protocol and psychological referral and support, as well as appropriate medical follow-up and evaluation for sexually transmitted diseases. Discusses incest and describes this as being more common than extrafamilial abuse.

Josephson, GW. The male rape victim: evaluation and treatment. *JACEP*. 1979;8: 13–15.

Introduction to the evaluation of male rape victims noting psychological and physical findings. Recommends therapy and legal considerations. Includes specific types of injuries, forensic evaluation, and treatment.

Krugman, R. Recognition of sexual abuse in children. *Pediatr Rev*. 1986;8:24–30.

Review article with overview of statistics, definitions, and behavioral and medical indicators. Advocates multidisciplinary approach and good history taking. Includes information on hymenal diameter, follow-up care, medical records, and false allegations. Stresses importance of therapy and prevention programs.

Kerns, DL, et al. Concave hymeneal variations in suspected child sexual abuse victims. *Pediatrics*. 1993.

Some 1,383 premenarchal and adolescent girls were evaluated for possible sexual abuse. Photocolposcopy was used for the anogenital examinations.

Ladson, S, CF Johnson, and RE Doty. Do physicians recognize sexual abuse? *Am J Dis Child*. 1987;141:411–415.

Review of results of questionnaires given to primary care physicians. Indicates that many physicians cannot identify normal anatomy and often do not include genital examinations as part of their examination. States that the normal hymenal diameter opening should be between 3 and 6 mm.

Landwirth, J. Children as witnesses in child sexual abuse trials. *Pediatrics.* 1987;80: 585–589.

A review article with the goal of presenting a better understanding of the issues pertaining to the role of children as witnesses. Reviews the competency and credibility of children as witnesses and notes that research in child psychology has shown that there is little correlation between age and honesty and that children do not tend to fantasize about things outside the realm of normal life experiences. It also states that children's short-term memory for facts may be as good as adults and that children appear to be no more suggestible than adults about events for which their memory is equally strong. The article goes on to review the process of litigation, the rights of the accused, and a variety of proposals for judicial reform, which make the system more child-friendly.

Lanktree, C, L Zaidi, J Briere, and V Gutierrez. Differential identification of sexually abused children in psychiatric outpatient chart. Abstract, American Psychological Association, New Orleans, August 1989.

A previous study by Briere and Zaida revealed that adult psychiatric patients randomly selected from a psychiatric emergency room gave histories of child sexual abuse in only 6% of the cases; however, when personnel directly asked about childhood sexual victimization, the percentage increased to 70%. A similar review of child psychiatric outpatient evaluations was done. Sixty-four cases were reviewed, 29 were randomly selected, and 35 clinicians were instructed to inquire as to the history of sexual abuse. Of the random cases, 6.9% reported sexual abuse; 31.4% of those asked directly about sexual abuse indicated that this had occurred. This is a 4.5–fold increase over those who were not asked directly. This is an important study, especially in light of the fact that these children were referred for evaluation because of emotional problems and they still did not report to the evaluator unless they were specifically asked. Perhaps even more interesting is a comparison of the adult and child statistics, where the adults had an 11-fold increase after being specifically asked about abuse compared to the 4.5–fold for the children.

Levitt, CJ. Sexual abuse in children: a compassionate yet thorough approach to evaluation. *Postgrad Med.* 1986;80:201–215.

Introduction with excellent color illustrations. Includes details of history taking and medical examination. Also includes information on normal genital anatomy and hymenal diameters, value of colposcopy, findings consistent with abuse, forensic examinations, and sexually transmitted diseases. Discusses the child's perception of abusive acts. Notes that often after the acute phase, there may be no physical findings.

Levitt, CJ. Medical evaluation of the sexually abused child. *Prim Car.* 1993 Jun; 20(2):343–54. Review Article. 25 REFS.

McCann, J. Use of the colposcope in childhood sexual abuse examinations. *Pediatr Clin North Am.* 1990;37:863–880.

A review article that discusses in depth the advantages and disadvantages of using a colposcope in the examination of child sexual abuse.

McCann, J, D Reay, J Seibert, B Stephens, and S Wirtz. Postmortem Perianal Findings in Children. *American Journal of Forensic Medicine and Pathology.* 1996 Dec; 17(4):289–298.

A multicenter, collaborative study was designed to help address the problem of postmortem findings of anal dilation or an exposed pectinate line in children who have died under suspicious circumstances. It is suggested that anal dilatation alone cannot be used as a marker for prior sexual abuse and that exposure of the pectinate line should not be confused with tears or fissures of the anal vergue. Further studies of children known to have been sodomized prior to death are required.

McCann, J, and J Voris. Perianal injuries resulting from sexual abuse: A longitudinal study. *Pediatrics.* 1993 Feb; 91(2):390–7.

Report on four cases of children with Perianal injuries. Followed from 1 week to 14 months.

McCann, J, J Voris, M Simon, and R Wells. Comparison of genital examination techniques in prepubertal girls. *Pediatrics.* 1990;85:182–187.

A review of 172 girls who were all examined using three positions: (1) supine with labial separation, (2) supine with labial traction, and (3) prone. Both the supine with traction and the prone were superior to the separation techniques for visualization of the vaginal introitus. The authors measured both the horizontal and vertical diameters. The greatest transverse diameters were found using the supine traction technique. The largest antero-posterior measurements were found in the prone position. No additional findings were discussed.

McCann, J, J Voris, M Simon, and R Wells. Perianal findings in prepubertal children selected for nonabuse: a descriptive study. *Child Abuse Neglect.* 1989;13: 179–193.

A review of 161 girls and 106 boys between the ages of 2 months and 11 years. Children were selected as nonabused after questionnaires were filled out by parents, and children with possible indicators of abuse were eliminated. No interviews of the children were undertaken. Half of the girls were evaluated with the use of the colposcope and the others were not. The study documented the presence of erythema; pigmentation, venous congestion (three times during exam); anal dilatation, intermittent anal dilatation (fluttering), configuration during dilatation, smooth areas, dimple/depressions, skin tags (actually skin folds anterior to anus), and scars (no scars were noted after the colposcope was used so no verification of any scarring in these children is possible). **Commonly found:** Erythema (41%), increased pigmentation (30%), venous engorgement (52%), wedge-shaped smooth areas (26%), skin tags/folds (11% and all anterior). Forty-nine percent had some anal dilatation, which fluctuated in 62%. Flattening of anal verge during dilatation in 44% and 34%. **Infrequently:** Other skin tags/folds (0%); scars (1%), anal dilatation greater than 20 mm (1.2%), irregularity of the anal orifice after dilatation (3%), and prominence of the anal verge (3%). No abrasions, hematomas, fissures, or hemorrhoids were noted. Authors conclude that with the relatively high incidence of soft tissue changes, caution needs to be used in rendering an opinion on the significance of these medical findings. Authors also mention the need to understand that this group may include children who were sexually abused but remained undetected.

McCann, J, R Wells, M Simon, and J Voris. Genital findings in prepubertal girls selected for nonabuse: a descriptive study. *Pediatrics.* 1990;86:428–439.

A review of 93 cases selected from a general pediatric population for "non-abuse." The authors used all three of the examination positions discussed in their previous article. They noted that many of these "normals" demonstrated erythema, periurethral bands, labial adhesions, lymphoid follicles, and midline sparing of the posterior fourchette. They also documented hymenal mounds, projections, tags, and intravaginal ridges. An important article in documenting the presence of these congenital/normal variants and nonspecific changes seen frequently in the pediatric population. However, the significance of what was not found in this study is just as important as what was found. None of these children had hymenal scarring and/or attenuation. The article also reviews and compares hymenal opening sizes of groups.

McCann, J, J Voris, and M Simon. Genital injuries resulting from sexual abuse: a longitudinal study. *Pediatrics*. 1992;89:307–317.

A 14-month to 3-year followup of 3 girls with genital injuries from sexual abuse, showing phases of healing and techniques of examination.

McCauley, J, RL Gorman, and G Guzinski. Toluidine blue in the detection of perineal lacerations in pediatric and adolescent sexual abuse victims. *Pediatrics*. 1986;78:1039–1043.

A study of 49 cases of sexual abuse. All patients were examined within 24 hours from the onset of symptoms. There were 25 adolescent and 24 preadolescent girls in the study. All of the adolescent girls gave a history of attempted vaginal penetration (84% with actual penetration). The use of dye in this group increased the rate of detecting lacerations of the posterior fourchette from 4% to 28%. The pediatric age group divided into three groups: (1) no history from child but parents suspected child was previously abused, (2) history from child of fondling or rubbing, and (3) history positive for possible penetration. In the pediatric age group the detection rate of posterior fourchette lacerations improved from 16.5% to 33% with the use of dye. Control groups were also studied. The adolescent control group was made up of girls who had engaged in voluntary coitus during the previous 48 hours. Dye increased detection rate of lacerations from 0% to 28%. In the pediatric control group of 25 there were no lacerations noted with or without dye.

Mok, JY. When is HIV an issue after child sexual abuse? *Archives of Disease in Childhood*. 1996 Jul; 75(1):85–7.

Muram, D, PM Speck, and M Dockter. Child sexual abuse examination: Is there a need for routine screening for *N. gonorrhoeae? Journal of Pediatric And Adolescent Gynecology*. 1996 Apr; 9(2):79–80.

Results of a study involving 865 prepubertal girls seen within 72 hours following an assault revealed that vaginal cultures in asymptomatic prepubertal girls may not be indicated as part of the initial evaluation. All 12 prepubertal children who had positive vaginal cultures for *N. gonorrhoeae* reveled that they had signs of acute vulvovaginitis.

Muram, D. Genital tract injuries in the prepubertal child. *Pediatr Annals*. 1986;15: 616–620.

General overview of genital injuries including accidental and nonaccidental trauma. Discusses the mechanism of injury for both blunt force vulvar injuries and penetrating injuries involving the hymen and vagina.

Muram, D. Child sexual abuse—genital tract findings in prepubertal girls: the unaided medical examination. *Am J Obstet Gynecol*. 1989;160:328–333.

A prospective study of 206 prepubertal girls who were victims of sexual abuse. Thirty-two percent of the victims had normal-appearing genitalia changes. Normal-appearing genitalia were most often observed in those reporting digital assault, and specific findings were more commonly found in those describing genitogenital assault. The most common pattern of injury in this study was a linear laceration of the hymen posteriorly.

Muram, D. Child sexual abuse: relationship between sexual acts and genital findings. *Child Abuse Neglect*. 1989;13:211–216.

A comparison study between the findings observed during examination of female victims of sexual abuse compared to the sexual acts that the perpetrator confessed to having performed. Mean age of the girls was 9.1 years. Thirty-one cases were reviewed and in 18 cases the offender admitted to vaginal penetration. Specific findings were observed in 11 of these 18 (61%). Complaints of sexual abuse can be valid even if the physical examination fails to detect abnormalities.

Muram, D. Anal and perianal abnormalities in prepubertal victims of sexual abuse. *Am J Obstet Gynecol.* 1989;161:278–281.

A review of 310 prepubertal children who were determined to be victims of child sexual abuse. Sixty-six percent had normal examinations. Abnormal findings were found in 104, including anal gaping, skin tags, rectal tears, sphincter tears, HPV, perianal scarring, and bite marks.

Muram, D. Child sexual abuse—genital tract findings in prepubertal girls: comparison of colposcopic and unaided examinations. *Am J Obstet Gynecol.* 1989; 160:333–335.

Prospective study of 130 sexually abused girls. All victims were evaluated with and without a colposcope. Ninety-two of 130 girls were found to have abnormal findings. These findings were noted during the unaided examination in 96% of the cases. Concluded that in most cases the unaided examination is adequate for the evaluation.

Muram, D. Child sexual abuse. *Curr Opin Obstet Gyn.* 1993 Dec; 5(5):784–90. Review Article. 43 References.

Norvell, MK, GI Benrubi, and RJ Thompson. Investigation of microtrauma after sexual intercourse. *J Reprod Med.* 1984;29:269–271.

A report of a prospective study to determine if the colposcope could be valuable in documenting vaginal intercourse. Eighteen adult volunteers in the study were examined after 72 hours of sexual abstinence and again within 6 hours of vaginal intercourse. Positive colposcopic findings were found in 61.2% of patients after consensual vaginal intercourse as compared with 11.1% of patients after abstinence.

Oates, RK, DL Lynch, AE Stern, BI O'Toole, and G Cooney. The criminal justice system and the sexually abused child: Help or hindrance? *Med J Aust.* 1995 Feb; 162(3):126–30.

Prospective study of the progress of 59 sexually abused children through the criminal justice system to determine whether there were any effects on their self-esteem or behavior, whether it resulted in depression, and what their parents perceptions of the process were. Results: thirty-three cases were sent to trial or sentencing, resulting in 20 convictions. Twenty-two children testified in court. 55 percent of the parents expressed dissatisfaction with the legal system, thinking it was too stressful on their children. A comparison of the differences between children who testified with those who did not indicated no significant differences on indices of depression, self-esteem, or behavior. Most of the families participated in court-preparation programs, and most mothers were supportive of their children. Paper emphasizes importance of attempts to minimize stress through court-preparation and closed-circuit television.

Orr, DP, and SV Prietto. Emergency management of sexually abused children. *Am J Dis Child.* 1979;133:628–631.

Review of 100 cases of sexual abuse of children, evaluated by pediatric residents. Describes protocols including the history taken from the child and parent. Uses drawings and dolls and emphasizes the need for directed questioning. Describes nature of abuse in 100 cases, relationship of abuser, and physical findings. Sixty-five percent of children had normal examinations. Recommends multidisciplinary approach to case management.

Orr, CJ, MA Clark, DA Hawley, JE Pless, LR Tate, and PM Fardal. Fatal anorectal injuries; A series of four cases. *J Forensic Sci*. 1995 Mar; 40(2):219–21.

Review of four cases of fatal anorectal assault. Although anorectal injuries are commonly reported in cases of sexual abuse of children, fatalities are very rare. Included in this report is one case of a fatal child abuse resulting from anal intercourse. Article reports on two additional cases of anal "fisting" of adult females and one case of homosexual attack with a threaded pipe.

Paradise, JE. Predictive accuracy and the diagnosis of sexual abuse: a big issue about a little tissue. *Child Abuse Neglect*. 1989;13:169–176.

Commentary on the study by White and Ingram as to whether measuring the hymenal introital diameter has any positive predictive value in the diagnosis of sexual abuse. Results show that if this was used as a screening test, 35% would be true positive and 65% would be false positive. Conclusions: The overreliance on these measurements can result in not protecting the abused child without an enlarged hymenal introital diameter. Diagnosis of sexual abuse depends on the history from the child, not on genital measurements.

Paradise, JE. The medical evaluation of the sexually abused child. *Pediatr Clin North Am*. 1990;37:839–862.

Review article on the complete assessment of the sexually abused child. Includes information on presenting complaints, interviewing, medical examination, sexually transmitted diseases, reporting responsibilities, and referral to therapy. Article includes very little detailed information on medical findings diagnostic of sexual abuse. States that transverse hymenal diameters should not be taken as a reliable indicator of abuse.

Paradise, J, and M. Finkel. Assessments of girls' genital findings and the likelihood of sexual abuse. *Arch Pediatr Adolesc Med*. 151 Sep; 151(9):883–891.

This article measured agreement about genital examination findings among physicians who rated themselves as skilled in evaluating children for suspected sexual abuse. Results indicated that these assessments differ, although very experienced physicians conform more closely to consensus standards. Note: Caution should be used regarding the reliability of the assessments because the criteria used to measure experience, was based on 100 examinations.

Parra, JM, and ND Kellogg. Repair of a recto-vaginal fistula as a result of sexual assault. *Semin Perioper Nurs*. 1995 Apr; 4(20):140–5.

Case report of a four year old who sustained severe penetrating trauma of the vagina and rectum resulting in a recto-vaginal fistula. She presented two months after the assault and required anogenital reconstruction with a temporary colostomy. Article recommends a thorough examination of all children who present with significant perineal and/or vaginal trauma.

Paul, DM. The medical examination in sexual offenses. *Med Sci Law*. 1975;15: 154–162.

Early introduction to the evaluation of the rape victim during the acute postrape period. Includes general protocols for the examining physician. Details importance of history and forensic examination. Introduces the concept of documenting injuries using the "face-of-a-clock" technique. Describes postrape genital findings of the vaginal and anal areas. Examination should note the size or laxity of the hymenal opening, recent and old tears, length of vagina, condition of vaginal rugae, bruising, scratches, lacerations, and splits. Vaginal penetration may occur without trauma, when rape occurs through an elastic hymen or when rape occurs via fear not force. Anal injury of some kind is usually present with first time anal rape. More severe injuries present with the younger vicim. Examination may return to normal after a few days to a week. Chronic abuse may result in changed anal tone and thickening of the anal mucosa and/or skin.

Paul, DM. The medical examination in sexual offences against children. *Med Sci Law.* 1977;17:251–258.

General introduction to the problem of the child as a victim of sexual assault. Primary focus is on the acute postrape evaluation. Patterns of injuries vary depending on (1) size and type of the penetrating object, (2) size of the victim's pelvic outlet, and (3) the use of force. Describes pattern of injuries with attempted penetration versus actual penetration. Vaginal penetration results in (1) circumferential tears of the vestibular mucosa, (2) posterior linear tears of hymen which may extend into vagina or posteriorly to perineum, and (3) lacerations to vaginal walls. Digital penetration may cause linear tears of the hymen. Accidental injury to the vaginal area may be by penetration or stretching. Penetrating injury is usually lateral to the hymenal margin. Anal injuries: Any injury to skin, mucosa, or muscles is significant. Anal hematomas may heal, causing skin tag. Fissures may result (may also be due to constipation). Chronic penetration causes changes in tone and the skin folds, as well as thickening of the anal skin/mucosa. The history is very important to the evaluation. Children may be too frightened to respond during examination. In rape cases where the assailant is known to the child there is often an absence of findings.

Persaud, D, and J Squires. Use of Foley catheter to examine estrogenized hymens for evidence of sexual abuse. *J Pediatr Adolesc Gynecol.* 1997 May; 10(2):83–5.

This article discusses a unique technique to examine the landmarks of the hymen in adolescent females, enabling better delineation of the hymenal edge.

Pokorny, SF, et al. Acute genital injury in the prepubertal girl. *Am J Obstet Gynecol.* 1992; (166):1461–1466.

Retrospective review of 32 cases of acute injury which were either straddle, nonpenetrating, penetrating, or torque. No photographs were taken. Cases reviewed include sexual assault that caused hymeneal injuries as well as other "nonpenetrating injuries" that also damaged the hymen. These injuries include damage caused by tree stump, bicycle part, doctor's finger, and a toy.

Rimsza, ME, and EH Niggemann. Medical evaluation of sexually abused children: a review of 311 cases. *Pediatrics.* 1982;69:8–14.

Retrospective review of 311 patients medically evaluated for sexual abuse. Eighteen percent were assaulted by strangers, 42% by relatives, and 30% reported abuse by more than one assailant. Only 23% showed no abnormalities. Mean age was 9.2 years. Ages ranged from 2 months to 17 years. Eighty-six percent were females. The younger the child, the more likely the child described only genital fondling and the exam would be normal. When examined within 24 hours of the assault, 36% had findings. By history, 125 of the girls reported vaginal penetration. Correlations are made between the nature of the abuse by history and the physical findings. Stranger assault is more likely to cause physical findings.

Ross, JD, GR Scott, and A Busuttil. *Trichomonas vaginalis* infection in pre-pubertal girls. *Med Sci Law.* 1993 Jan; 33(1):82–5.

Short paper discusses the implications of infection of the genital tract in children in respect to suspected child abuse. Two case reports are described to illustrate the problems that can arise in the investigation of such cases. *T. vaginalis* is usually transmitted sexually, but the potential for non-sexual transmission does exist.

Sanfilippo, JS. Identifying the sexually molested preadolescent girl. *Pediatr Annals.* 1986;15:621–624.

> Overview of sexual abuse including information on incidence, recognition, and reporting. Psychological support very important. Review of behavioral changes and indicators of abuse. History taking and genital and anal findings described. Hymenal diameters discussed with significance of enlarged hymenal diameter. Discusses anal findings and hymenal trauma and location of findings.

Sarles, RM. Sexual abuse and rape. *Pediatr Rev.* 1982;4:3.

> Overview article with information on incidence, reporting, behavioral and physical presentations, and medical management. History taking is important and may go from nondirect to direct with specific questioning. Literature review shows that anywhere from 35% to 75% of cases may have physical findings. Family support is important to the outcome of the case. Discusses forensic examination and medical treatment of possible injuries or disease. Counseling recommended for all cases.

Seidel, JS, SL Elvik, CD Berkowitz, and C Day. Presentation and evaluation of sexual misuse in the emergency department. *Pediatr Emer Care.* 1986;2:157–164.

> Fifty-seven of the patients discussed did not present with complaints of sexual abuse. Results are given for age, sex, chief complaint, physical findings, protocol for triage, history taking, and physical examination. Techniques for genital examination with a drawing of normal anatomy also included. Discusses genital and anal trauma and its significance.

Sicoli, RA, JD Losek, JM Hudlett, and D Smith. Indications for *Neisseria gonorrhoeae* cultures in children with suspected sexual abuse. *Arch Pediatr Adolesc Med.* 1995 Jan; 149(1):86–9.

> Review of a prospective management plan within a large pediatric emergency department. Records of all children less than 12 years-of-age examined for suspected sexual abuse were reviewed. 316 children received vaginal/urethral, oral, and anal cultures. Seven children had a total of 12 positive cultures, seven vaginal/urethral, four rectal, and one oral. Evidence of vaginal/urethral discharge on physical examination was the best predictor of GC. Historical and physical evidence of discharge was present in all cases with a positive culture. Conclusion: Children less than 12 years-of-age who are examined for sexual abuse but who did not have evidence of vaginal or urethral discharge were found to have a 100 percent probability of having a negative culture. Routine cultures for GC in asymptomatic children are not recommended.

Siegel, RM, CJ Schubert, PA Myers, and RA Shapiro. The prevalence of sexually transmitted diseases in children and adolescents evaluated for sexual abuse in Cincinnati: Rational for limited STD testing in prepubertal girls. *Pediatrics.* 1995 Dec; 96(6);1090–4.

> Prospective study of the prevalence of *Chlamydia trachomatis, Neisseria gonorrhoeae, Trichomonas vaginalis,* syphilis, and human immunodeficiency virus (HIV) in sexually abused children. Review of 855 children referred for sexual abuse. AAP Guidelines for STD testing were followed Results: Twelve children were determined to have *N. gonorrhoeae* infection, 11 had *C. trachomatis* infection, and four had *Trichomonas* infection. Overall, the prevalence of STDs in prepubertal girls was 3.2 percent and 14.6 percent in pubertal girls. The prevalence of *N. gonorrhoeae* in prepubertal girls with

vaginal discharge was 11.1 percent and 0 percent in prepubertal girls without discharge. *C. trachomatis* infection was diagnosed in 0.8 percent of prepubertal girls compared with 7.0 percent of pubertal girls. None of the children tested positive for syphilis or HIV, and no males had a STD. Conclusions: *N. gonorrhoeae* testing in prepubertal girls can be limited to those with a vaginal discharge on examination unless other risk factors are present. The prevalence of *C. trachomatis* and *Trichomonas* in prepubertal girls is low and may be omitted from routine evaluations. All pubertal girls evaluated for sexual abuse should be tested for STDs.

Simon, HK, and DW Steele. Varicella: Pediatric genital/rectal vesicular lesions of unclear origin. *Ann Emerg Med.* 1995 Jan; 25(1):111–4.

Report of three cases of varicella which present with localized vesicular rash in the diaper area. This rash might be easily confused with HSV-1 or -2 infections. Appropriate testing should be done to differentiate.

Sinal, S, M Lawless, and RM Soderstrom. Clinical agreement on physical findings in child sexual abuse cases. *Archives of Pediatrics and Adolescent Medicine.* 1997 May; 151(5):497–501.

This article measures the agreement among experienced clinicians regarding the interpretation of physical findings in child sexual abuse cases and found that clinicians do not agree perfectly when viewing photographs of female Tanner stage 1 or 2 genital findings. Note: Caution should be used regarding the reliability of the examinations since the criteria used for expertise was based on 100 examinations.

Soderstrom, RM. An objective approach to assessing sexual abuse of girls. *Journal of Reproductive Medicine.* 1994 Jan; 39(1):6–8.

Validates that the use of the colposcope in association with simultaneous photographs of the measuring device allows for accurate assessment of findings for medical-legal purposes.

Spencer, MJ, and P Dunklee. Sexual abuse of boys. *Pediatrics.* 1986;78:133–138.

Retrospective review of 140 boys who were evaluated for sexual abuse. Boys made up 9% of the referrals. Ages ranged from 1 to 17 years. Most gave a positive history of abuse. Physical evidence of abuse was present in 68% of cases. Includes information on perpetrators, type of abuse by history, erythema and abrasion, lacerations, fissures, hyperpigmentation, venous dilatation and hematomas, sphincter tone, scars (including skin tags), and sexually transmitted diseases.

Starling, S, and C Jenny. Forensic examination of adolescent female genitalia: The Foley catheter technique. *Arch Pediatr Adolesc Med.* 1997 Jan; 151:102–103.

This article discusses a unique technique to examine the landmarks of the hymen in adolescent females, compares this procedure to utilization of the cotton-tipped swab, and suggests that it can overcome excessive redundancy and allow full delineation of the hymenal edge.

Steward, MS, K Bussey, GS Goodman, and Saywitz. Implications of developmental research for interviewing children. *Child Abuse Negl.* 1993 Jan/Feb; 17(1):25–37. Review Article: 60 REFS.

Provides a brief review of recent research to update the investigative interviewer on children's development of cognition, memory, and language. Results of studies that have focused on the development of children's specific knowledge about the legal system.

Teixeira, RG. Hymenal colposcopic examination in sexual offenses. *Am J Forensic Med Pathol.* 1981;2:209–214.

Review of 500 cases referred for evaluation of hymenal integrity. Of these patients, 102 were under the age of 14. Reports on the usefulness of the colposcope in clarifying the diagnosis in 11.8% of the cases. Compares the diagnosis made with and without magnification. Discusses complete versus incomplete rupture of the hymen which may occur with vulvar coitus. In addition, author documented the healing process, which may occur as quickly as 9 days, but varies depending on the severity of injury. He also compared congenital notches versus posttraumatic ruptures (with healing). The article raises the issue of "hymenal complacency" in which penetration may occur without lacerations; the author notes that this is particularly true with fimbriated hymens. With fimbriated hymens (to age 10: 33 cases in this series) colposcopic examinations were helpful in 72% of the cases. Also documented the location of hymenal ruptures with 63% occurring in the posterior (5- to 7-o'clock position) hymen.

   Concludes that colposcopy is irreplaceable in cases such as incomplete ruptures, fringed, fimbriated hymens, infantile hymens, healing hymens, and whenever the forensic doctors feel that diagnosis is difficult or impossible.

Terezhalmy, GT, and GD Naylor. Oral manifestations of selected sexually related conditions. *Dermatologic Clinics.* 1996 Apr; 14(2):303–17.

It is prudent for health care personnel to acknowledge the presence of many sexually transmitted diseases in the oropharynx and to consider them in the differential diagnosis of many well—established conditions.

Tilelli, J. Sexual abuse of children. *N Engl J Med.* 1980;302:319–323.

Retrospective review of 130 cases of sexual abuse, ages 2–16 years, including 113 females and 17 males. Thirty presented with medical and social problems. Forty-three of the children had physical trauma. Physical findings ranged from bruises and nuchal petechiae to oral and perineal laceration. Only four children less than 12 years of age had signs of chronic physical abuse. Younger children (<8) were more likely to know the assailant, be victims of recurrent abuse, report crimes not involving intercourse, and to present with abused siblings. Incest victims were younger than other victims. Also notes that these victims were more likely to be abused. Recommends evaluation by trained specialist rather than emergency room personnel.

Tipton, AC. Child sexual abuse: physical examination techniques and interpretation of findings. *Adoles Pediatr Gynecol.* 1989;2:10–25.

An in-depth review article with general introductory information on child sexual abuse. Further information on the clinical interview with specifics that the medical professional may want to document during the course of the interview. Tipton also describes various examination techniques, hymenal diameters, and different abusive acts. Article includes a list of physical findings that are strongly indicative of sexual abuse, including hymenal damage or disruptions, damage to the posterior fourchette, and anal dilatation greater than 15 mm with traction on the buttocks. There are well-organized sections on sexually transmitted diseases and forensic evidence collection. Treatment, follow-up, and testifying guidelines are also included. Excellent section discussing the developmental issues surrounding children as witnesses and historians.

Underhill, RA, and J Dewhurst. The doctor cannot always tell: medical examination of the "intact hymen." *Lancet.* 1978;2:375–376.

Brief communication describing how difficult it is for trained physicians examining a postpubertal woman to determine whether she is virginal. Includes 28 women volunteers who were examined before a history of sexual activity was taken. In some cases the volunteers were examined by two different physicians and their findings compared.

Waterman, J, and R Lusk. Psychological testing in evaluation of child sexual abuse. *Child Abuse Negl.* 1993 Jan/Feb; 17(1):145–59. Review Article: 60 REFS.

West, R, A Davies, and T Fenton. Accidental vulvar injuries in childhood. *Br Med J.* 1989;298:1002–1003.

A review of 13 cases in which girls sustained accidental trauma. Even with penetrating trauma, there were no cases of damage to the hymen.

White, ST, DL Ingram, and PR Lyna. Vaginal introital diameter in the evaluation of sexual abuse. *Child Abuse Neglect.* 1989;13:217–224.

Prospective study of 242 prepubertal females to determine if vaginal introital diameter is useful in evaluating a child for sexual abuse. Three groups were established: group 1 had a history of sexual contact or *N. gonorrheae;* group 2 had no history but was at risk; group 3 was nonabused. A vaginal introital transverse diameter greater than 4 mm was more prevalent in group 1 (94%) than in group 2 (5%) or in group 3 (0%). Their conclusion is that a vaginal introital diameter greater than 4 mm is highly associated with sexual contact in children less than 13 years of age.

Woodling, BA. Sexual abuse and the child. *Emer Med Ser.* 1986;15:17–25.

Review article includes information on incidence of abuse, type of abuse, and relationship of abuser. Possible indicators of child sexual abuse both behaviorial and physical. Details of sexually transmitted diseases, hymenal diameter, and physical and laboratory evaluation.

Woodling, BA, and A Heger. The use of the colposcope in the diagnosis of sexual abuse in the pediatric age group. *Child Abuse Neglect.* 1986;10:111–114.

A brief communication documenting the usefulness of the colposcope for the diagnosis of sexual abuse in the pediatric age group. Reports that diagnosis of an additional 10% of pediatric cases of sexual abuse may be clarified through the use of the colposcope.

Woodling, BA, and PD Kossoris. Sexual misuse: rape, molestation and incest. *Pediatr Clin North Am.* 1981;28:481–499.

General introduction to sexual misuse of children. Includes information on definitions, pedophilia, victims, incidence, emotional trauma, and physical injuries. Discusses both acute and chronic cases of sexual abuse and the nature of the injuries. Outline of medical management of a sexual abuse case with the importance of history taking and a nontraumatizing physical examination. Includes: Outline of physical findings on the genital examination with locations using the "clock face" technique; discusses digital versus penile penetration, accidental injuries, and the use of tampons; medicolegal evaluation including laboratory analysis and test for sexually transmitted diseases; patient management and preparation of the medical report; and information on preparing for and testifying in court.

Wynne, JM. Injuries to the genitalia in female children. *SA Med J.* 1980;57: 47–50.

Review of 33 girls who had sustained injury to the genitalia. Twenty-four had been raped, seven had fallen, and two were involved in auto accidents. Reviews findings in these types of genital injuries. In rape victims, average age was 6. Recommended management and procedures are discussed. The pattern of injury for the rape victim is described as being either (1) without penetration—bruising and minor lacerations of the vulvar region or (2) with penetration—posterior midline lacerations of varying severity.

Young, SJ, DL Wells, and EJ Ogden. Lichen sclerosis, genital trauma, and child sexual abuse. *Aust Fam Phys.* 1993 May; 22(95):729, 732–3.

Lichen sclerosus affecting the genitalia of prepubertal females is an uncommon condition that may be mistaken for trauma associated with sexual abuse.

Appendices

A. State of California Sexual Abuse Protocol

State of California

Office of Criminal Justice Planning (OCJP) 925

MEDICAL REPORT—SUSPECTED CHILD SEXUAL ABUSE

<u>Record examination findings:</u> Penal Code § 13823.5 requires every physician who conducts a medical examination for evidence of child sexual abuse to use this form to record findings. Complete each part of the form and if an item is inapplicable, write N/A.

<u>Child abuse reporting law:</u> Penal Code § 11166 requires all professional medical personnel to report suspected child abuse, defined by Penal Code § 11165, immediately by telephone and submit a written report (DOJ SS 8572) within 36 hours to the local law enforcement agency, county department of social services or probation department. Professional medical personnel means any physician and surgeon, psychiatrist, psychologist, dentist, resident, intern, podiatrist, chiropractor, licensed nurse, dental hygienist, or any other person who is currently licensed under Division 2 (commencing with Section 500) of the Business and Professions Code.

<u>Minors:</u> Civil Code § 34.9 permits minors, 12 years of age or older, to consent to medical examination, treatment, and evidence collection related to a sexual assault without parental consent. Physicians are required, however, to attempt to contact the parent or legal guardian and note in the treatment record the date and time the attempted contact was made including whether the attempt was successful or unsuccessful. This provision is not applicable if the physician reasonably believes the parent or guardian committed the sexual assault on the minor. If applicable, check here (   ) and note date and time attempt to contact parents was made in the treatment record.

<u>Liability and release of information:</u> No civil or criminal liability attaches to filling out this form. Confidentiality is not breached by releasing this form or other relevant information contained in the medical records to law enforcement or child protective agencies (Penal Code § 11167).

A.   AUTHORIZATION FOR EXAM REQUESTED BY PATIENT/PARENT/GUARDIAN (Note: Parental consent for an evidential examination is not required in cases of known or suspected child abuse. Contact a law enforcement or child protective service agency.)

I hereby request a medical examination for evidence of sexual abuse and treatment for injuries. I understand that collection of evidence may include photographing injuries and these photographs may include the genital area. I further understand that hospitals and physicians are required to notify child protective authorities of known or suspected child abuse and if child abuse is found or suspected, this form and any evidence obtained will be released to a child protective agency.

Patient/Parent/Guardian (circle)

I have been informed that victims of crime are eligible to submit crime victim compensation claims to the State Board of Control for out-of-pocket medical expenses, loss of wages, and job retraining and rehabilitation. I further understand that counseling is also a reimbursable expense.

Patient/Parent/Guardian (circle)

B.   AUTHORIZATION FOR EVIDENTIAL EXAM REQUESTED BY CHILD PROTECTIVE AGENCY

I request a medical examination and collection of evidence for suspected sexual abuse of the patient at public expense.

Law enforcement officer or child protective services	Agency	ID number	Date

C.   GENERAL INFORMATION
(print or type)   Name of Hospital:

1. Name of patient   Patient ID number

2. Address   City   County   State   Phone

3. Age	DOB	Sex	Race	Date/time of arrival	Date/time of exam	Date/time of discharge

4. Name of: (   ) Mother   (   ) Stepmother   (   ) Guardian   Address   City   County   State   Phone (W) (H)

5. Name of: (   ) Father   (   ) Stepfather   (   ) Guardian   Address   City   County   State   Phone (W) (H)

6. Siblings: Name	DOB	Name	DOB	Name	DOB

7. Phone report made to: (   ) Law enforcement agency

Name   Agency   ID number   Phone

(   ) Child protective services

Name   Agency   ID number   Phone

8. Responding officer   Agency   ID number   Phone

DISTRIBUTION OF OCJP 925 | **HOSPITAL IDENTIFICATION INFORMATION**

**ORIGINAL TO CHILD PROTECTIVE AGENCY REQUESTING EXAM;
PINK COPY TO CRIME LAB (SUBMIT WITH EVIDENCE);
YELLOW COPY TO HOSPITAL RECORDS**

D. OBTAIN PATIENT HISTORY. RECORDER SHOULD ALLOW PATIENT OR OTHER PERSON PROVIDING HISTORY TO DESCRIBE INCIDENT(S) TO THE EXTENT POSSIBLE AND RECORD THE ACTS AND SYMPTOMS DESCRIBED BELOW. DETERMINE AND USE TERMS FAMILIAR TO THE PATIENT. FOLLOW-UP QUESTIONS MAY BE NECESSARY TO ENSURE THAT ALL ITEMS ARE COVERED.

1. Name of person providing history	Relationship to child	Address	City	County	State	Phone (W) (H)

2. Chief complaint(s) of person providing history

3. Chief complaint(s) in child's own words

4. ☐ Less than 72 hours since incident(s) took place   Date/time/location   ☐ Over 72 hours since incident(s) took place   Date(s) or time frame/location

5. Identity of alleged perpetrator(s), if known	Age	Sex	Race	Relationship to child

6. Acts described by patient and/or other historian

Described by patient / Described by historian (Yes No Unk / Yes No Unk)

Vaginal contact
  Penis
  Finger
  Foreign object
  Describe the object
Anal contact
  Penis
  Finger
  Foreign object
  Describe the object
Oral copulation of genitals
  of victim by assailant
  of assailant by victim
Oral copulation of anus
  of victim by assailant
  of assailant by victim
Masturbation
  of victim by assailant
  of assailant by victim
  other
Did ejaculation occur
  outside a body orifice?
If yes, describe the location
  on the body:
Foam, jelly, or condom used
  (circle)
Lubricant used
Fondling, licking or kissing
  (circle)
If yes, describe the location
  on the body:
Other acts:

Was force used upon patient?
If yes, describe:

7. Post-assault hygiene/activity
(   ) Not applicable if over 72 hours

Described by patient / Described by historian (Yes No Unk / Yes No Unk)

Urinated
Defecated
Genital wipe/wash
Bath/shower
Douche
Removed/inserted tampon
Brushed teeth
Oral gargle/swish
Changed clothing

8. Symptoms described by patient and/or other historian

Described by patient / Described by historian (Yes No Unk / Yes No Unk)

Physical symptoms
  Abdominal/pelvic pain
  Vulvar discomfort or pain
  Dysuria
  Urinary tract infections
  Enuresis (daytime or nighttime)
  Vaginal itching
  Vaginal discharge
  Describe color, odor and
    amount below.
  Vaginal bleeding
  Rectal pain
  Rectal bleeding
  Rectal discharge
  Constipation
  Incontinent of stool
    (daytime or nighttime)
  Lapse of consciousness
  Vomiting
  Physical injuries, pain, or
    tenderness. Describe below.

Behavioral/emotional symptoms
  Sleep disturbances
  Eating disorders
  School
  Sexual acting out
  Fear
  Anger
  Depression
  Other symptoms

Additional information:

HOSPITAL IDENTIFICATION INFORMATION

OCJP 925   —2—   86 96690

270

E. OBTAIN PERTINENT PAST MEDICAL HISTORY

1. Menarche age ( ) N/A	Date of last menstrual period ( ) N/A	Use of tampons ( ) Yes ( ) No ( ) N/A	History of Vaginitis ( ) Yes ( ) No ( ) N/A

2. Note pre-existing physical injuries ( ) N/A

3. Pertinent medical history of anal-genital injuries, surgeries, diagnostic procedures, or medical treatment? ( ) Yes ( ) No   If yes, describe

4. Previous history of child abuse? ( ) Yes ( ) No ( ) Unknown.   If known, describe

F. CONDUCT A GENERAL PHYSICAL EXAM AND RECORD FINDINGS. COLLECT AND PRESERVE EVIDENCE FOR EVIDENTIAL EXAM.

1. Blood pressure	Pulse	Temperature	Respiration	Include percentiles for children under six
				Height Weight

2. Record general physical condition noting any abnormality   ( ) Within normal limits

* Record injuries and findings on diagrams: erythema, abrasions, bruises (detail shape), contusions, induration, lacerations, fractures, bites, and burns.
* Record size and appearance of injuries. Note swelling and areas of tenderness.
* Examine for evidence of physical neglect.
* Take a GC culture from the oropharynx as a base line. Take other STD cultures as indicated. Provide prophylaxis.
  IF EXAMINED WITHIN 72 HOURS OF ALLEGED INCIDENT(S):
* Note condition of clothing upon arrival (rips, tears, or foreign materials) if applicable. Use space below to record observations.
* Collect outer and underclothing if worn during or immediately after the incident.
* If applicable, collect fingernail scrapings.
* Collect dried and moist secretions, stains, and foreign materials from the body including the head, hair, and scalp. Identify location on diagrams.
* Scan the entire body with a Wood's Lamp. Swab each suspicious substance or fluorescent area with a separate swab. Label Wood's Lamp findings "W.L."
* Examine the oral cavity for injury and the area around the mouth for seminal fluid. Note frenulum trauma. If indicated by history: Swab the area around the mouth. Collect 2 swabs from the oral cavity up to 6 hours post-assault for seminal fluid. Prepare two dry mount slides.
* Collect saliva and head hair reference samples at the time of the exam if required by crime lab and if there is a need to compare them to a suspect.
* Record specimens collected on Section 7.

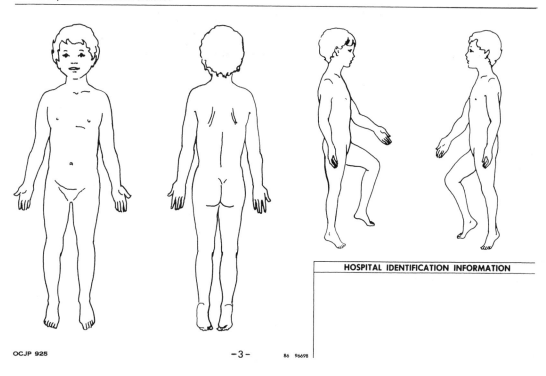

HOSPITAL IDENTIFICATION INFORMATION

271

Optional: Take photographs of genitals before and after exam.

Record injuries and findings on anal-genital diagrams: abrasions, erythema, bruises, tears/transections, scars, distortions or adhesions, etc. Use anal-genital chart on next page to record additional descriptive information.

3. External genitalia
* Examine the external genitalia and perianal area including inner thighs for injury.
* For boys, take a GC culture from the urethra. Take other STD cultures as indicated. Provide prophylaxis.
  IF EXAMINED WITHIN 72 HOURS OF INCIDENT:
* Collect dried and moist secretions and foreign materials. Identify location on diagrams.
* Pubertal children: Cut matted pubic hair. Comb pubic hair to collect foreign materials. Collect pubic hair reference samples at time of exam if required by crime lab and if there is a need to compare them to a suspect.
* Scan area with Wood's Lamp. Swab each suspicious substance or fluorescent area. Label Wood's Lamp findings "W.L."
* For boys, collect 2 penile swabs if indicated. Collect one swab from the urethral meatus and one swab from the glans and shaft. Take a GC culture from the urethra. Take other STD cultures as indicated. Provide prophylaxis.
* Record specimens collected on Section 7.
4. Vagina
* Examine for injury and foreign materials.
* Pre-pubertal girls with intact hymen/normal vaginal orifice: No speculum exam necessary.
* Pre-pubertal girls with non-intact hymen and/or enlarged vaginal orifice: Only conduct a speculum exam if major trauma is suspected and use pediatric speculum.
* Take a GC culture from the vaginal introitus in pre-pubertal girls with intact hyman/normal vaginal orifice; from the vagina in pre-pubertal girls with non-intact hymen and/or enlarged vaginal orifice; and, the endocervix in adolescents. Take other STD cultures as indicated. Provide prophylaxis.
* Obtain pregnancy test (blood or urine) from pubertal girls.
  IF EXAMINED WITHIN 72 HOURS OF INCIDENT:
* Pre-pubertal girls with intact hymen/normal vaginal orifice: Collect 2 swabs from the vulva.
* Adolescents or pre-pubertal girls with non-intact hymen and/or enlarged vaginal orifice: Collect 3 swabs from vaginal pool. Prepare 1 wet mount and 2 dry mount slides. Examine wet mount for sperm and trichomonas.
* Record specimens collected on Section 7.
5. Anus and rectum
* Examine the buttocks, perianal skin, and anal folds for injury.
* Conduct an anoscopic or proctoscopic exam if rectal injury is suspected.
* Take a GC culture from the rectum. Take other STD cultures as indicated. Provide prophylaxis.
* Take blood for syphilis serology. Provide prophylaxis.
  IF EXAMINED WITHIN 72 HOURS OF ALLEGED INCIDENT:
* Collect dried and moist secretions and foreign materials. Foreign materials may include lubricants and fecal matter.
* If indicated by history and/or findings: Collect 2 rectal swabs and prepare 2 dry mount slides. Avoid contaminating rectal swabs by cleaning the perianal area and relaxing the anus using the lateral or knee-chest position prior to insertion of swabs.
* Record specimens collected on Section 7.

DRAW SHAPE OF ANUS AND ANY LESIONS ON GENITALIA, PERINEUM, AND BUTTOCKS

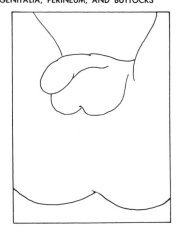

DRAW SHAPE OF HYMEN AND ANUS AND ANY LESIONS ON GENITALIA, PERINEUM, OR BUTTOCKS

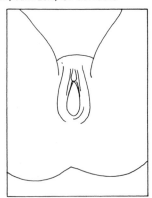

HOSPITAL IDENTIFICATION INFORMATION

6. Anal-genital chart

Female/Male General	WNL	ABN	Describe
Tanner stage			
Breast 1 2 3 4 5	☐	☐	_____
Genitals 1 2 3 4 5	☐	☐	_____
Inguinal adenopathy	☐	☐	_____
			_____
Medial aspect of thighs	☐	☐	_____
			_____
Perineum	☐	☐	_____
			_____

	Yes	No	
Vulvovaginal/urethral discharge	☐	☐	_____
			_____
Condyloma acuminata	☐	☐	_____

Female	WNL	ABN	Describe
Labia majora	☐	☐	_____
			_____
Clitoris	☐	☐	_____
			_____
Labia minora	☐	☐	_____
			_____
Periurethral tissue/ urethral meatus	☐	☐	_____
			_____
Perihymenal tissue (vestibule)	☐	☐	_____
			_____
Hymen	☐	☐	_____
Record diameter of hymen and check measurement used:			_____
☐ Horizontal			_____
☐ Vertical			_____
Posteriour fourchette	☐	☐	_____
			_____
Fossa Navicularis	☐	☐	_____
			_____
Vagina	☐	☐	_____
			_____
Other			_____
			_____

Exam position used:
☐ Supine
☐ Knee chest

Male	WNL	ABN	Describe
Penis	☐	☐	_____
Circumcised			_____
☐ Yes ☐ No			
Urethral Meatus	☐	☐	_____
			_____
Scrotum	☐	☐	_____
			_____
Testes	☐	☐	_____
			_____

Female/Male Anus	WNL	ABN	Describe
Buttocks	☐	☐	_____
			_____
Perianal skin	☐	☐	_____
			_____
Anal verge/ folds/rugae	☐	☐	_____
			_____
Tone	☐	☐	_____

Anal spasm
☐ Yes ☐ No
Anal laxity
☐ Yes ☐ No
Note presence of stool in rectal ampulla
☐ Yes ☐ No
Method of exam for anal tone (discretion of examiner)
☐ Observation
☐ Digital exam
Exam position used:
☐ Supine
☐ Prone
☐ Lateral recumbent
Anoscopic exam
☐ Yes ☐ No ☐ N/A
Proctoscopic exam
☐ Yes ☐ No ☐ N/A
Genital exam done with:
Direct visualization ☐
Colposcope ☐
Hand held magnifier ☐

HOSPITAL IDENTIFICATION INFORMATION

OCJP 925   –5–   86 96698

273

7. Record evidential and specimens collected.

FOR EVIDENTIAL EXAMS CONDUCTED WITHIN 72 HOURS OF ALLEGED INCIDENT

ALL SWABS AND SLIDES MUST BE AIR DRIED PRIOR TO PACKAGING (PENAL CODE § 13823.11). AIR DRY UNDER A STREAM OF COOL AIR FOR 60 MINUTES. Swabs and slides must be individually labeled, coded to show which slides were prepared from which swabs, and time taken. All containers (tubes, bindles, envelopes) for individual items must be labeled with the name of the patient, contents, location of body where taken, and name of hospital. Package small containers in a larger envelope and record chain of custody. See the State of California Medical Protocol for Examination of Sexual Assault and Child Sexual Abuse Victims published by the state Office of Criminal Justice Planning, 1130 K Street, Sacramento, California 95814 (916) 324-9100 for additional information.

SPECIMENS FOR PRESENCE OF SEMEN, SPERM MOTILITY, AND TYPING TO CRIME LAB

	Swabs	Dry Mount Slides	Yes	No	N/A	Taken by	Time
Oral							
Vaginal							
Rectal							
Vulvar							
Penile							

Vaginal wet mount slide examined for spermatozoa and trichomonas, dried, and submitted to crime lab			
Motile sperm observed			
Non-motile sperm observed			

OTHER EVIDENCE TO CRIME LAB

	Yes	No	N/A	Taken by
Clothing				
Fingernail scrapings				
Foreign materials on body				
Blood				
Dried secretions				
Fiber/loose hair				
Vegetation				
Dirt/gravel/glass				
Matted pubic hair cuttings				
Pubic hair combings				
Comb				
Swabs of bite marks				
Control swabs				
Photographs				
Area of body ___				
Type of camera ___				
Other ___				

REFERENCE SAMPLES AND TOXICOLOGY SCREENS TO CRIME LAB

Reference samples can be collected at the time of the exam or at a later date according to crime lab policies if there is a need to compare them to a suspect. Toxicology screens should be collected at the time of the exam upon the recommendation of the physical examiner, law enforcement officer, or child protective services.

Reference samples	Yes	No	N/A	Taken by
Blood typing (yellow top tube)				
Saliva				
Head hair				
Pubic hair				
Toxicology screens				
Blood/alcohol toxicology (grey top tube)				
Urine toxicology				

OCJP 925

CLINICAL EVIDENCE TO HOSPITAL LAB

	Yes	No	N/A	Taken by
Syphilis serology (red top tube)				
STD culture				
Oral				
Vaginal				
Rectal				
Penile				
Pregnancy test Blood (red top tube) or urine				

PERSONNEL INVOLVED (print)	PHONE
History taken by:	
Physical examination performed by:	
Specimens labeled and sealed by:	
Assisting nurse:	
Family assessment taken by: ( ) N/A ( ) Report attached	
Additional narrative prepared by physician: ( ) N/A ( ) Report attached	

FINDINGS AND FOLLOW-UP

Report of child sexual abuse, exam reveals:

☐ PHYSICAL FINDINGS   ☐ NO PHYSICAL FINDINGS
  ☐ Exam consistent with history   ☐ Exam consistent with history
  ☐ Exam inconsistent with history   ☐ Exam inconsistent with history

SUMMARY OF PHYSICAL FINDINGS:

☐ Oral trauma   ☐ Genital trauma
☐ Perineal trauma   ☐ Anal trauma
☐ Hymenal trauma
☐ Other findings consistent/inconsistent (circle one) with history as follows:

___
___
___

Follow-up arranged: ( ) Yes ( ) No

Child released to: ___

PHYSICAL EXAMINER

Print name of examiner

Signature of examiner

License number of examiner

LAW ENFORCEMENT/CHILD PROTECTIVE SERVICES

I have received the indicated items of evidence and the original of this report.

___
Law enforcement officer or child protective services

Agency	ID number	Date

HOSPITAL IDENTIFICATION INFORMATION

86 96698

-6-

274

B. Memphis, Tennessee Sexual Abuse Protocol

2 copies to Police Officer
1 copy to Clinic

CHILDREN

Case # _____
Sibling Case # _____

**FORENSIC EXAMINATION
OF
ALLEGED SEXUAL ASSAULT**

1. Identifying Information:
   Name _____
   Guardian ☐ Parent ☐ _____
   DOB _____ Age _____ Sex _____ Race _____
   Address _____
   City/State _____ Zip Code _____
   Phone (home) _____ (other) _____

Alleged Assault:
Unknown: ☐
Date: _____
Time: _____

Forensic Exam:
Date: _____
Time: _____

2. Anal-genital chart

Female/Male General	WNL	ABN	Describe
Tanner stage			
Breast 1 2 3 4 5	☐	☐	_____
Genitals 1 2 3 4 5	☐	☐	_____
Medial aspect of thighs	☐	☐	_____
Perineum	☐	☐	_____

	Yes	No	
Vulvovaginal/urethral discharge (describe)	☐	☐	
Flat plaques/growths (describe)	☐	☐	

Female	WNL	ABN	Describe
Labia Majora	☐	☐	_____
Clitoris	☐	☐	_____
Labia minora	☐	☐	_____
Periurethral tissue/ urethral meatus	☐	☐	_____
Perihymenal tissue (vestibule)	☐	☐	_____
Hymen	☐	☐	_____
☐ Cresent			
☐ Annular			
☐ Other (describe)			
☐ Unable to determine (describe)			
Diameter of hymenal lumen			
☐ Horizontal _____ mm.			
☐ Vertical _____ mm.			
Posterior fourchette	☐	☐	_____
Vagina	☐	☐	_____
Other			_____

Exam position used for genital evaluation:
☐ Supine ☐ Mother's lap
☐ Knee chest

Male	WNL	ABN	Describe
Penis	☐	☐	
☐ circumcised ☐ uncircumcised			_____
Urethral meatus	☐	☐	_____
Scrotum	☐	☐	_____
Testes	☐	☐	_____

Female/Male Anus	WNL	ABN	Describe
Buttocks	☐	☐	_____
Perianal skin	☐	☐	_____
☐ feces present			
Anal verge/folds	☐	☐	_____
Anal shape (describe)	☐	☐	_____
☐ linear			
☐ circular			
☐ irregular (describe)			
Anal tone	☐	☐	

Method of exam: ☐ Observation ☐ Digital exam
Anal dilation ☐ ☐
☐ No dilation noted ☐ Funneling present
☐ External ☐ Internal Sphincter relaxation
☐ Horizontal _____ mm. in _____ seconds
☐ Vertical _____ mm. in _____ seconds
☐ Feces in rectal ampulla

Anal tags Location: _____
☐ Yes ☐ No
Anal fissures Location: _____
☐ Yes ☐ No

Exam position used for anal evaluation:
☐ Supine ☐ Lateral recumbent ☐ Mother's lap
☐ Prone ☐ Knee chest

Summary of Evidence Released to:
☐ Kit collected _____
☐ No kit _____
☐ Clothing _____
☐ Other _____

Genital exam done with:
Direct visualization ☐
Colposcope ☐
Pictures taken ☐ # _____

275

3. PERTINENT PAST MEDICAL HISTORY
Menarche age .... ☐ N/A _____
Date of last menstrual period .... ☐ N/A _____
Note history of physical injuries   ☐ Yes ☐ No ☐ N/A _____

Pertinent medical history of ☐ anal-genital injuries, ☐ surgeries
☐ diagnostic procedures, or ☐ medical treatment? If yes, describe:

_____
_____

Previous child abuse investigation? ☐ Yes ☐ No   ☐ Physical
(describe when and where)   ☐ Sexual
_____   ☐ Neglect

5. Check behaviors observed during exam:

☐ tearful   ☐ fidgeting
☐ sobbing   ☐ trembling
☐ yelling   ☐ controlled
☐ loud   ☐ agitated
☐ quiet   ☐ listless
☐ tense   ☐ fearful
☐ cooperative   ☐ other _____

_____
_____
responds to questions:
☐ readily ☐ briefly ☐ reluctantly

4. Symptoms described by patient: ☐ _____
by historian: ☐ _____
not evaluated: ☐ _____
Physical symptom/hx:
☐ Abdominal/pelvic pain   _____
☐ Vulvar discomfort or pain   _____
☐ Dysuria   _____
☐ Urinary tract infection   _____
☐ Enuresis (daytime or nighttime) _____
☐ Vaginal itching   _____
☐ Vaginal discharge   _____
  Describe color, odor, amount   _____

☐ Vaginal bleeding   _____
☐ Rectal pain   _____
☐ Rectal bleeding   _____
☐ Rectal discharge   _____
☐ Constipation   _____
☐ Incontinent of stool (day/night) _____

Other: _____
_____
_____

6. Additional Observation or Remarks: _____
_____
_____
_____
_____
_____
_____
_____
_____
_____
_____
_____
_____
_____
_____
_____
_____
_____
_____
_____

7. Treatment:
Hospitalization:
  location _____
Prophylaxis:
  pregnancy _____
  gonorrhea _____

Testing:
  pregnancy _____   VDRL _____
  GC culture _____
  Referral _____

8. Testing: Sperm

	SEEN	MOTILE	NON-MOTILE	NOT SEEN	NOT DONE
Vaginal					
Oral					
Anal					

9. Instructions for Follow-up

	Yes	No
A. ORAL	☐	☐
B. WRITTEN		
Agency brochures	☐	☐
Medical follow-up inst.	☐	☐

This report of the examination is an investigative report used as evidence by Memphis Police Services, Shelby County law enforcement agencies, Tennessee Department of Human Services, and other cooperating agencies.

Investigating
Agency _____
DHS Social
Counselor _____
Date _____
MRCC Counselor _____

MRCC Forensic
Evaluator _____
Police
Officer _____
R&I # _____
CPT # _____

PREPUBERTAL FEMALE GENITAL and ANAL FORENSIC EXAMINATION

CASE NO. ____________________

NAME OF VICTIM ____

DATE OF COLLECTION ________________ TIME __________ AM - PM

NURSE/CLINICIAN ____

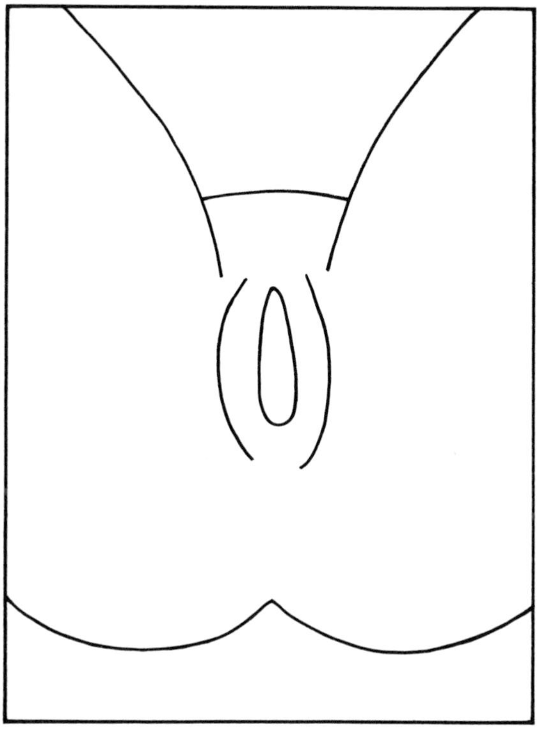

Comments: ____

☐ Refused ☐ Full Cooperation ☐ Partial Cooperation

F-2100 549G

Rev 8/89

MALE GENITAL and ANAL FORENSIC EXAMINATION

CASE NO. ____________________

NAME OF VICTIM ____

DATE OF COLLECTION ________________ TIME __________ AM - PM

NURSE/CLINICIAN ____

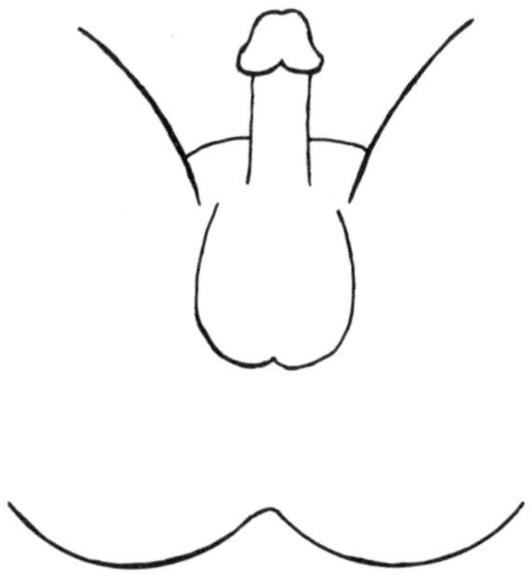

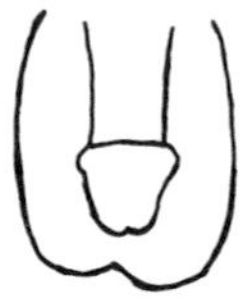

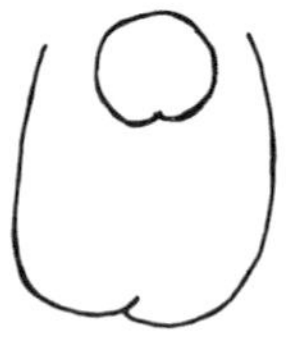

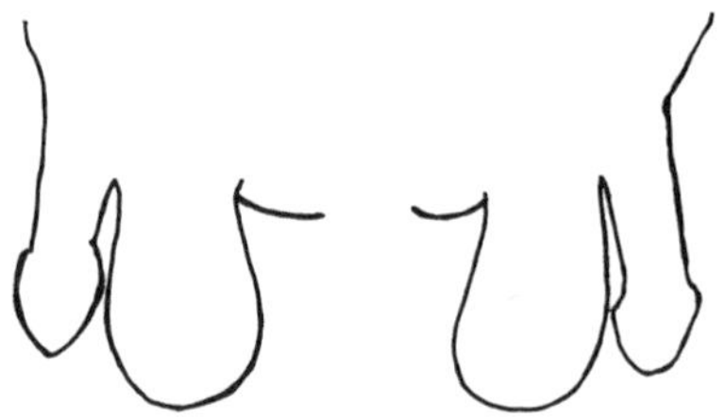

Left Right

Comments: ____

____

____

____

____

____

☐ Refused ☐ Full Cooperation ☐ Partial Cooperation

F-2100 549M Rev. 8/89

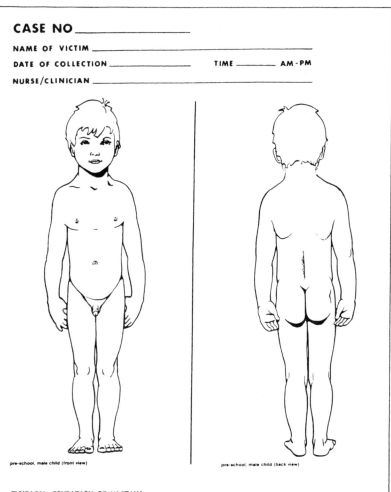

CASE NO _____

NAME OF VICTIM _____

DATE OF COLLECTION _____ TIME _____ AM-PM

NURSE/CLINICIAN _____

pre-school, male child (front view)

pre-school, male child (back view)

PHYSICAL CONDITION OF VICTIM:

INDICATE ALL SIGNS OF PHYSICAL TRAUMA - E.G., BRUISES, SCRATCHES, MARKS, DIS-
COLORATIONS (SIZE AND COLOR), OR BITE MARKS ON ANY PART OF THE BODY. (NOTE ALL
SIGNS OF TRAUMA ON THE APPROPRIATE ANATOMICAL DRAWING).

2100.550

New 6/85

279

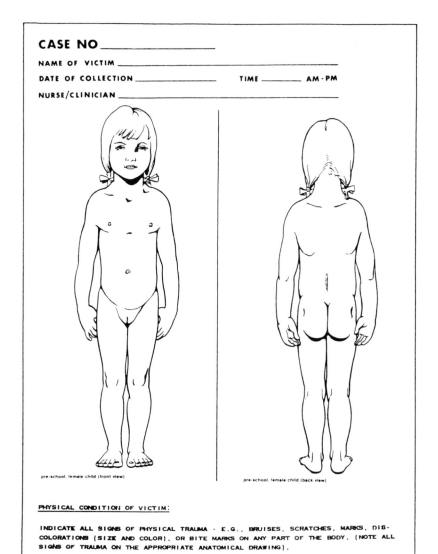

CASE NO _____

NAME OF VICTIM _____

DATE OF COLLECTION _____   TIME _____ AM - PM

NURSE/CLINICIAN _____

pre-school, female child (front view)

pre-school, female child (back view)

PHYSICAL CONDITION OF VICTIM:

INDICATE ALL SIGNS OF PHYSICAL TRAUMA - E.G., BRUISES, SCRATCHES, MARKS, DIS-
COLORATIONS (SIZE AND COLOR), OR BITE MARKS ON ANY PART OF THE BODY. (NOTE ALL
SIGNS OF TRAUMA ON THE APPROPRIATE ANATOMICAL DRAWING).

C. Commonwealth of Massachusetts Sexual Abuse Protocol

COMMONWEALTH OF MASSACHUSETTS
SEXUAL ASSAULT EVIDENCE COLLECTION KIT INSTRUCTIONS

This kit is designed to assist the examining physician and nurse in the collection of evidentiary specimens for analysis by the crime laboratory serving your local police agency. The hospital is not requested or encouraged to analyze any of the specimens/evidence collected in this kit. Any specimens required by the hospital are to be collected with hospital supplies.

If the case history and/or patient's symptoms warrant, i.e. the patient indicates that there were periods that they experienced unconsciousness, or lack of motor control, or their belief that they were drugged prior to or during the assault, then obtain patient's consent and collect a urine sample for drug testing. Please note that items collected with this kit are not routinely analyzed for drugs. Samples collected for the purpose of drug testing may be submitted, along with the kit, to the investigating police agency.

STEP 1   **HOSPITAL REPORTS ENVELOPE**

> Note: This envelope contains five Hospital Report forms. Retain Forms 1, 2, 3 and 4 along with white copy of Form 5 for hospital records. Please note that Form 5 consists of carbon copy forms; therefore, use care to prevent inscribing the writing from other forms onto Form 5.

Form 1   Fill out all information requested and have patient and witness sign and date where indicated.

Forms 2, 3 and 4   Fill out all information requested then sign and date where indicated.

Form 5   Fill out all information requested and return yellow copy to Step 1 envelope.

STEP 2   **ORAL SWABS, SMEARS AND FLOSS** (Collect only if oral assault occurred within the past 24 hours)

> Note: Do not stain or chemically fix smears. Do not moisten swabs prior to sample collection.

Remove folded paper from the envelope and use the dental floss provided to collect debris from between the patient's teeth. Place the used dental floss into the center of the paper and refold to retain floss. Return to envelope. Using both swabs simultaneously, carefully swab the upper and lower areas between the lips and gums, and along the tooth and gum lines. Using both swabs, prepare two smears. Allow swabs (2) and smears (2) to air dry. Return swabs to their original paper sleeve and smears to slide holder. Return swabs and smears to envelope, then seal and fill out all information requested on envelope. Affix kit number label where indicated.

Using hospital-supplied swab(s), collect the appropriate culture(s) at this time.

STEP 3   **SALIVA SAMPLE** (For Secretor Status - collect even if no oral contact)

> Notes: 1. If patient was/is bleeding from the oral cavity, do not collect saliva sample.
> 2. The patient should not have anything to eat, drink or smoke for a minimum of 15 minutes prior to saliva sample collection.

Have patient remove folded filter paper disk from SALIVA SAMPLE envelope and saturate inner circle with saliva. Allow sample to air dry. Return disk to SALIVA SAMPLE envelope being careful not to touch the inner circle. Seal and fill out all information requested on envelope. Affix kit number label where indicated.

STEP 4   **FINGERNAIL SCRAPINGS** (Collect only if patient scratched assailant's skin or clothing)

LEFT HAND: Remove one of the folded papers and fingernail scrapers provided in envelope, and unfold and place on flat surface. Hold patient's left hand over paper and scrape under all five fingernails allowing any debris present to fall onto paper. Place used scraper in center of paper and refold paper to retain debris and scraper. Mark folded paper "Left Hand".

RIGHT HAND: Follow same procedure for right hand.

Return both folded papers to FINGERNAIL SCRAPINGS envelope. Seal and fill out all information requested on envelope. Affix kit number label where indicated.

STEP 5   **CLOTHING** (10 paper bags provided)

> Notes: 1. If patient is not wearing the clothing worn at the time of the assault, collect only the items that are in direct contact with patient's genital area.
> 2. If patient changed clothing after assault, inform officer in charge so that the clothing worn at the time of the assault will be collected by the police as soon as possible.
> 3. Do not cut through any existing holes, rips or stains in patient's clothing.
> 4. Do not shake out patient's clothing or microscopic evidence will be lost.
> 5. If additional clothing bags are required, use only new paper (grocery-type) bags.
> 6. If foreign material is present, see Steps 16A and 16B.

Unfold and place a clean bed sheet on floor. Remove paper sheet from DEBRIS COLLECTION envelope, unfold and place over bed sheet. Instruct patient to stand in center of sheet and carefully disrobe. Collect each item as removed and place in a separate CLOTHING bag. Collect patient's underpants and place in UNDERPANTS bag. Staple all bags shut. Refold DEBRIS COLLECTION SHEET to retain any foreign material present and return to DEBRIS COLLECTION envelope and seal envelope. Fill out all information requested and affix kit number label on all bags and the DEBRIS COLLECTION envelope. Return bed sheet to hospital laundry.

STEP 6   **HEAD HAIR COMBINGS**

Remove paper towel and comb provided in HEAD HAIR COMBINGS envelope. Place paper under patient's head. Using comb provided, comb head hair so that any loose hairs and/or debris will fall onto paper towel. Carefully remove towel from under patient's head. Place used comb in center of towel. Fold towel to retain both comb and any evidence present. Return to HEAD HAIR COMBINGS envelope, seal and fill out all information requested on envelope. Affix kit number label where indicated.

STEP 7   **HEAD HAIR STANDARD (Pulled hairs are preferred)**

Remove one of the five (5) folded papers from the HEAD HAIR STANDARD envelope, unfold and place on a flat surface. From the front of the head, individually grasp 2-3 hairs as close to the scalp as possible and using swift force, pluck and place them in the center of the paper. Then cut, as close to the scalp as possible, approximately 20 full-length hairs and place them in the center of the paper. Refold the paper to retain the hairs. Label the paper "Front" and return the paper to the envelope. Repeat the above procedure for the remaining scalp locations: Top, Back, Right Side, and Left Side, labeling each paper as appropriate. Seal the envelope and fill out all information requested on envelope. Affix kit number label where indicated.

STEP 8   **PUBIC HAIR COMBINGS**

Remove paper towel and comb provided in PUBIC HAIR COMBINGS envelope with patient in lithotomy position, place towel under patient's buttocks. Using comb provided, comb pubic hair in downward strokes so that any loose hairs and/or debris will fall onto paper towel. Fold towel to retain both comb and any evidence present. Return to PUBIC HAIR COMBINGS envelope. Seal and fill out all information requested on envelope. Affix kit number label where indicated.

RE1MA INS 3 4/98

STEP 9   <u>PUBIC HAIR STANDARD</u> **(Pulled hairs are preferred)**

Remove folded paper from PUBIC HAIR STANDARD envelope, unfold and place on flat surface. Individually grasp 2-3 hairs as close to the skin as possible and using swift force, pluck and place them in the center of the paper. Then cut, <u>as close to the skin as possible</u>, approximately 25 <u>full-length</u> pubic hairs from various locations. Place all hairs in center of paper and refold to retain hairs. Return folded paper to envelope, seal and fill out all information requested on envelope. Affix kit number label where indicated.

STEP 10   <u>EXTERNAL GENITAL SWABBINGS</u> (Collect only if the patient's external genitalia was involved in the assault)

> Note: Lightly moisten both swabs with a sterile saline solution prior to swabbing.

Using both swabs simultaneously, carefully swab the genital area and inner thighs. Allow both swabs to air dry. Return swabs to their original paper sleeve then return swabs to envelope. Seal and fill out all information requested on envelope. Affix kit number label where indicated.

STEP 11   <u>VAGINAL SWABS AND SMEARS</u> (Collect only if within 5 days of assault)

> Note: Do not stain or chemically fix smears. Do not moisten swabs prior to sample collection.

Using two swabs simultaneously, carefully swab the vaginal vault, then put used swabs aside to air dry. Using the two additional swabs provided, repeat the swabbing procedure. Then prepare two smears on the slides provided. Allow swabs (4) and smears (2) to air dry. Return swabs to their original paper sleeve and smears to cardboard slide holder. Return swabs and smears to envelope, seal and fill out all information requested on envelope. Affix kit number label where indicated. Using hospital-supplied swab(s), collect the appropriate culture(s) at this time.

STEP 12   <u>PERIANAL SWABBINGS</u> (Collect only if anorectal assault occurred within the past 24 hours.
                                        Collect even if bowel movement has occurred since time of assault.)

> Note: Lightly moisten both swabs with a sterile saline solution prior to swabbing.

Using both swabs simultaneously, carefully swab the perianal area. Allow both swabs to air dry. Return swabs to their original paper sleeve, then return swabs to envelope. Seal and fill out all information requested on envelope. Affix kit number label where indicated.

STEP 13   <u>ANORECTAL SWABS AND SMEARS</u> (Collect only if anorectal assault occurred within the past 24 hours.
                                            Collect even if bowel movement has occurred since time of assault.)

> Note: Do not stain or chemically fix smears. Do not moisten swabs prior to sample collection.

Using both swabs simultaneously, carefully swab the rectal canal. Using both swabs, prepare two smears. Allow swabs (2) and smears (2) to air dry. Return swabs to their original paper sleeve and smears to cardboard slide holder. Return swabs and smears to envelope, then seal and fill out all information requested on envelope. Affix kit number label where indicated.

Using hospital-supplied swab(s), collect the appropriate culture(s) at this time.

STEP 14   <u>CONTROL SWABS</u>

Lightly moisten both swabs provided with the same sterile saline solution used for Steps 10, 12 and 16B. Allow both swabs to air dry. Return swabs to their original paper sleeve, then return swabs to envelope. Seal and fill out all information requested on envelope. Affix kit number label where indicated.

STEP 15   <u>KNOWN BLOOD SAMPLE</u> (For DNA testing)

> **Note: The expiration date on the kit box applies to blood tube only.**

Using the blood collection tube provided, draw sample from patient and allow tube to fill to maximum volume. Affix a kit number label onto blood tube. Return filled and labeled blood tube to envelope. Seal and fill out all information requested on envelope. Affix kit number label where indicated on envelope as well.

> Note: Steps 16A and 16B are provided for collection of additional evidence, not specified elsewhere, when indicated.

STEP 16A <u>FOREIGN MATERIAL COLLECTION</u> (2 envelopes supplied)

Remove folded paper from FOREIGN MATERIAL COLLECTION envelope. Unfold and place on flat surface. Collect any foreign material found on patient's body (leaves, fibers, hair, etc.) and place in center of paper. Refold paper to retain debris, and return to envelope. Note location from which sample was taken on anatomical drawings on envelope. Seal and fill out all information requested on envelope. Affix kit number label where indicated.

STEP 16B <u>ADDITIONAL SWABBINGS</u>

This envelope is provided for the collection of dry or damp blood, semen, saliva, etc. which may be present on the patient's body. Lightly moisten both swabs provided with sterile saline solution. Using both swabs simultaneously, collect the specimen. Note location from which specimen was taken on anatomical drawings on envelope. Return swabs to their original paper sleeve, then return swabs to envelope. Seal and fill out all information requested on envelope. Affix kit number label where indicated.

STEP 17   <u>HOSPITAL REPORT ENVELOPE</u> (See Step 1 envelope)

<u>Forms 3 and 4</u> Fill out all information requested and then sign Form 4 where indicated.

<u>Form 5</u>   Fill out all information requested on form, then separate the two pages. Place 2nd page of Form 5 in kit box. Return all other forms to HOSPITAL RECORDS envelope (Step 1) and retain this envelope for hospital records.

FINAL INSTRUCTIONS

1) Make sure all envelopes and bags are sealed and kit number labels have been affixed.
2) With the exception of the sealed and labeled CLOTHING and UNDERPANTS bags, return all other evidence collection envelopes, used or unused, to kit box.
3) Affix kit number label on kit box where indicated, then fill out all information requested under "For Hospital Personnel".
4) Initial and affix police evidence seals where indicated on sides of box, then affix biohazard label where indicated.
5) Fill out all information requested on EVIDENCE TRANSPORT bag and affix kit number label where indicated.
6) Place all CLOTHING and UNDERPANTS bags and sealed kit box in EVIDENCE TRANSPORT bag and staple.
7) Make first entry on Chain of Possession label on EVIDENCE TRANSPORT bag and hand bag to investigating officer.

> Note: If officer is not present at this time, place sealed kit and sealed bags in secure and refrigerated area (if possible), and hold for pick up by investigating officer.

RE1MA: INS.3 4/98

282

FORM 1

RECORD OF REPORTED SEXUAL ASSAULT

```
AFFIX KIT NUMBER LABEL HERE
```

PLEASE PRINT CLEARLY

PATIENT'S: NAME: _____

             ADDRESS: _____

             _____

             DATE OF BIRTH: _____ SEX: _____ RACE: _____

DATE OF ASSAULT: _____ TIME OF ASSAULT (APPROXIMATELY): _____

DATE OF ADMISSION: _____ TIME OF ADMISSION: _____

CLINICIANS: _____

_____

MEDICAL FACILITY: _____

PATIENT'S CONSENT

I consent and authorize _____ and/or the medical staff of _____ Hospital to obtain history, to perform a physical examination, to administer appropriate medical treatment, and to collect and release evidence (including but not limited to specimens, clothing, and photographs) in connection with this reported sexual assault.

_____
Witness' Signature

_____
Signature of Patient (or guardian)

_____
Date

_____
Date

(RETAIN THIS FORM FOR HOSPITAL RECORDS)

RE1MA: FORM1.1 2/96

283

FORM 2

1. PATIENT'S REPORT OF INCIDENT

<u>NOTE</u>: TO BE COMPLETED BY ONE CLINICIAN

Brief description of assault in patient's own words (include physical surroundings, threats, force and trauma, sexual acts demanded and performed, penetration (or attempted penetration) by penis or other body part or object, ejaculation, suggestion or evidence of weapons):

_____
_____
_____
_____
_____
_____
_____
_____
_____
_____
_____
_____
_____
_____
_____
_____
_____
_____
_____
_____
_____
_____
_____
_____
_____

CLINICIAN'S SIGNATURE: _____

DATE: _____ TIME: _____

(RETAIN THIS FORM FOR HOSPITAL RECORDS)

RE1MA: FORM2.1 2/96

284

FORM 3

MEDICAL HISTORY: Document major medical problems (allergies and medications, including contraceptives - DO NOT include prior STD, pregnancies, abortions, unless medically indicated):

_____
_____
_____
_____

EXAMINATION

A. GENERAL PHYSICAL APPEARANCE: _____
_____
_____

B. EMOTIONAL STATUS: _____
_____
_____

C. PHYSICAL EXAMINATION: Note all signs of trauma (use diagrams if desired). Include notations of patient's indications of tenderness, if applicable:

			DESCRIBE ABNORMAL/SIGNIFICANT FINDINGS BELOW
Skin	NL	ABNL	
Hair	NL	ABNL	
Face	NL	ABNL	
Mouth	NL	ABNL	
Throat	NL	ABNL	
Breasts	NL	ABNL	
Abdomen	NL	ABNL	
Back	NL	ABNL	
Extremities	NL	ABNL	

RESULTS OF PELVIC/GENITAL EXAMINATION: Use non-lubricated, warm water-moistened speculum.

Include all signs of trauma (extent, location). Be certain to examine cervix for parity and signs of pregnancy, menstruation, trauma and infection. Document signs of foreign material and nature of fluid/discharge, if any:

_____
_____
_____
_____
_____
_____
_____
_____
_____
_____

CLINICIAN'S SIGNATURE: _____

(RETAIN THIS FORM FOR HOSPITAL RECORDS)   RE-1MA 1/93

285

FORM 4

D. LAB SPECIMENS OBTAINED FOR EVALUATION BY MEDICAL FACILITY:

NOTE: EXAMINATION OF STAINED, DRIED SMEARS WILL BE PERFORMED IN THE CRIME LABORATORY

GC Cultures ☐ cervix ☐ pharynx ☐ rectum ☐ other _____
- ☐ Pap smear
- ☐ Chlamydia   type: _____
- ☐ Urine for UCG
- ☐ Blood for RPR
- ☐ Blood for pregnancy test
- ☐ Blood for typing
- ☐ Other _____

IV. TREATMENT (this information may need to be included on other hospital forms)

Antibiotic therapy   ☐ YES   ☐ NO   drug _____

dose _____

drug _____

dose _____

Contraception medication   ☐ YES   ☐ NO   drug _____

dose _____

Other medications prescribed: _____

Other treatment: _____

V. DISPOSITION

1. Primary health care (site or clinical): _____

2. Patient's telephone number: _____ day _____ evening.

3. Discharge instructions and information regarding sexual assault given to patient ☐ YES ☐ NO

4. a. DSS involved   ☐ YES   ☐ NO
   b. 51A filed   ☐ YES   ☐ NO
   c. police involved   ☐ YES   ☐ NO

VI. SIGNATURES OF EXAMINING CLINICIANS:

_____

_____

(RETAIN THIS FORM FOR HOSPITAL RECORDS)

RE1MA: FORM4.1 2/96

286

FORM 5

INFORMATION PERTAINING TO ASSAULT

KIT NUMBER (use same number that appears on labels):_____

PATIENT'S AGE:_____ SEX:_____ RACE:_____

DATE OF ASSAULT:_____ TIME OF ASSAULT (approximately):_____

DATE OF ADMISSION:_____ TIME OF ADMISSION:_____

1. Was victim menstruating at time of assault? ☐YES ☐NO

2. Were there multiple assailants? ☐ YES ☐ NO If yes, number:_____

3. Assailant's relationship to victim: ☐Stranger ☐Acquaintance ☐other:_____

4. Race of assailant, if known: ☐Caucasian ☐Hispanic ☐African American ☐other:_____

5. Lacerations on patient resulting in bleeding? ☐YES ☐NO

6. Lacerations on assailant resulting in bleeding? ☐YES ☐NO ☐UNCERTAIN

7. Penetration occurred (check all that apply):.........................Ejaculation occurred (check all that apply):

	yes	no	uncertain
vaginally			
orally			
anally			

	yes	no	uncertain
vaginally			
orally			
anally			
externally			

8. Did assailant use lubricant? (Note: Saliva is a lubricant) ☐YES ☐NO ☐UNCERTAIN

9. Did assailant insert foreign object(s)? ☐YES ☐NO If yes, type of object:_____

10. Was a condom worn by the assailant? ☐YES ☐NO ☐UNCERTAIN

11. Does the patient suspect having been drugged by another? ☐YES ☐NO ☐UNCERTAIN

12. Has the patient used any of the following products within 24 hours of the assault?

	yes	no	uncertain		yes	no	uncertain
spermicidal gel/cream				lubrication products			
contraceptive sponge				powder (talc or cornstarch)			

13. Since the assault, has the patient:

	yes	no	uncertain		yes	no	uncertain
wiped/washed off				defecated			
bathed/showered				vomited			
douched				brushed teeth			
urinated				changed clothes			

other, explain:_____

14. Was there voluntary, consensual intercourse within 5 days of the assault?

☐ YES ☐ NO ☐ UNCERTAIN Approximate date:_____

15. Was a condom used within 5 days of the assault?

☐YES ☐NO ☐ UNCERTAIN Approximate date:_____

(FIRST PAGE, RETAIN FOR HOSPITAL RECORDS - RETURN SECOND PAGE TO KIT BOX)

RE1MA: FORM5.2 4/98

D. Pilot Sexual Abuse Protocol, Children's Hospital, Boston

MEDICAL REPORT   Hospital Stamp

A. <u>GENERAL INFORMATION</u>

Name (Victim)	Address	City/State	Zip Code	Phone ( )

DOB (mm/dd/yy)	Age	Sex M F	Race	1=White 2=Black 3=Hispanic 4=American Indian 5=Oriental 6=Other

	Name	DOB	Address	Phone	Race
O 1.Mother					
O 2.Stepmother					
O <u>3.Guardian</u>					
O 1.Father					
O 2.Stepfather					
O <u>3.Guardian</u>					

Siblings
_____
_____
_____

Alleged Perpetrator(s)	Name	DOB	Sex	Race	Address/Phone
	1.				
	2				

Relationship to Victim:
1. _____
2. _____

Completed By:_____ M.S.W.

Page 1 of 11

288

NAME/TITLE _____
_____ M.D.
_____ R.N.
_____ M.S.W.
_____

**Please "sign in" and
initial as you document.**   Hospital Stamp

_____
              ***
       **O Less than 72 hours since
          incident(s) took place.
          USE RAPE KIT AND FORMS**
       O Over 72 hours since incident(s)
          took place <u>use this protocol.</u>
          <u>DATE/TIME/LOCATION</u>
       _____
       _____

B.   <u>OBTAIN PATIENT HISTORY.</u> Recorder should allow patient or
      other person providing the history to describe incident(s)
      to the extent possible and record the acts and symptoms
       described below. Determine and use terms familiar to the
      patient. Follow-up questions may be necessary to ensure
      that all items are covered.

      NARRATIVE HISTORY.

      O Chief complaint (s) or description of event(s) in child's
        "own words". (Verbatim quotes)._____

      _____

      _____

      _____

      _____

      _____

      _____

      _____

      _____

      _____

                              Initials_____

                    Page 2 of 11

                                                              289

O Description of event(s) from caretaker's report of child
  disclosure statement.

  Person providing history: NAME: _____
                           PHONE: __(___)_____
              RELATIONSHIP TO VICTIM: _____

_____

_____

_____

_____

_____

_____

_____

_____

_____

_____

_____

_____

_____

_____

_____

_____

_____

_____

_____

_____

_____

_____

                    Initials_____   MSW

290

C. OBTAIN PERTINENT PAST MEDICAL HISTORY   <u>Allergies</u>

    1. If pubertal female:
       Menarche age:____   LMP:____   Uses Tampons:
       <u>___( )N/A_____( )Yes ( )No_____</u>
       <u>History of Vaginitis: ( )Yes ( )No ( )N/A_____</u>
       <u>Previous Sexual Activity: ( )Yes ( )No ( )N/A</u>
       <u>Use of Birth Control: ( )Yes ( )No ( )N/A____</u>
       <u>   If yes, which form:_____</u>
    2. Pre-existing physical injuries (i.e. scars) ( )N/A.
      <u>   </u>
      <u>   </u>
      <u>   </u>

    3. Pertinent medical history of ano-genital injuries,
       surgeries, diagnostic procedures, or medical treatment?
       ( )No   ( )Yes   DESCRIBE:
      <u>   </u>
      <u>   </u>
      <u>   </u>

    4. Previous history of child abuse? ( )No ( )Yes ( )Unknown
       If known, describe:<u>_____</u>
      <u>   </u>
      <u>   </u>
      <u>   </u>

D. <u>SUMMARY OF ACTS DESCRIBED BY PATIENT AND/OR HISTORIAN</u>
   <u>DURING INTERVIEW.</u> **(Indicate whether reported by patient or**
   historian).

   Genital contact (with penis, finger, foreign objects, etc.)

   <u>   </u>

   <u>   </u>

   <u>   </u>

   Anal contact (with penis, finger, foreign objects, etc.)

   <u>   </u>

   <u>   </u>

291

Indicate whether reported by patient or historian.
Oral copulation of genitals (of victim by assailant, of assailant by victim)._____

_____

_____

Oral copulation of anus (of victim by assailant, of assailant by victim)._____

_____

_____

Physical symptoms (pain, enuresis, bleeding, discharge, etc.)

_____

_____

_____

Behavioral symptoms(sleep, aggressiveness, sexual acting out).

_____

_____

_____

Additional information (other symptoms)._____

_____

_____

_____

_____

_____ M.D.

Page 5 of 11

292

E. CONDUCT A GENERAL PHYSICAL EXAMINATION AND RECORD FINDINGS.
    COLLECT AND PRESERVE EVIDENCE FOR EVIDENTIAL EXAM IF INDICATED

    Blood Pressure   Pulse   Temperature   Weight
         /   /min.   kg.
    Record general physical condition, noting any abnormality.
    Record injuries and findings on diagrams: erythema, abrasions
     bruises, contusions, induration, lacerations, fractures,
     bites, burns.
    Record size and appearance of injuries/findings.

GENERAL EXAMINATION:
    General:_____

    HEENT: _____

    Skin: _____

    Resp/CV:_____

    M-S: _____
    Neuro: _____
    GI: _____
    Comments:

    Genitalia Exam- Next Page   Initials _____

                    Page 6 of 11

                                                            293

TANNER STAGING

Tanner Stage Breasts_____   Tanner Stage Genitalia_____

Genitalia Exam/Female. General exam done with:
   O Direct Visualization   O Colposcope   O Hand held Magnifier
   Exam position used: O Supine   O Knee Chest

Labia Majora: WNL O ABN O   Describe:_____

Clitoris: WNL O ABN O   Describe:_____

Labia Minora: WNL O ABN O   Describe:_____

Periurethral tissue/ urethral meatus:
              WNL O ABN O   Describe:_____

DRAW SHAPE OF HYMEN (CRESCENT,
ANNULAR, REDUNDANT) AND ANUS
AND ANY LESIONS ON GENITALIA,
PERINEUM, OR BUTTOCKS. **(DO NOT
USE "INTACT" OR "NOT INTACT").
*** Prepubertal child-external
exam only (speculum not used).**
Hymen:_____

Position(Supine or knee-chest):

Retraction: Lateral O   or
 Traction with labia pulled
 toward examiner O
Diameter (mm) transverse:_____

Posterior Fourchette: WNL O   ABN O Describe:_____

        Vagina: WNL O   ABN O Describe:_____

        Cervix: WNL O   ABN O Describe:_____

              Initials_____
              Page 7 of 11

294

	WNL	ABN	DESCRIBE
Buttocks:	O	O	
Perianal skin:	O	O	
Anal verge/folds/rugae:	O	O	
Tone:	O	O	

Tags: O No O Yes Location:
Anal spasm: O No O Yes
Fissures: O No O Yes
Anal laxity: O No O Yes
Presence of stool in vault: O No O Yes
Method of exam for anal tone:
    O Observation   O Digital Exam
Exam position used: O Supine O Prone
                    O Lateral Recumbent
Anoscopic exam: O No O Yes O N/A
Protoscopic exam: O No   O Yes O N/A

★★
GENITALIA EXAM- MALE

Genital Exam done with:
    O Direct visualization O Colposcope O Hand held magnifier

DRAW SHAPE OF ANUS AND ANY LESIONS ON GENITALIA, PERINEUM, AND
BUTTOCKS.

Tanner Staging___

	WNL	ABN	DESCRIBE
Penis:	O	O	
Circumcised:			
O Yes O No			
Urethral Meatus:	O	O	
Scrotum:	O	O	
Testes	O	O	

Initials _____

LABORATORY COLLECTION: In prepubertal girls, cultures are usually taken from the throat, vagina, and rectum for GC and the vagina for chlamydia. In post menarcheal adolescents, cultures are usually taken from the throat, endocervix and rectum for GC and endocervix for chlamydia. In boys, cultures from the throat, urethra and rectum are taken for GC and the rectum and urethra are cultured for chlamydia. The following tests do not have to be performed on all patients. When the history and/or physical exam suggests the possibility of oral, genital, or rectal contact or no reliable history can be obtained, cultures and serologies should be done.

	Check if Done	Results +/-
GC		
Vaginal	_____	_____
Cervix	_____	_____
Rectal	_____	_____
Urethral	_____	_____
Oral/pharynx	_____	_____
Chlamydia **(Culture, NOT EIA)**		
Cervical	_____	_____
Vaginal	_____	_____
Urethral	_____	_____
Rectal	_____	_____
Oral/pharynx	_____	_____
RPR	_____	_____
HIV	_____	_____
Hepatitis B	_____	_____
Wet Mount	_____	_____
Sperm	_____	_____
Trichomonas	_____	_____
Frozen Serum	_____	_____
Pregnancy		
Urine	_____	_____
Serum	_____	_____
Toxicology Screen		
Urine	_____	_____
Serum	_____	_____

Other:

_____ M.D.

TREATMENT FOR **ACUTE SEXUAL ASSAULT:**

STD prophylaxis is indicated for almost all adolescents girls (need to treat for GC <u>AND</u> chlamydia). Most boys and prepubertal girls are not treated unless significant symptoms are present or the patient is the victim of an acute rape.

* Circle treatment.   ? ALLERGIES_____

<u>Gonococcal prophylaxis:</u>   Ceftriaxone 250 mg IM (> 45 kg.)
                                      125 mg IM (< 45 kg.)
                          Other_____

                    PLUS

<u>Chlamydia prophylaxis:</u>   Doxycycline 100 mg p.o. BID for 7 days
                                    OR
                          Erythromycin 500 mg p.o. QID for 7 days
                          Children < 9yrs. erythromycin 50 mg/kg/d

_____

Post-coital contraception:
    (<72 hours from assault, post-pubertal girl)
            _____Yes   _____No

    Ovral: Two tablets orally immediately **plus** two tablets 12
hours later
    (* Ovral is 0.5 mg norgestrel + 0.05 mg ethinyl estradiol)

_____

Td Booster: O Yes   O No

Other medications/treatments prescribed:_____

_____

_____

_____

_____

                                                          M.D.
                    _____

NOTE: Antibiotic doses and emergency contraception options have changed. See Chapters 5 and 9.

IMPRESSIONS: (FINDINGS)

_____

_____

_____

_____

_____

_____

_____

_____

_____

_____

_____

PLAN:

    Follow-up arranged:

        Yes_____ On (Date)_____With_____ M.D.

        No _____ Explain who is to arrange:_____

                _____

    Child released to:_____

    Follow-up information sheet given to:_____

                    Completed by:_____

                    Reviewed by:_____

Page 11 of 11

298

FOLLOW-UP INFORMATION SHEET

Name: _____

Was examined on_____ to:
1. determine if any injuries were present which required
   treatment;
2. do a number of lab tests which can provide medical and
   legal information.

MEDICATION:
   - Your child received_____medication
     against venereal disease (syphilis, gonorrhea, chlamydia).
   - Your child received_____medication to aid
     in pregnancy prevention.
   - Your child received_____medication for
     _____.
   - Your child needs no medication at this time.

FOLLOW-UP VISITS:
   The Social Worker you had contact with today is_____.
   The Physician you had contact with today is_____.
   The nurse you had contact with today is_____.

Please call either your primary care provider or the Emergency Room
(617-735-6611) for advice if your child exhibits:

1. Signs of infection (fever, pain, sores, vaginal discharge).
2. Urinary Symptoms (painful urination, blood in urine,
   frequency of urination).
3. GYN Symptoms (unusual bleeding from the vagina, late
   period, or if your child does not have a period within 1
   week of completing the medicine given to prevent pregnancy.
4. Rectal bleeding.

Please note:
   Behavioral changes such as changes in eating and sleeping
patterns, nausea, vomiting, bedwetting, nightmares, unusual fears
and sexualized behaviors are commonly associated with sexual
trauma. Questions and concerns should be addressed with the
child's pediatrician or discussed at follow up appointments.

YOUR FOLLOW-UP APPOINTMENT IS VERY IMPORTANT.
Please return to: The Medical Follow-up Clinic on : Fegan 6

to see Dr. Vandeven on (Date/Time)_____.

The results of your child's tests will be discussed.

SPECIAL INSTRUCTIONS:
                    Completed by: _____

E. Preappointment Questionnaire, University of California, Irvine

Pre-appointment Questionnaire

Deborah C. Stewart, M.D.
University of California, Irvine Medical Center

___Patient Identification Stamp___

You/your child has an appointment for a medical evaluation for possible sexual molestation/assault. A very important part of this process is to obtain pertinent medical history. Please fill out this form as thoroughly as possible and bring it with you when you see Dr. Stewart.

Name of person filling out form: _____

Relationship to patient: Mother   Father   Other _____

What is the name, and if known, the address and/or phone number of the patient's doctor?

_____

_____

_____

_____

Is the patient currently in counseling?   Yes   No

Has the patient been in the past?   Yes   No

What is the name, and if known, the address and/or phone number of the patient's counselor/therapist?

_____

_____

_____

_____

_____

Has the patient ever had any other medical evaluation for possible sexual molestation?   Yes   No

If so, where and when?

_____

_____

_____

Is the patient under medical care for any ongoing medical or psychological condition?   Yes   No

Has the patient ever had any accidents or injuries to the vaginal or genital area?   Yes   No

Has the patient ever had any accidents or injuries to the rectal area?   Yes   No

300

Has the patient ever had any medical treatments, operations or procedures to the vaginal, rectal or genital area?

         Yes   No   Not Applicable

Has the patient begun her menstrual periods yet?

         Yes   No   Not Applicable

If so, does she wear tampons?

         Yes   No   Not Applicable

Has the patient ever had any vaginal infection?

         Yes   No

Has the patient ever had any skin infection around the vagina or the rectum?

         Yes   No

Does the patient have any bowel or stomach problems or diseases?

         Yes   No

Has the patient ever had any rectal suppositories or enemas?

         Yes   No

Have there ever been any other concerns about previous physical abuse or sexual molestation?

         Yes   No

Has the patient experienced any of the following symptoms or medical problems at any time in the past or present?

	Yes	No	Don't Know
Abdominal (stomach) pain			
Vulvar (the lips of the vagina) pain			
Pain on urination			
Urinary tract infection			
Daytime or nighttime wetting			
Vaginal itching			
Vaginal discharge			
Vaginal bleeding			
Rectal Pain			
Rectal bleeding			
Rectal discharge			
Constipation			
Accidents with bowel movements			
Unconsciousness			
Vomiting			
Physical injuries or pain due to the alleged episodes			
Sleeping problems			
Eating problems			
School problems			
Excessive sexual behavior			
Fearfulness			
Unusual/excessive anger			
Depression/suicidal thoughts/feelings			

Any other physical or behavioral concerns?

_____

Do you have any further concerns?   Yes   No

_____

Please discuss with the doctor any questions which you do not understand or if you would like further explanation.

F. Practice Guidelines

Descriptive Terminology in Child Sexual Abuse Medical Evaluations

Published by the American Professional Society on the Abuse of Children (AP-SAC), the nation's largest interdisciplinary professional society for those who work in the field of child maltreatment. APSAC's aim is to ensure that everyone affected by child maltreatment receives the best possible professional response. APSAC provides ongoing professional education in the form of publications and conferences and, through the media and legislative advocacy, educates the public about the complex issues involved in child maltreatment. For further information contact APSAC at 407 S. Dearborn St., Suite 1300, Chicago, IL 60605.

JET LIBRARY

INTRODUCTION

The forensic medical evaluation of suspected child sexual abuse victims has developed into a specialized field of practice in the last ten years. Pediatricians, gynecologists, nurse practitioners, and physician assistants may all be called upon to examine children for suspected sexual abuse and describe their findings. The records of such examinations then become medico-legal documents.

Precision in documentation is critical for all who must communicate and understand medical findings. These terminology Guidelines were developed to assist professionals actively involved in the medical diagnosis and treatment of child sexual abuse to establish a shared vocabulary which is clear, precise, and easily communicated. This shared vocabulary will enable those in child protection, law enforcement, and the courts to understand previously confusing and, at times, inconsistent terminology. Consistency in terminology will also assist in the development of a research language.

The terminology presented in these Guidelines emanates primarily from medical dictionary definitions, anatomy texts, and clinicians actively involved in the care of sexually abused children. Unless otherwise noted, definitions are from Stedman's [Medical Dictionary]. As experience and scientific knowledge expand, further revision of these guidelines is expected.

ANATOMICAL STRUCTURES

1. ANAL SKIN TAG - A protrusion of anal verge tissue which interrupts the symmetry of the perianal skin folds.

2. ANAL VERGE - The tissue overlying the subcutaneous external anal sphincter at the most distal portion of the anal canal (anoderm) and extending exteriorly to the margin of the anal skin.

3. ANTERIOR COMMISSURE - The union of the two labia minora anteriorly (toward the clitoris).

4. ANUS - The anal orifice, which is the lower opening of the digestive tract, lying in the fold between the buttocks, through which feces are extruded.

5. CLITORIS - A small cylindrical, erectile body situated at the anterior (superior) portion of the vulva, covered by a sheath of skin called the clitoral hood; homologous with the penis in the male.

6. FOSSA NAVICULARIS/POSTERIOR FOSSA - Concavity on the lower part of the vestibule situated posteriorly (inferiorly) to the vaginal orifice and extending to the posterior fourchette (posterior commissure).

7. GLANS PENIS - The cap-shaped expansion of the corpus spongiosum at the end of the penis; also called balanus. It is covered by a mucous membrane and sheathed by the prepuce (foreskin) in uncircumcised males.

8. GENITALIA (External) - The external sexual organs. In males, includes the penis and scrotum. In females, includes the contents of the vulva.

9. HYMEN - This membrane (external vaginal plate or urogenital septum) partially or rarely completely covers the vaginal orifice. This membrane is located at the junction of the vestibular floor and the vaginal canal.

10. LABIA MAJORA - ("outer lips") Rounded folds of skin forming the lateral boundaries of the vulva.

11. LABIA MINORA - ("inner lips") Longitudinal thin folds of tissue enclosed within the labia majora. In the pubertal child, these folds extend from the clitoral hood to approximately the mid point on the lateral wall of the vestibule. In the adult, they enclose the structures of the vestibule.

12. MEDIAN RAPHE - A ridge or furrow that marks the line of union of the two halves of the perineum.

13. MONS PUBIS - The rounded, fleshy prominence, created by the underlying fat pad which lies over the symphysis pubis (pubic bone) in the female.

14. PECTINATE/DENTATE LINE - The saw-toothed line of demarcation between the distal (lower) portion of the anal valves and the pectin, the smooth zone of stratified epithelium which extends to the anal verge. This line is apparent when the external and internal anal sphincters relax and the anus dilates.

15. PENIS - Male sex organ composed of erectile tissue through which the urethra passes (homologous with the clitoris in the female).

16. PERIANAL FOLDS - Wrinkles or folds of the anal verge skin radiating from the anus, which are created by contraction of the external anal sphincter. (Definition not found in Stedman's.)

17. PERINEAL BODY - The central tendon of the perineum located between the vulva and the anus in the female and between the scrotum and anus in the male.

18. PERINEUM - The external surface or base of the perineal body, lying between the vulva and the anus in the female, and the scrotum and the anus in the male [Stedman's]. Underlying the external surface of the perineum is the pelvic floor and its associated structures occupying the pelvic outlet, which is bounded anteriorly by the public symphysis (pubic bone), laterally by the ischial tuberosity (pelvic bone) and posteriorly by the coccyx (tail bone).

19. POSTERIOR COMMISSURE - The union of the two labia majora posteriorly (toward the anus).

20. POSTERIOR FOURCHETTE - The junction of two labia minora posteriorly (inferiorly). This area is referred to as a posterior commissure in the prepubertal child, as the labia minora are not completely developed to connect inferiorly until puberty, when it is referred to as the fourchette.

21. SCROTUM - The pouch which contains the testicles and their accessory organs.

22. URETHRAL ORIFICE - External opening of the canal (urethra) from the bladder.

23. VAGINA - The uterovaginal canal in the female. This internal structure extends from the uterine cervix to the inner aspect of the hymen.

24. VAGINAL VESTIBULE - An anatomic cavity containing the

opening of the vagina, the urethra and the ducts of Bartholin's glands. Bordered by the clitoris anteriorly, the labia laterally and the posterior commissure (fourchette) posteriorly (inferiorly). The vestibule encompasses the fossa navicularis immediately posterior (inferior) to the vaginal introitus.

25. VULVA - The external genitalia or pudendum of the female. Includes the clitoris, labia majora, labia minora, vaginal vestibule, urethral orifice, vaginal orifice, hymen, and posterior fourchette (or commissure).

HYMENAL MORPHOLOGY

1. ANNULAR - Circumferential. Hymenal membrane tissue extends completely around the circumference of the entire vaginal orifice.
2. CRIBRIFORM - Hymen with multiple small openings.
3. CRESCENTIC - Hymen with attachments at approximately the 11 and 1 o'clock positions without tissue being present between the two attachments.
4. IMPERFORATE - A hymenal membrane with no opening.
5. SEPTATE - The appearance of the hymenal orifice when it is bisected by a band of hymenal tissue creating two or more orifices.

DESCRIPTIVE TERMS RELATING TO THE HYMEN

1. ESTROGENIZED - Effect of influence by the female sex hormone estrogen resulting in changes to the genitalia. The hymen takes on as a result a thickened, redundant, pale appearance. These changes are observed in neonates, with the onset of puberty and the result of exogenous estrogen.
2. FIMBRIATED/DENTICULAR - Hymen with multiple projections and indentations along the edge, creating a ruffled appearance.
3. NARROW/WIDE HYMENAL RIM - The width of the hymenal membrane as viewed in the coronal plane, i.e., from the edge of the hymen to the muscular portion of the vaginal introitus.
4. REDUNDANT - Abundant hymenal tissue which tends to fold back on itself or protrude.

5. MEMBRANE THICKNESS - The relative amount of tissue between the internal and external surfaces of the hymenal membrane.

OTHER STRUCTURES/FINDINGS

1. ACUTE LACERATION - A tear through the full thickness of the skin or other tissue.
2. ATTENUATED - This term has been used to describe areas where the hymen is narrow. However, the term should be restricted to indicate a documented change in the width of the posterior portion of the hymen following an injury.
3. DIASTASIS ANI - A congenital midline smooth depression which may be V-shaped or wedge shaped, located either anterior or posterior to the anus, that is due to a failure of fusion of the underlying of the corrugator external anal sphincter muscle.
4. ERYTHEMA - Redness of tissues.
5. EXTERNAL HYMENAL RIDGE - A midline longitudinal ridge of tissue on the external surface of the hymen. May be either anterior or posterior. Usually extends to the edge of the membrane.
6. FRIABILITY OF THE POSTERIOR FOURCHETTE/COMMISSURE - A superficial breakdown of the skin in the posterior fourchette (commissure) when gentle traction is applied, causing slight bleeding.
7. HYMENAL CYST - A fluid-filled elevation of tissue, confined within the hymenal tissue.
8. HYMENAL CLEFT - An angular or V-shaped indentation on the edge of the hymenal membrane. When curved, it creates a hollowed or U-shaped depression on the edge of the membrane which has been referred to as a "concavity."
9. LABIAL AGGLUTINATION (labial adhesion) - The result of adherence (fusion) of the adjacent edges of the mucosal surfaces of the labia minora. This may occur at any point along the length of the vestibule although it most commonly occurs posteriorly (inferiorly).
10. LINEA VESTIBULARIS - A vertical, pale/avascular line across the posterior fourchette and/or fossa, which may be accentuated by putting lateral traction on the labia majora.

11. O'CLOCK DESIGNATION - A method by which the location of structures or findings may be designated by using the numerals on the face of a clock. The 12 o'clock position is always superior (up). The 6 o'clock position is always inferior (down). The position of a patient must be indicated when using this designation.

12. PERINEAL GROOVE - Developmental anomaly, also called "Failure of Midline Fusion". This skin and mucosal defect may be located anywhere from the fossa to anus.

13. PROJECTIONS -
    a. Mound/bump - A solid elevation of hymenal tissue which is wider or as wide as it is long, located on the edge of the hymenal membrane. This structure may be seen at the site where an intravaginal column attaches to the hymen.
    b. Hymenal Tag - An elongated projection of tissue rising from any location on the hymenal rim. Commonly found in the midline and may be an extension of a posterior vaginal column.

14. SCAR - Fibrous tissue which replaces normal tissue after the healing of a wound.

15. SYNECHIA - Any adhesion which binds two anatomic structures through the formation of a band of tissue [Stedman's]. A synechia can result in the healing process following an abrasion of tissues.

16. TRANSECTION OF HYMEN (Complete) - A tear or laceration through the entire width of the hymenal membrane extending to (or through its attachment) to the vaginal wall.

17. TRANSECTION OF HYMEN (Partial) - A tear or laceration through a portion of the hymenal membrane not extending to its attachment to the vaginal wall.

18. VAGINAL COLUMNS (columnae rugarum vaginae) - Raised (sagittally oriented) columns most prominent on the anterior wall with less prominence on the posterior wall. May also be observed laterally.

19. VAGINAL RUGAE (rugae vaginales) - Folds of epithelium (rugae) running circumferentially from vaginal columns. These rugae account in part for the ability of the vagina to distend.

20. VASCULARITY (increased) - Dilatation of existing superficial blood vessels.

21. VESTIBULAR BANDS-
    a. Periurethral bands - Small bands lateral to the urethra that connect the periurethral tissues to the anterior lateral wall of the vestibule. These bands are usually symmetrical and frequently create a semi-lunar shaped space between the bands on either side of the urethral meatus. Also called urethral supporting ligaments.
    b. Perihymenal bands (pubo vaginal) - Bands lateral to the hymen connecting to the vestibular wall.

DESCRIPTIVE TERMS FOR VARIATIONS IN PERIANAL ANATOMY

1. ANAL DILATATION - Opening of the external and internal anal sphincters with minimal traction on the buttocks.
2. ANAL FISSURE - A superficial break (split) in the perianal skin which radiates out from the anal orifice.
3. FLATTENED ANAL FOLDS - A reduction or absence of the perianal folds or wrinkles, noted when the external anal sphincter is partially or completely relaxed.
4. VENOUS CONGESTION - Pooling of venous blood in the perianal tissues resulting in a purple discoloration which may be localized or diffuse.

Adapted from APSAC Practice Guidelines, without accompanying illustrations and documentation of source material given in the original document.

Index

abdominal pain, in abused children, 5(t), 58

ABO blood group antigens, forensic detection of, 87, 88

abrasion, definition of, 241

abscess, definition of, 241

abuser(s), 3, 22
  as child's escort to medical interview, 43–44, 53
  as child's "only friend", 2
  dental impressions of, 83
  description of vaginal penetration by, 60
  DNA typing of, 88–89
  forensic characteristics of, 87–89
  hepatitis B virus in, 216
  incarceration of, 36
  interview questions about, 48(t)
  juveniles as, 4
  as member of extended family, 34
  prosecution of, 76, 193, 245(b)
  STDs in, 66, 190, 193
  threats by, 3
  undifferentiated perverse, 3–4
  victim's contact with genitalia of, 66

accidental injuries, to genital area, 65, 118(t), 119

accommodation, in child sexual abuse accommodation syndrome, 3

acetic acid, use to visualize genital warts, 210

acid phosphatase
  forensic detection of, 86
  laboratory tests for, 67, 248(b)
  persistence in vagina, 80
  in semen, 86, 194

acinobacter, diagnosis of, 191

acquaintance, as abuser, 178(p), 179(p)

"acting-out" behavior, in sexually abused children, 3

acyclovir, in herpes treatment, 206

adenopathy, examination for, 70

adhesions, of labia, 63, 118(t), 127(p), 137(p), 138(p), 295–296

adnexa, anatomy of, 241

adolescents
  bacterial vaginosis in, 206, 207
  chlamydial infections in, 66, 200, 202, 203
  consensual intercourse in, 66, 122, 127(p), 188, 247(b)
  genital injuries in, 121–122
  genital warts in, 209, 210, 212
  gonorrhea in, 195–196, 197, 198(t)
  growth spurt of, 107
  hymen in, 64–65, 73, 74, 127(p)128(p), 176(p), 252(b)
  longitudinal intravaginal ridge in, 137(p)
  medical interview of, 49(t)
  N. gonorrhoeae infections in, 195
  physical examination of, 57–78
    girls, 73–74
  sexual abuse of, 22, 115, 121–122, 245(b)
    regressed behavior from, 35
    symptoms, 25
  STDs in, 65–66, 122, 188, 190, 191
  T. vaginalis infections in, 215
  vaginal physiology of, 188(t)